ELEVENTH EDITION

THE ONLY EKG BOOK You'll Ever Need

ELEVENTH EDITION

THE ONLY EKG BOOK You'll Ever Need

MALCOLM S. THALER

Wolters Kluwer

Philadelphia • Baltimore • New York • London
Buenos Aires • Hong Kong • Sydney • Tokyo

Acquisitions Editor: Joseph Cho
Development Editor: Cindy Yoo
Lead Editorial Coordinator: Sean Hanrahan
Marketing Manager: Kirsten Watrud
Production Project Manager: Jennifer L. Harper
Manager, Graphic Arts & Design: Diane Drier, Stephen Druding
Art Director, Illustration: Jennifer Clements
Senior Manufacturing Coordinator: Lisa Bowling
Prepress Vendor: Aptara, Inc.

Eleventh Edition

9 8 7 6 5 4 3 2 1

Printed in Mexico

Cataloging-in-Publication Data available on request from the Publisher

ISBN: 978-1-9752-4661-7

---

shop.lww.com

QUADM0126

Dedication

To Nancy, Ali, Jon, Tracey, Ben, Eliana, Miles, Maia, and Greta with infinite love for the joy you bring to everything and everyone, and to each and every one of you involved in health care—whatever your role—the most humane calling of all.

Preface

You've picked up this book so presumably you want to learn how to read EKGs. Or perhaps you know the basics and want to get more comfortable with them. Or you feel—not without justification—that you are pretty good and just want to fill in the few remaining gaps in your knowledge. Or you are regarded by your admiring peers as something of a stalwart among electrocardiographers and are looking for a refresher. Whatever the reason, welcome to *The Only EKG Book You'll Ever Need* family of readers!

What is most remarkable is that over the years—despite all the advances in imaging technology and the exponential rise of artificial intelligence—the EKG, read by real humans in real human situations, remains among the most important tools in our clinical arsenal. Your patient has chest pain? Get an EKG. Palpitations? An EKG is your answer. Shortness of breath? Dizziness? You will want an EKG almost every time. Not only does the EKG take only minutes to run and interpret, but it costs only pennies and comes virtually free of adverse side effects.

The aims of this edition remain the same as ever—keep things simple, concise, clear, and—yes—fun. You will find illustrations, bulleted lists, tables, and EKG tracings on almost every page. New material has been added—including all-new sections on eating disorders and common electrical artifacts—and old material revised to keep you up to date. Perhaps most importantly, everything is presented within the relevant clinical context; at the end of each chapter, you will get to participate in actual clinical scenarios that will help you see the power of this tool in common (and often gripping) circumstances. In this way, you will learn how to use the EKG to its best advantage and retain the information you learn along the way.

Once again I want to thank the amazing Dr. Adam H. Skolnick, MD, Charles A. Poindexter Associate Professor of Medicine, Leon H. Chaney Division of Cardiology at the NYU Grossman School of Medicine for ensuring that everything in this book is current and accurate. Any mistakes are mine and mine alone. And of course I want to thank all the folks at Wolters Kluwer who always manage to produce an eye-catching, user-friendly text and who never skimp on quality; special kudos to Joseph Cho, Sean Hanrahan, and Cindy Yoo.

—Malcolm S. Thaler, MD

Contents

Getting Started

In this chapter, you will learn:

1 not a thing, but don't worry. There is plenty to come. Here is your chance to turn a few pages, take a deep breath or two, and get yourself settled and ready to roll. Relax. Pour some tea. Begin.

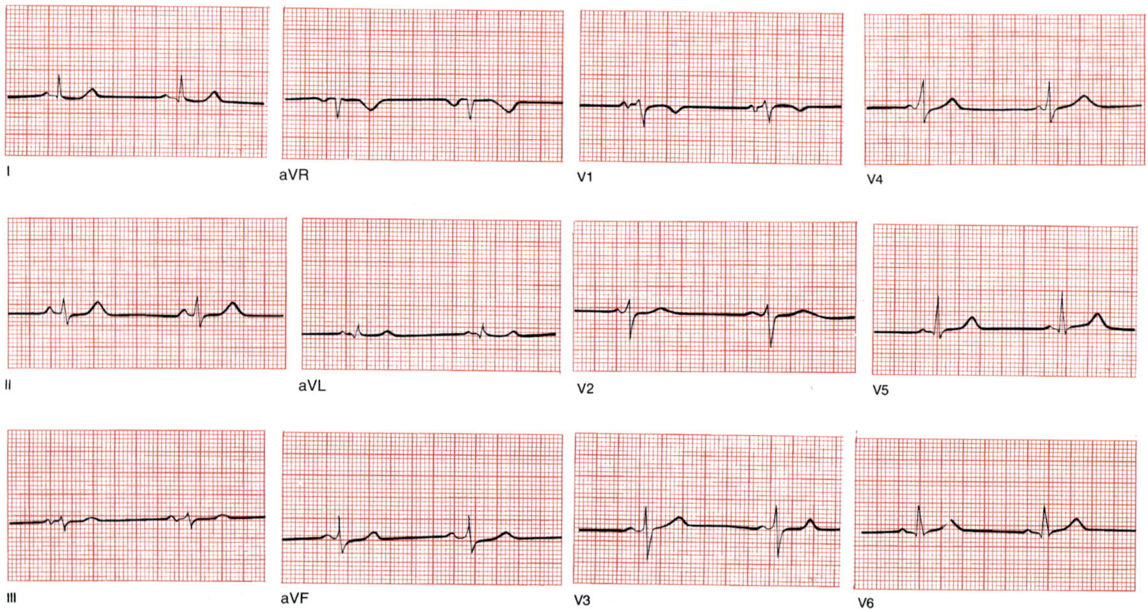
I
aVR
V1
V4
II
aVL
V2
V5
III
aVF
V3
V6

On the opposite page is a normal electrocardiogram, or EKG.* By the time you have finished this book—and it won't take you very much time at all—you will be able to recognize a normal EKG almost instantly. Even more importantly, you will have learned to spot all of the common abnormalities that can occur on an EKG, and you will be good at it!

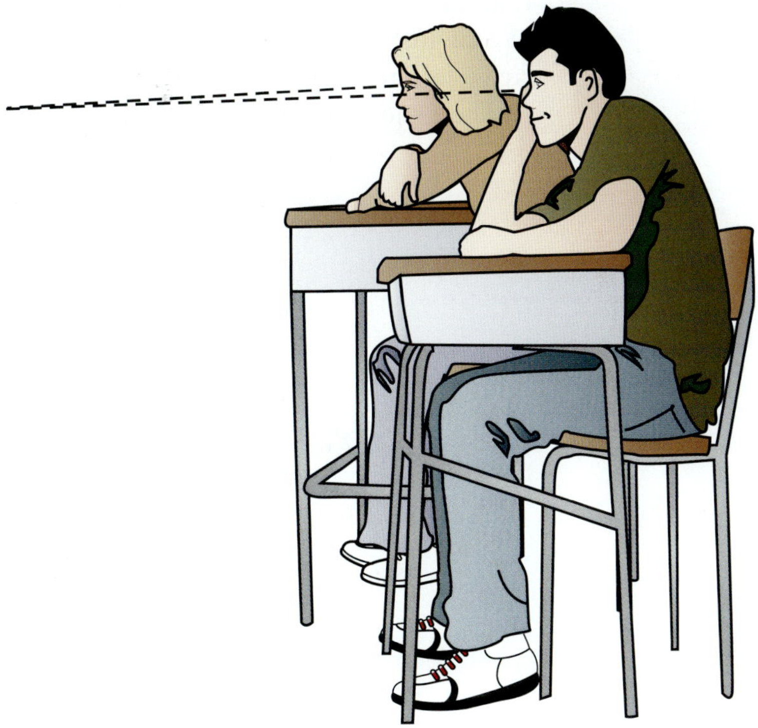

*Before going any further, we feel compelled to address one of the less monumental polarizing controversies of our time: EKG vs ECG. A little history may help. As much as we can give credit to any one person for inventing this amazing tool, that credit belongs to Willem Einthoven, the Dutch Nobel Laureate who created the first real Electrokardiogram machine. Did you notice the "k" stuck in the middle? Whereas most of the world has converted to the English spelling—electrocardiogram, hence ECG—in the United States, where obstinacy is too often viewed as a virtue, we have clung to the EKG acronym, although even here the bonds of tradition are loosening. So no worries. Either is OK. After all, you don't panic when you are invited to a barbecue instead of a barbeque, do you?

Some people have compared learning to read EKGs with learning to read music. In both instances, one is faced with a completely new notational system not rooted in conventional language and full of unfamiliar shapes and symbols.

But there really is no comparison. The simple lub-dub of the heart cannot approach the subtle complexity of a Beethoven string quartet (especially the late ones!), the multiplying tonalities and polyrhythms of Stravinsky's Rite of Spring, or the extraordinary jazz interplay of Keith Jarrett's Standards Trio.

There's just not that much going on.

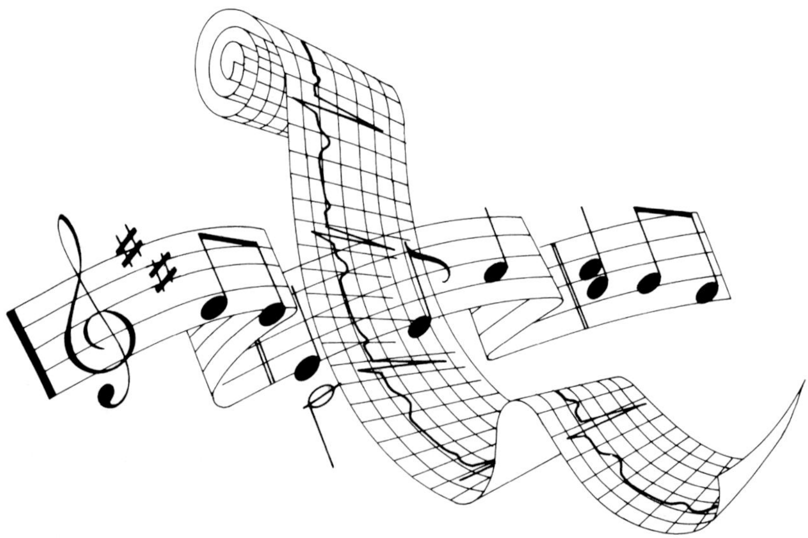

The EKG is a tool of remarkable clinical power, both because of the ease with which it can be mastered and because of the extraordinary range of situations in which it can provide helpful and often critical information. With one glance at an EKG, you can diagnose an evolving myocardial infarction, identify a potentially life-threatening arrhythmia, pinpoint the chronic effects of sustained hypertension, recognize the acute effects of a massive pulmonary embolus, or determine the likelihood of underlying coronary artery disease in a patient with chest pain.

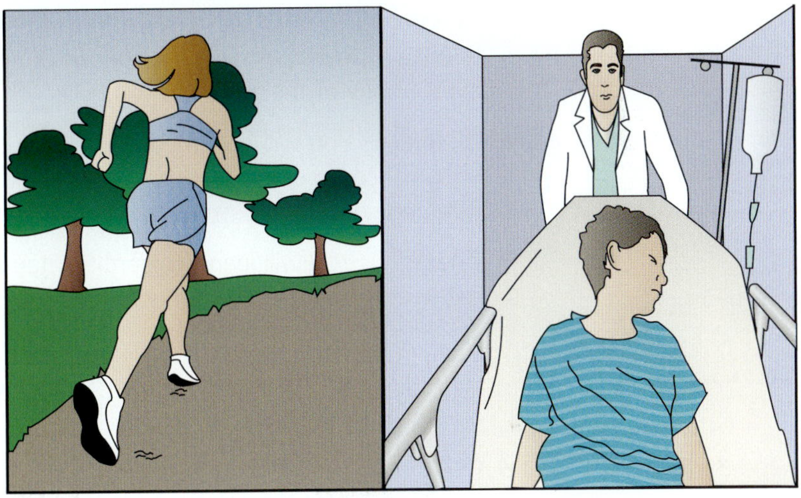

Remember, however, that the EKG is only a tool and, like any tool, is only as capable as its user. Put a chisel in my hand and you are unlikely to get Michelangelo's *David*.

The nine chapters of this book will take you on an *electrifying* voyage from ignorance to dazzling competence. You will amaze your friends and family (and, more importantly, yourself) and—the real point of this whole undertaking—help your patients. The road map you will follow looks like this:

- Chapter 1: You will learn about the electrical events that generate the different waves on the EKG, and—armed with this knowledge—you will be able to recognize and understand the normal 12-lead EKG.
- Chapter 2: You will see how simple and predictable alterations in certain waves permit the diagnosis of enlargement and hypertrophy of the atria and ventricles.
- Chapter 3: You will become familiar with the most common disturbances in cardiac rhythm and learn why some are life threatening, whereas others are benign or mere nuisances.
- Chapter 4: You will learn to identify interruptions in the normal pathways of cardiac conduction and be introduced to pacemakers.
- Chapter 5: You will see what happens when the heart's electrical current bypasses the usual channels of conduction and arrives more quickly at its destination.
- Chapter 6: You will learn to diagnose ischemic heart disease: myocardial infarctions (heart attacks) and angina (discomfort that results when regions of the heart are deprived of oxygen).
- Chapter 7: You will see how various other important cardiac and noncardiac phenomena can alter the EKG, and explore the current consensus on the utility of the EKG in evaluating patients before surgery and athletes before sports participation.
- Chapter 8: You will put all your newfound knowledge together into a simple method for reading any and all EKGs.
- Chapter 9: You will be able to test your knowledge by analyzing a panoply of practice strips, some simple, some challenging, and revel in your newly acquired skills.

The whole process is straightforward and should not be the least bit intimidating. Intricacies of thought and great leaps of creative logic are not required.

This is not the time for deep thinking.

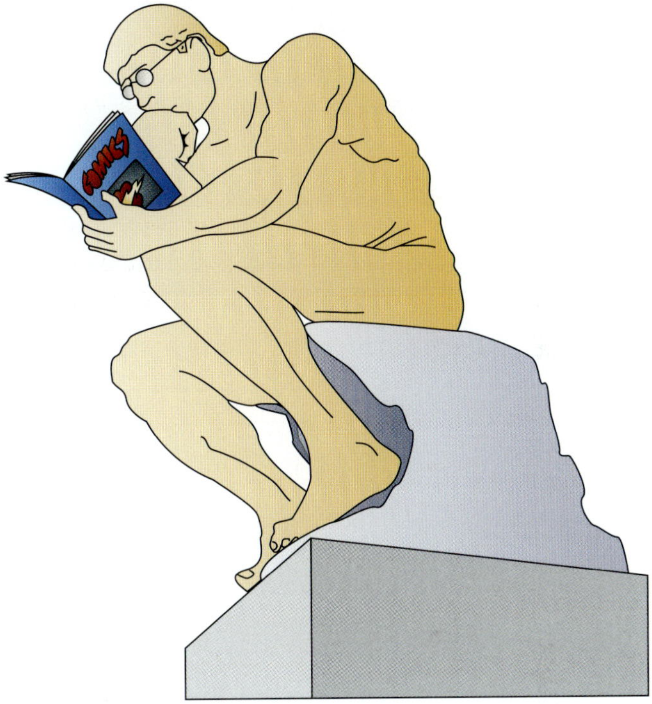

1 The Basics

In this chapter, you will learn:

1. how the electrical current in the heart is generated
2. how this current is propagated through all four chambers of the heart
3. that the movement of electricity through the heart produces predictable wave patterns that we are able to detect and whose height, width, and shape we can measure
4. how the EKG machine records these waves
5. that the EKG looks at the heart from 12 different perspectives, providing a remarkable three-dimensional electrical map of the heart
6. to *understand* what all the lines and waves on the 12-lead EKG represent
7. that trusting the EKG machine to interpret your patient's EKG is nothing but an invitation to trouble!

Electricity and the Heart

Electricity, an innate biologic electricity, is what makes the heart go. The EKG is nothing more than a recording of the heart's electrical activity, and it is through perturbations in the normal electrical patterns that we are able to diagnose many different cardiac and noncardiac disorders.

All You Need to Know About Cellular Electrophysiology in a Few Brief Paragraphs

Cardiac cells, in their resting state, are electrically polarized; their insides are negatively charged with respect to their outsides. This electrical polarity is maintained by membrane pumps that ensure the appropriate distribution of ions (primarily potassium, sodium, chloride, and calcium) necessary to keep the insides of these cells relatively electronegative. These ions pass into and out of cells through special ion channels in the cellular membrane.

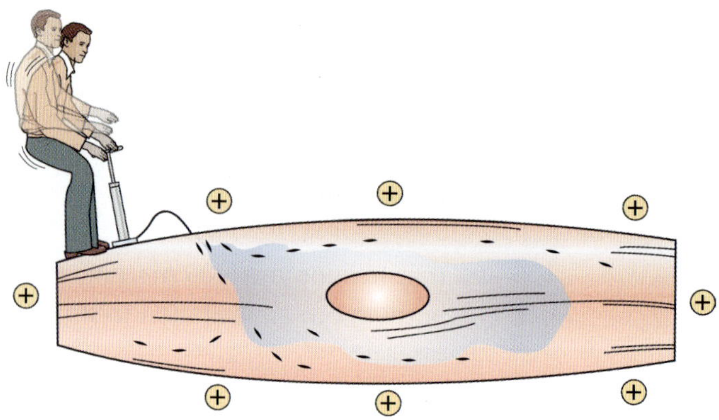

The resting cardiac cell maintains its electrical polarity by means of a membrane pump. This pump requires a constant supply of energy, and the gentleman above, were he real rather than a metaphor, would soon be flat on his back.

Sometimes lethal disturbances in the conduction of electricity through the heart can occur because of an inherited disorder affecting these transmembrane ion channels. We will encounter some of these *channelopathies* as we progress through this book. Many different genetic mutations affecting the cardiac ion channels have been identified, and more are being discovered every year. Various medications and toxins can also alter the normal function of these cardiac ion channels.

Cardiac cells can lose their internal negativity in a process called *depolarization*. **Depolarization is the fundamental electrical event of the heart**. In some cells, known as pacemaker cells, it occurs spontaneously. In others, it is initiated by the arrival of an electrical impulse that causes positively charged ions to cross the cell membrane.

Depolarization is propagated from cell to cell, producing a wave of depolarization that can be transmitted across the entire heart (see the illustration on the next page). This wave of depolarization represents a flow of electricity, an electrical current, that can be detected by electrodes placed on the surface of the body.

After depolarization is complete, the cardiac cells restore their resting polarity through a process called *repolarization*. Repolarization is accomplished by the membrane pumps, which reverse the flow of ions. Just like depolarization, this process can also be detected by recording electrodes.

All of the different waves that we see on an EKG are manifestations of these two processes: depolarization and repolarization.

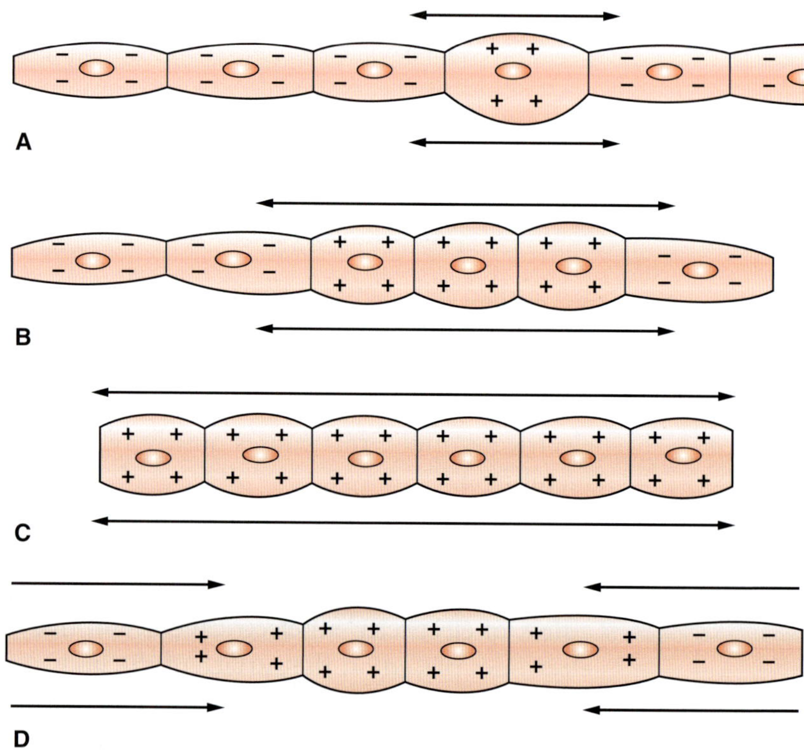

In (*A*), a single cell has depolarized. A wave of depolarization then propagates from cell to cell (*B*) until all are depolarized (*C*). Repolarization (*D*) then restores each cell's resting polarity.

Some people like to visualize the flow of electricity through the heart by using the analogy of a pond. Toss a pebble into a pond; a wave will originate at that single point and then spread out through the entire body of water. Do you like analogies? Here's another example for thinking about depolarization and repolarization. Picture a row of dominos. With depolarization, once the initial impetus has been applied to the first domino, they will all fall down one after another until they are all flat on their backs. Repolarization is when they all flip back and are upright again, ready to restart the process.

The Cells of the Heart

From the standpoint of the electrocardiographer, the heart consists of three types of cells:

- *Pacemaker cells*—under normal circumstances, the electrical power source of the heart
- *Electrical conducting cells*—the hard wiring of the heart
- *Myocardial cells*—the contractile machinery of the heart; unlike the first two cell types, myocardial cells lack specialized conducting properties

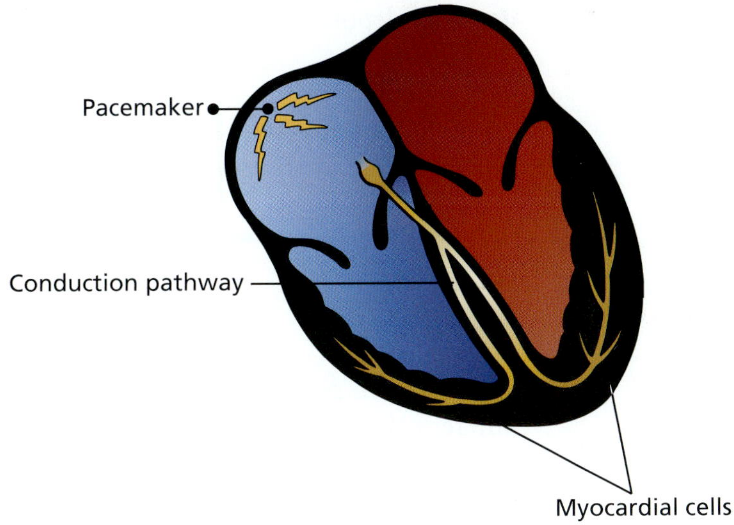

Pacemaker Cells

Pacemaker cells are small cells ~5–10 μm long, about the same as the width of a single strand of a spider's web. These cells are able to depolarize spontaneously over and over again. The rate of depolarization is determined by the innate electrical characteristics of the cell and by external neurohormonal input. Each spontaneous depolarization serves as the source of a wave of depolarization that initiates one complete cycle of cardiac contraction and relaxation.

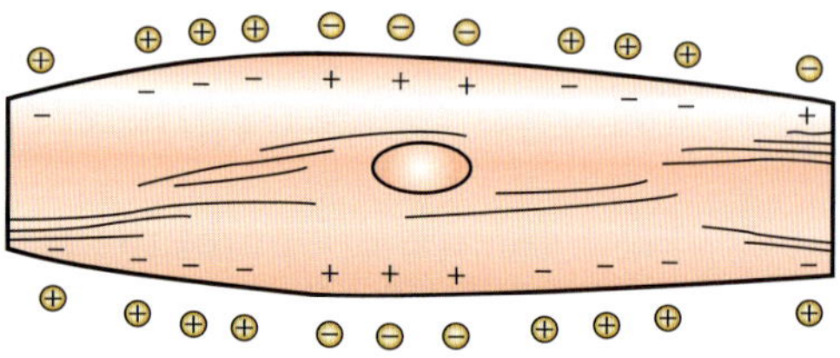

A pacemaker cell depolarizing spontaneously.

If we record the electrical activity from a single cell, we can obtain an electrical tracing called an **action potential**. With each spontaneous depolarization, a new action potential is generated, which in turn stimulates neighboring cells to depolarize and generate their own action potential, and so on and on, until the entire heart has been depolarized.

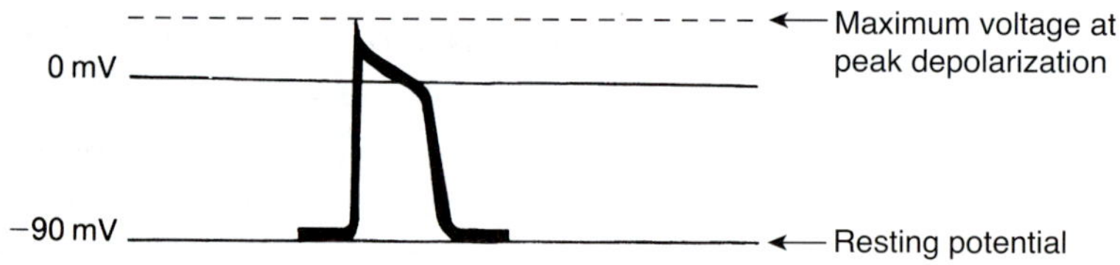

A typical myocyte action potential.

The action potential of a cardiac pacemaker cell looks a little different than the generic action potential shown above. A pacemaker cell does *not* have a true fixed resting potential. Its electrical charge drops to a minimal negative potential of approximately −60 mV, which it maintains for just a moment (it does not rest there), and then gradually rises until it reaches the threshold for another sudden depolarization, that is, another action potential. These events are illustrated on the following tracing.

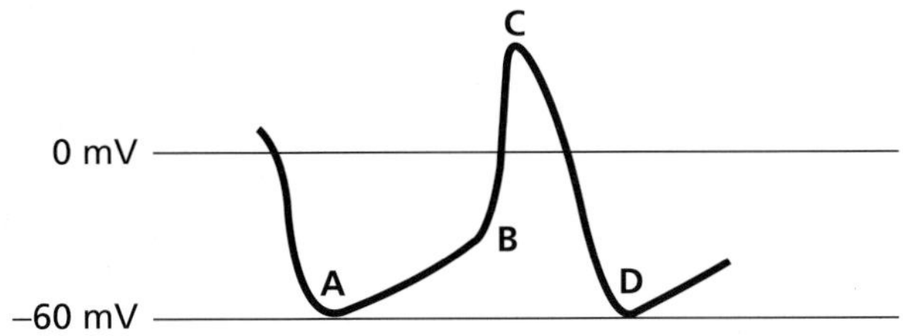

The electrical depolarization–repolarization cycle of a cardiac pacemaker cell. Point *A* is the minimal negative potential. The gentle rising slope between points *A* and *B* represents a slow, gradual depolarization. At point *B*, a threshold is crossed and the cell dramatically depolarizes (as seen between points *B* and *C*); that is, an action potential is produced. The downslope between points *C* and *D* represents repolarization. This cycle will repeat over and over for, let us hope, many, many years.

The dominant pacemaker cells in the heart are located high up in the right atrium. This group of cells is called the **sinoatrial (SA) node**, or **sinus node** for short. These cells typically fire at a rate of 60–100 times per minute, but the rate can rise or fall far outside this range depending upon the activity of the autonomic nervous system (thus, eg, sympathetic stimulation from catecholamines [the "fight-or-flight" component of the nervous system], such as epinephrine and norepinephrine, accelerates the sinus node, whereas vagal stimulation ["rest or digest"] slows it) and the demands of the body for increased cardiac output (exercise raises the heart rate, whereas a well-deserved and restful afternoon nap lowers it). Vagal stimulation is dominant at rest.

It is important to know that we do not rely on just a single pacemaker cell to drive the heart, but rather a group of pacemaker cells—that is, a node of cells, specifically the sinus node. For this reason, we refer to the normal rhythm of the heart as **sinus rhythm**.

Pacemaker cells are really good at what they do. They will continue firing in a donor heart even after it has been harvested for transplant and before it has been connected to the new recipient. The transplanted heart, devoid of normal vagal stimulation (the nerves are cut when the new heart is implanted), beats at an average rate of 100 beats per minute (bpm).

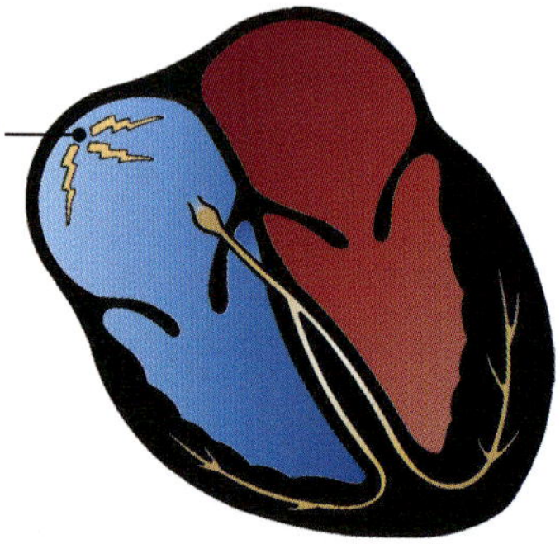

In a resting individual, the sinus node typically fires 60–100 times per minute, producing a regular series of action potentials, each of which initiates a wave of depolarization (depicted here as little lightning bolts) that will spread through the heart.

Actually, *every* cell in the heart has the ability to behave like a pacemaker cell. This so-called *automatic ability,* often referred to as automaticity, generates a rate that is normally slower than that of the sinus node and is therefore suppressed unless (1) the dominant cells of the sinus node fail or slow down below the intrinsic rate of other cells in the heart or (2) if something in the internal or external environment (sympathetic stimulation, cardiac disease, etc.) of a nonsinus cell stimulates its automatic behavior. This topic will assume great importance later on when we discuss *Ectopic Rhythms* in Chapter 3.

Electrical Conducting Cells

Like the wires of an electrical circuit, *electrical conducting cells* carry current rapidly and efficiently to distant regions of the heart. They are, in effect, the heart's electrical highway.

The electrical conducting cells of the ventricles form distinct electrical pathways that are remarkably consistent anatomically from one person to the next. The ventricular conducting fibers constitute what is called the *Purkinje system.*

The conducting pathways in the atria have more anatomic variability; prominent among these are fibers at the top of the intra-atrial septum in a region called the Bachmann bundle that allow for rapid activation of the left atrium from the right.

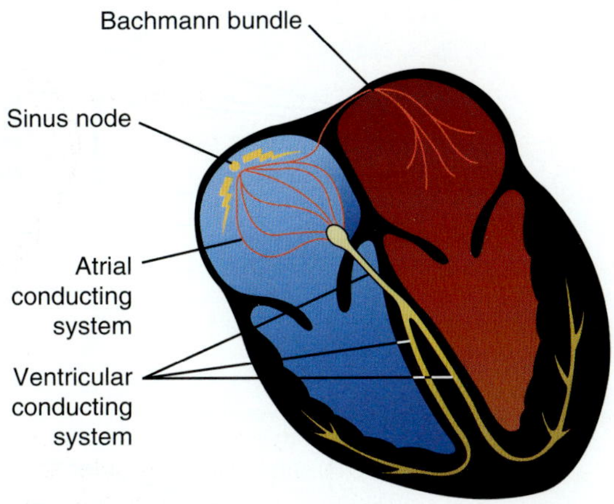

The hard wiring of the heart.

Myocardial Cells

The *myocardial cells* constitute by far the largest part of the heart. They are responsible for the heavy labor of repeatedly contracting and relaxing, thereby delivering blood to the rest of the body. These cells are about 50–100 μm in length and contain an abundance of the contractile proteins, actin and myosin.

When a wave of depolarization reaches a myocardial cell, calcium is released within the cell, causing the cell to contract. This process, in which calcium plays the key intermediary role, is called *excitation–contraction coupling*. Keep in mind that the electrical activity must precede the mechanical activity of the myocardium; hence, a disturbance in the heart's electrical activity can be life threatening.

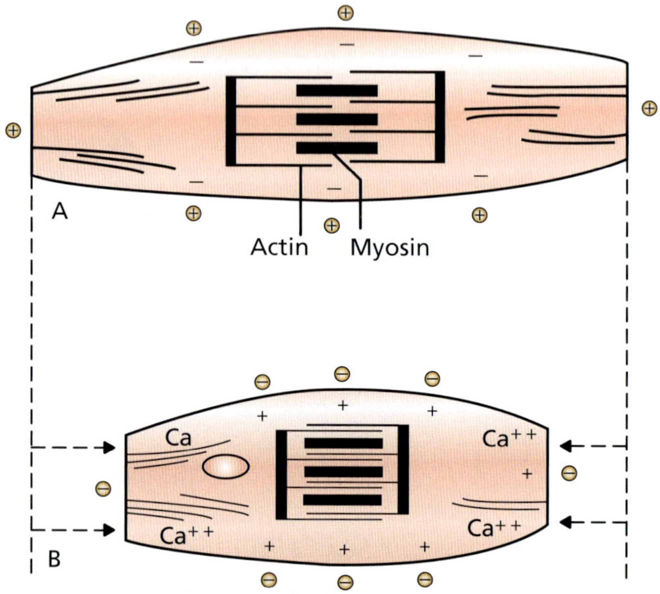

Depolarization causes calcium to be released within a myocardial cell. This influx of calcium allows actin and myosin, the contractile proteins, to interact, causing the cell to contract. (*A*) A resting myocardial cell. (*B*) A depolarized, contracted myocardial cell.

Myocardial cells can transmit an electrical current just like electrical conducting cells, but they do so far less efficiently. Thus, a wave of depolarization, upon reaching the myocardial cells, will spread slowly across the entire myocardium.

Time and Voltage

The waves that appear on an EKG primarily reflect the electrical activity of the *myocardial cells*, which make up the vast bulk of the heart. Pacemaker activity and transmission by the conducting system are generally not seen on the EKG; these events simply do not generate sufficient voltage to be recorded by the surface electrodes used to generate the standard 12-lead EKG that we will be discussing.

The waves produced by myocardial depolarization and repolarization are recorded on EKG paper and, like any wave, have three chief characteristics:

1. *Duration*, measured in fractions of a second
2. *Amplitude*, measured in millivolts (mV)
3. *Morphology*, a more subjective criterion referring to the shape and appearance of a wave

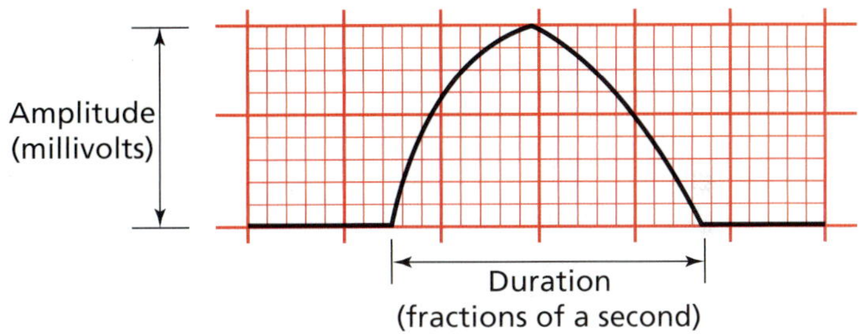

A typical wave that might be seen on any EKG. It is two large squares (or 10 small squares) in amplitude, three large squares (or 15 small squares) in duration, and slightly asymmetric in configuration.

EKG Paper

EKG paper is a long, continuous roll of graph paper, usually pink (although any color will do), with light and dark lines running vertically and horizontally. The light lines circumscribe small squares of 1×1 mm; the dark lines delineate large squares of 5×5 mm.

The horizontal axis measures time. When run at standard paper speed, the distance across one small square represents 0.04 seconds (or 40 milliseconds). The distance across one large square is five times greater, or 0.2 seconds (200 milliseconds).

The vertical axis measures voltage. The height of one small square represents 0.1 millivolts (mV), and along one large square, 0.5 mV.

You will need to memorize these numbers at some point, so you might as well do it now.

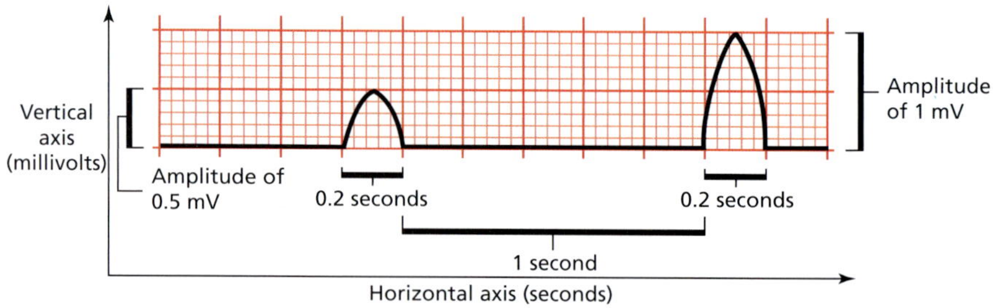

Both waves are one large square in duration (0.2 seconds), but the second wave is twice the voltage of the first (1 mV compared with 0.5 mV). The flat segment connecting the two waves is five large squares (5 × 0.2 seconds = 1 second) in duration.

P Waves, QRS Complexes, T Waves, and Some Straight Lines

Let's follow one cycle of cardiac contraction (systole) and relaxation (diastole), focusing on the electrical events that produce the basic waves and lines of the standard EKG.

Atrial Depolarization

The sinus node fires spontaneously (an event not visible on the EKG), and a wave of depolarization begins to spread along the atrial conducting system (also not visible on the EKG) into the atrial myocardium (now we can start to see things happening on the EKG), much as if a pebble were dropped into a calm body of water (yes, we are back to the pond analogy).

Depolarization of the atrial myocardial cells results in atrial contraction.

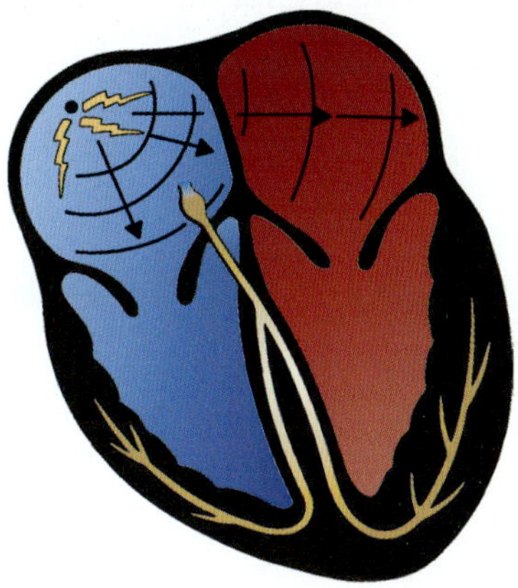

Each cycle of normal cardiac contraction and relaxation begins when the sinus node depolarizes spontaneously. The wave of depolarization then propagates through both atria, causing them to contract.

During atrial depolarization and contraction, electrodes placed on the surface of the body record a small burst of electrical activity lasting a fraction of a second. This is the *P wave*. It is a recording of the spread of depolarization through the atrial myocardium from start to finish.

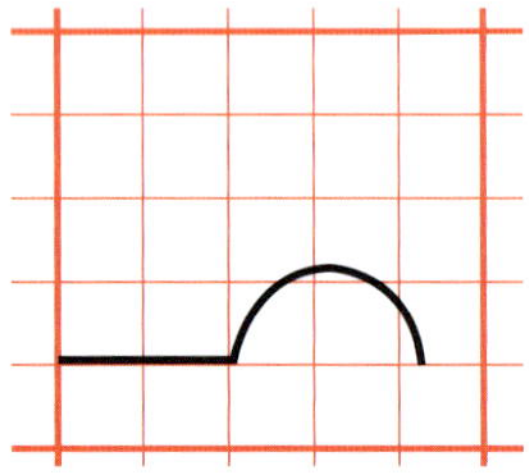

With atrial depolarization, the EKG records a small deflection, the P wave.

Because the sinus node is located in the right atrium, the right atrium begins to depolarize before the left atrium and finishes earlier as well. In normal conduction, the delay between left and right atrial depolarization is so small that we see only a single wave. However, it is important to recognize that the first part of the P wave predominantly represents right atrial depolarization and the second part left atrial depolarization.

Once atrial depolarization is complete, the EKG again becomes electrically silent.

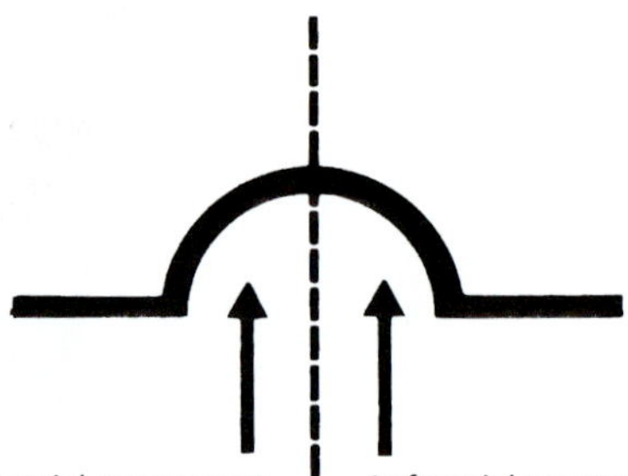

The components of the P wave.

A Pause Separates Conduction From the Atria Into the Ventricles

The wave of depolarization, having completed its journey through the atria, is prevented from communicating with the ventricles by the heart valves that separate the atria and ventricles. Electrical conduction must therefore be funneled along the interventricular septum, the wall that separates the right and left ventricles. Here, a structure called the *atrioventricular* (*AV*) *node* slows conduction to a crawl. This pause lasts only a fraction of a second.

This physiologic delay in conduction at the AV node is essential to allow the atria to finish contracting before the ventricles begin to contract. This simple but clever electrical wiring of the heart permits the atria to empty their volume of blood completely into the ventricles before the ventricles contract. The AV node also protects the ventricles from overstimulation should the atria start firing rapidly (as can occur with, for example, atrial fibrillation, see page 152). Think of the AV as a filter.

Like the sinus node, the AV node is also under the influence of the autonomic nervous system. Vagal stimulation slows the current even further, prolonging the delay, whereas sympathetic stimulation accelerates the current through the AV node.

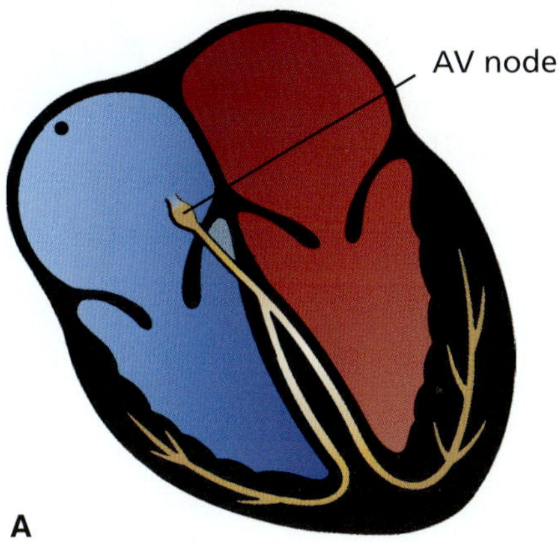

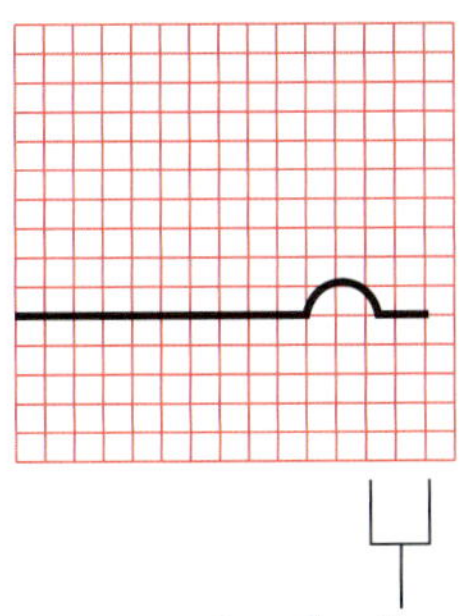

(*A*) The wave of depolarization is briefly held up at the AV node. (*B*) During this pause, the EKG falls silent; there is no detectable electrical activity.

Ventricular Depolarization

After about one-tenth of a second, the depolarizing wave escapes the AV node and is swept rapidly down the ventricles along specialized electrical conducting cells.

This ventricular conducting system has a complex anatomy but essentially consists of three parts:

1. Bundle of His
2. Bundle branches
3. Terminal *Purkinje fibers*

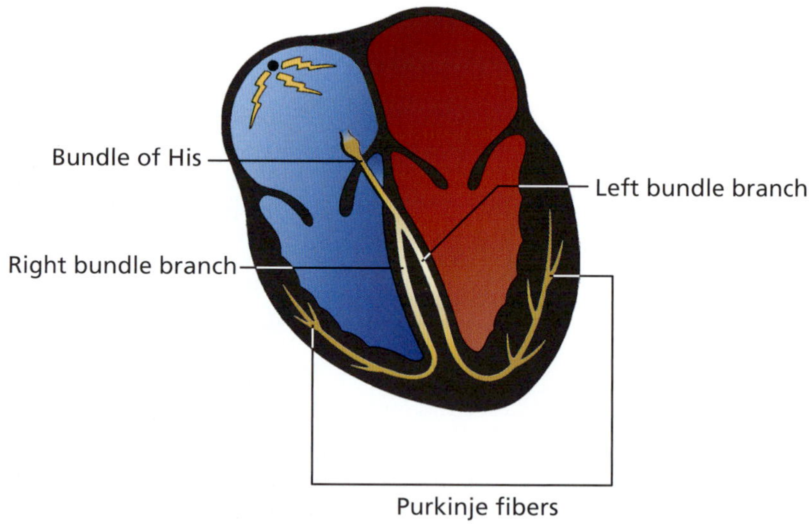

The *bundle of His* emerges from the AV node and almost immediately divides into right and left bundle branches. The *right bundle branch* carries the current down the right side of the interventricular septum all the way to the apex of the right ventricle. The *left bundle branch* is more complicated. It divides into three major fascicles:

1. *Septal fascicle*, which depolarizes the interventricular septum (the wall of muscle separating the right and left ventricles) in a left-to-right direction

2. *Anterior fascicle*, which runs along the anterior wall (ie, the part of the heart closest to the chest) of the left ventricle
3. *Posterior fascicle*, which sweeps over the posterior wall of the left ventricle

The right bundle branch and the left bundle branch and their fascicles terminate in countless tiny Purkinje fibers, which resemble little twigs coming off the branches of a tree. These fibers deliver the electrical current into the ventricular myocardium.

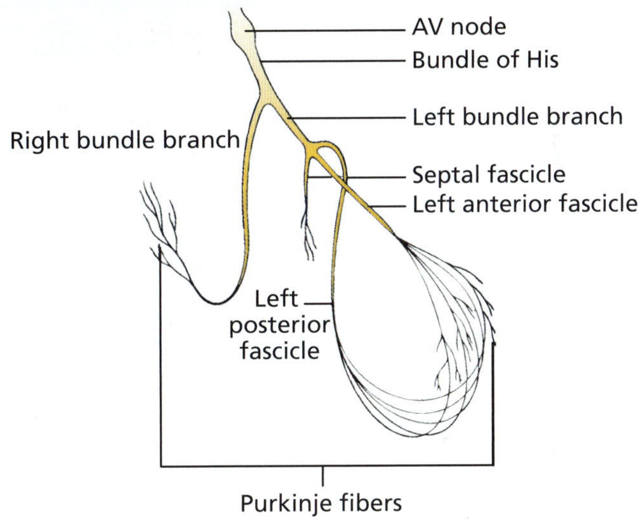

The ventricular conduction system, shown in detail. Below the bundle of His, the conduction system divides into right and left bundle branches. The right bundle branch remains intact, whereas the left divides into three separate fascicles.

Ventricular myocardial depolarization causes ventricular contraction. It is marked by a large deflection on the EKG called the *QRS complex*. Why does it take three letters to name this deflection, unlike the more straightforward P wave? Because each letter stands for a different component, that is, wave, of the complete complex as you will see in just a moment.

The amplitude of the QRS complex is much greater than that of the atrial P wave because the ventricles have so much more muscle mass than the atria. The QRS complex is also more complicated and variable in shape than the P wave, reflecting the greater intricacy of the pathway of ventricular depolarization.

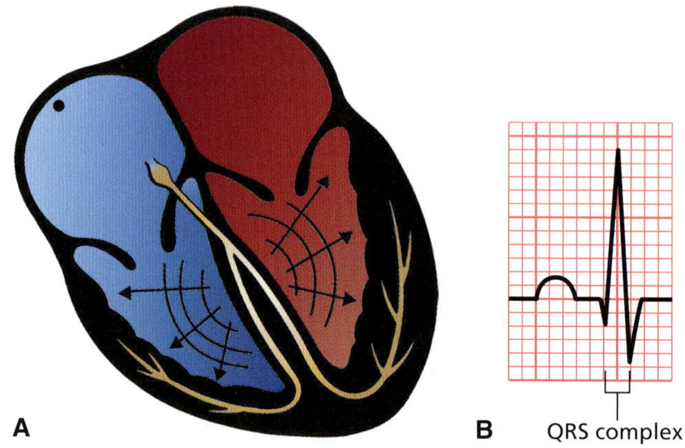

(*A*) Ventricular depolarization generates (*B*) a large, complicated waveform on the EKG called the QRS complex.

The Parts of the QRS Complex

The QRS complex consists of several distinct waves, each of which has a name. Because the precise configuration of the QRS complex can vary so greatly, a standard format for naming each component has been devised. It may seem a bit arbitrary to you right now, but it actually makes good sense.

1. If the first deflection is downward, that part of the QRS complex is called a *Q wave.*
2. The first upward deflection is called an *R wave.*
3. If there is a second upward deflection, it is called *R′* ("R-prime").
4. The first downward deflection following an upward deflection is called an *S wave*. Therefore, if the first wave of the complex is an R wave, the ensuing downward deflection is called an S wave, not a Q wave. A downward deflection can only be called a Q wave if it is the first wave of the complex. Any other downward deflection is called an S wave.
5. If the entire configuration consists solely of one downward deflection, the wave is called a *QS wave.*

Here are several of the most common QRS configurations, with each wave component named.

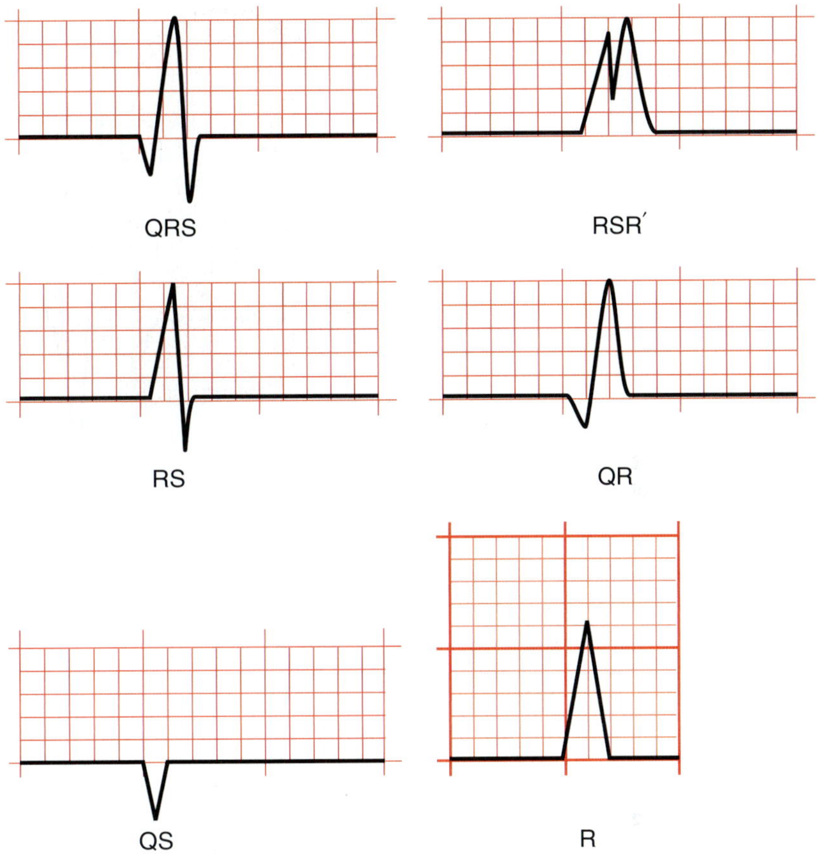

The earliest part of the QRS complex represents depolarization of the interventricular septum by the septal fascicle of the left bundle branch. The right and left ventricles then depolarize at about the same time, but most of what we see on the EKG represents left ventricular activation because, in normal healthy hearts, the muscle mass of the left ventricle is about three times that of the right ventricle.

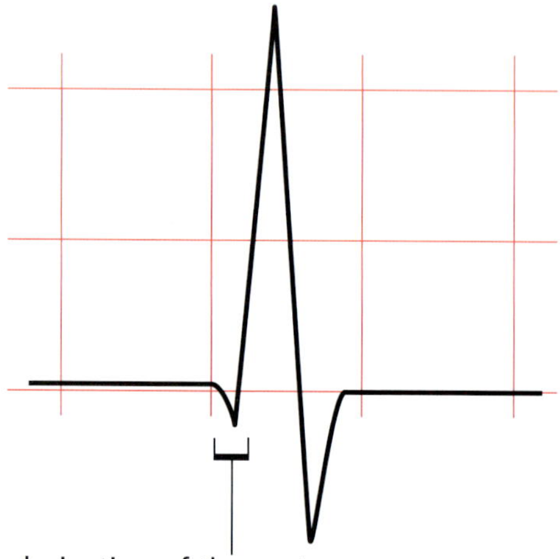

The initial part of the QRS complex represents septal depolarization. Sometimes, this septal depolarization may appear as a small, discrete, negative deflection, a Q wave.

Repolarization

After myocardial cells depolarize, they pass through a brief refractory period during which they are resistant to further stimulation. They then *repolarize*; that is, they restore the electronegativity of their interiors so that they can be restimulated (feel free to revisit the domino analogy on page 12).

Just as there is a wave of depolarization, there is also a wave of repolarization. This, too, can be seen on the EKG. Ventricular repolarization inscribes a third wave on the EKG, the *T wave*.

Note: There is a wave of atrial repolarization as well, but it coincides with ventricular depolarization and is almost always hidden by the much more prominent QRS complex.

Ventricular repolarization is a slower process than ventricular depolarization. Therefore, the T wave is broader than the QRS complex. Its configuration is also simpler and more rounded, like the silhouette of a gentle hill compared to the sharp, jagged, and often intricate contour of the QRS complex. Except in certain pathologic conditions, which we will explore later, the amplitude of the T wave is less than that of the QRS complex.

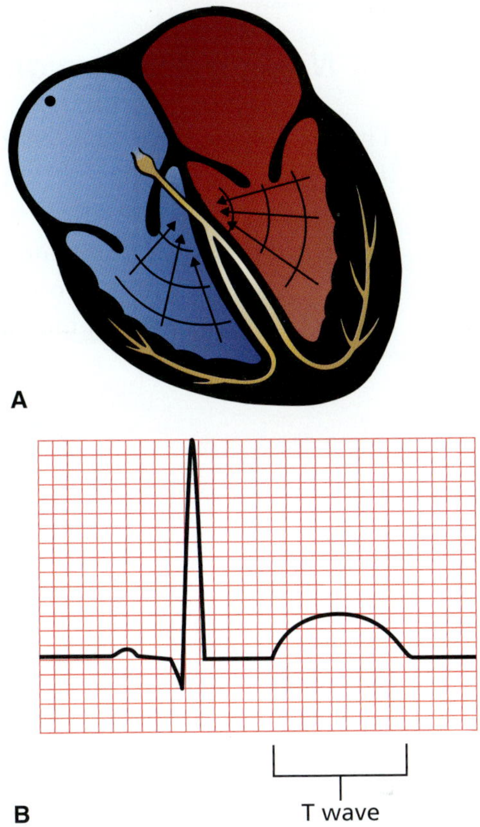

(*A*) Ventricular repolarization generates (*B*) a T wave on the EKG.

Naming the Straight Lines

The different straight lines connecting the various waves have also been given names. Thus, we speak of the *PR interval*, the *ST segment*, the *QT interval*, and so on.

What differentiates a segment from an interval? A segment is a straight line connecting two waves, whereas an interval encompasses at least one wave plus, in most instances, the connecting straight line.

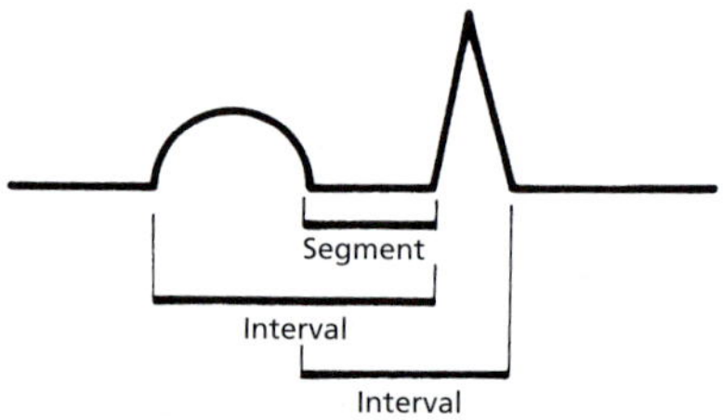

The *PR interval* includes the P wave and the horizontal line connecting it to the QRS complex. It therefore measures the time from the start of atrial depolarization to the start of ventricular depolarization.

The *PR segment* is the horizontal line running from the end of the P wave to the start of the QRS complex. It therefore measures the time from the end of atrial depolarization to the start of ventricular depolarization.

You might be wondering: if the QRS complex has a Q wave, shouldn't the PR segment be called the PQ segment, and the PR interval the PQ interval? Well, yes, but they're not. These straight lines are always called the PR segment and PR interval, no matter what the configuration of the QRS complex.

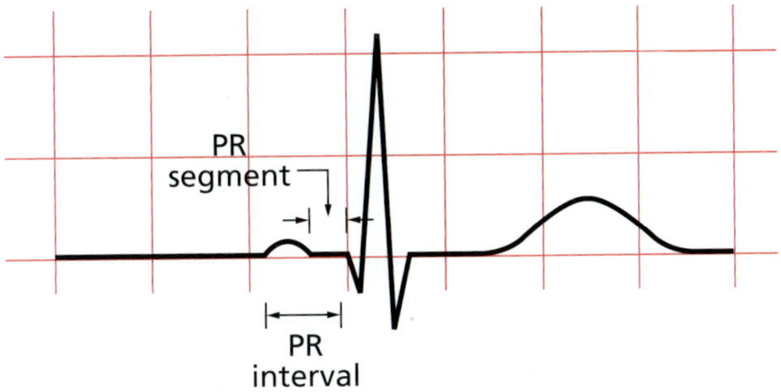

The *ST segment* is the straight line connecting the end of the QRS complex with the beginning of the T wave. It measures the time from the end of ventricular depolarization to the start of ventricular repolarization.

The *QT interval* includes the QRS complex, the ST segment, and the T wave. It therefore measures the time from the beginning of ventricular depolarization to the end of ventricular repolarization. And, yes, the term QT interval is used even if a particular QRS complex does not have a Q wave.

The term *QRS interval* is used to describe the duration of the QRS complex alone without any connecting segments. It measures the duration of ventricular depolarization.

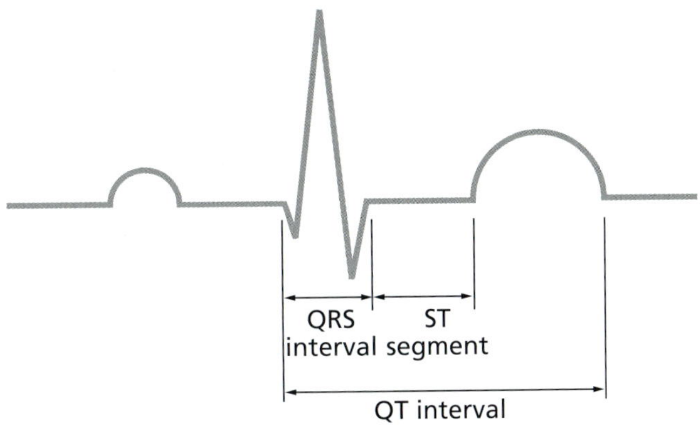

SUMMARY The Waves and Straight Lines of the EKG

1. Each cycle of cardiac contraction and relaxation is initiated by spontaneous depolarization of the sinus node. This event is not seen on the EKG.
2. The P wave records atrial depolarization and contraction. The first part of the P wave reflects right atrial activity; the second part reflects left atrial activity.
3. There is a brief pause when the electrical current reaches the AV node and the EKG falls silent (the PR segment).
4. The wave of depolarization then spreads along the ventricular conducting system (bundle of His, bundle branches, and Purkinje fibers) and out into the ventricular myocardium. The first part of the ventricles to be depolarized is the interventricular septum. Ventricular depolarization generates the QRS complex.
5. The T wave records ventricular repolarization. Atrial repolarization is not seen.
6. Various segments and intervals describe the time between these events:
   a. The PR interval measures the time from the **start** of atrial depolarization to the **start** of ventricular depolarization.
   b. The PR segment measures the time from the **end** of atrial depolarization to the **start** of ventricular depolarization.
   c. The ST segment records the time from the **end** of ventricular depolarization to the **start** of ventricular repolarization.
   d. The QT interval measures the time from the **start** of ventricular depolarization to the **end** of ventricular repolarization.
   e. The QRS interval measures the time of ventricular depolarization.

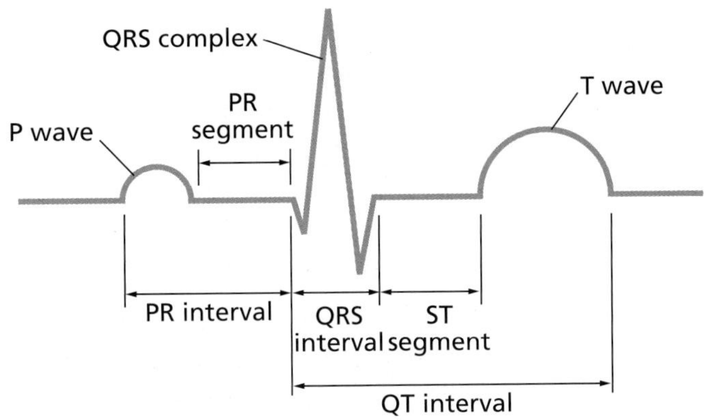
QRS complex
PR
segment
P wave
T wave
PR interval
QRS
interval
ST
segment
QT interval

Making Waves

Electrodes can be placed anywhere on the surface of the body to record the heart's electrical activity. If we do this, we quickly discover that the waves recorded by a positive electrode on the left arm look very different from those recorded by a positive electrode on the right arm (or right leg, left leg, etc.).

It's easy to see why. A wave of depolarization moving *toward* a positive electrode causes a *positive* deflection on the EKG. A wave of depolarization moving *away* from a positive electrode causes a *negative* deflection.

Look at the figure below. The wave of depolarization is moving left to right, *toward* the electrode. The EKG records a positive deflection.

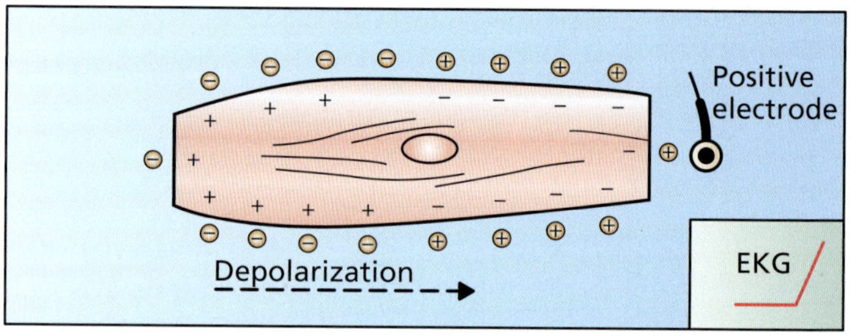

A wave of depolarization moving toward a positive electrode records a positive deflection on the EKG.

Now look at the following figure. The wave of depolarization is moving right to left, *away* from the electrode. The EKG therefore records a negative deflection.

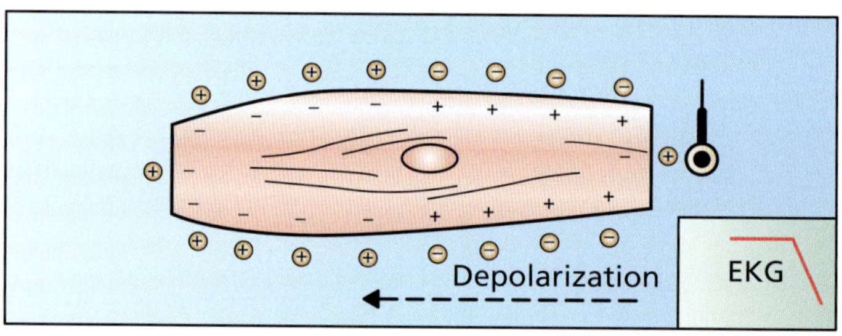

A wave of depolarization moving away from a positive electrode records a negative deflection on the EKG.

What will the EKG record if the positive electrode is placed near the middle of the cell?

Initially, as the wavefront approaches the electrode, the EKG records a positive deflection.

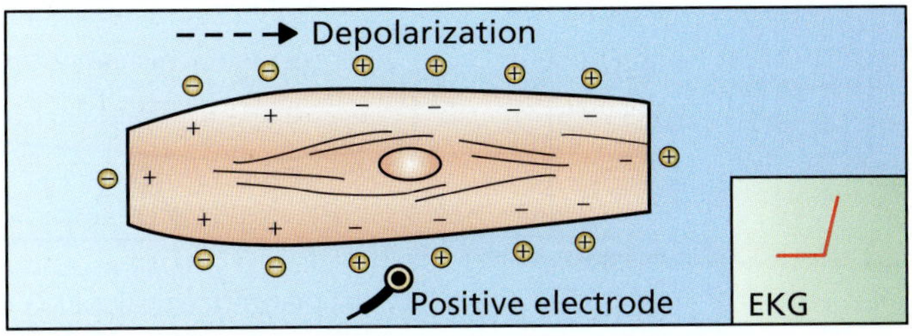

Depolarization begins, generating a positive deflection on the EKG.

Then, at the precise moment that the wave reaches the electrode, the positive and negative charges are balanced and essentially cancel each other out. The EKG recording returns to baseline.

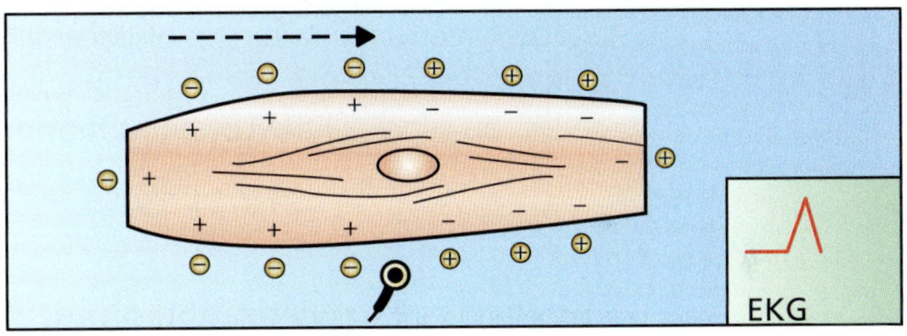

The wavefront reaches the electrode. The positive and negative charges are balanced, and the EKG returns to baseline.

As the wave of depolarization recedes, a negative deflection is inscribed.

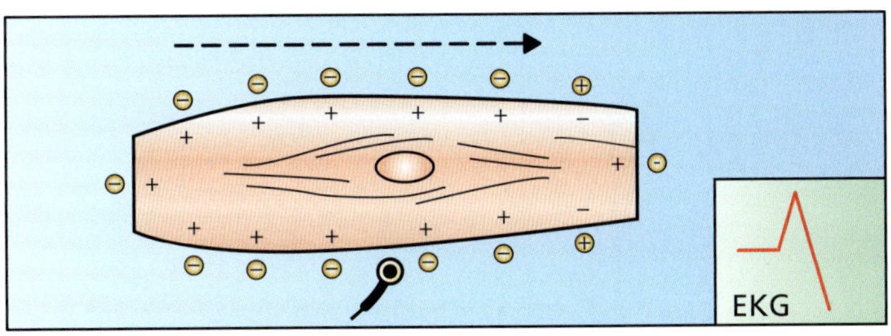

The wave of depolarization begins to recede from the electrode, generating a negative deflection.

The EKG finally returns to baseline once again when depolarization is complete.

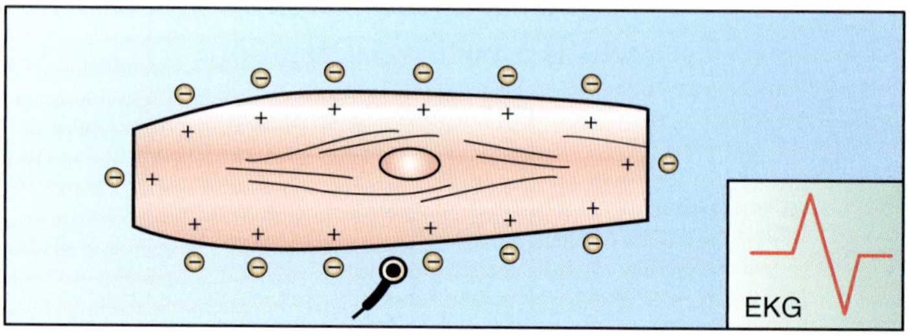

The cell is fully depolarized, and the EKG once again returns to baseline.

The final inscription of a depolarizing wave moving perpendicularly to a positive electrode is therefore a *biphasic wave*.

What would the tracing look like if the recording electrode was placed directly over a region of pacemaker cells sufficient to generate a detectable current? The tracing would show a downward, negative deflection, since all the current is moving away from the origin where you are recording.

The effects of repolarization on the EKG are similar to those of depolarization, except that the charges are reversed. A wave of repolarization moving *toward* a positive electrode inscribes a *negative* deflection on the EKG. A wave of repolarization moving *away* from a positive electrode produces a *positive* deflection on the EKG. A perpendicular wave produces a *biphasic wave*; however, the negative deflection of the biphasic wave now *precedes* the positive deflection.

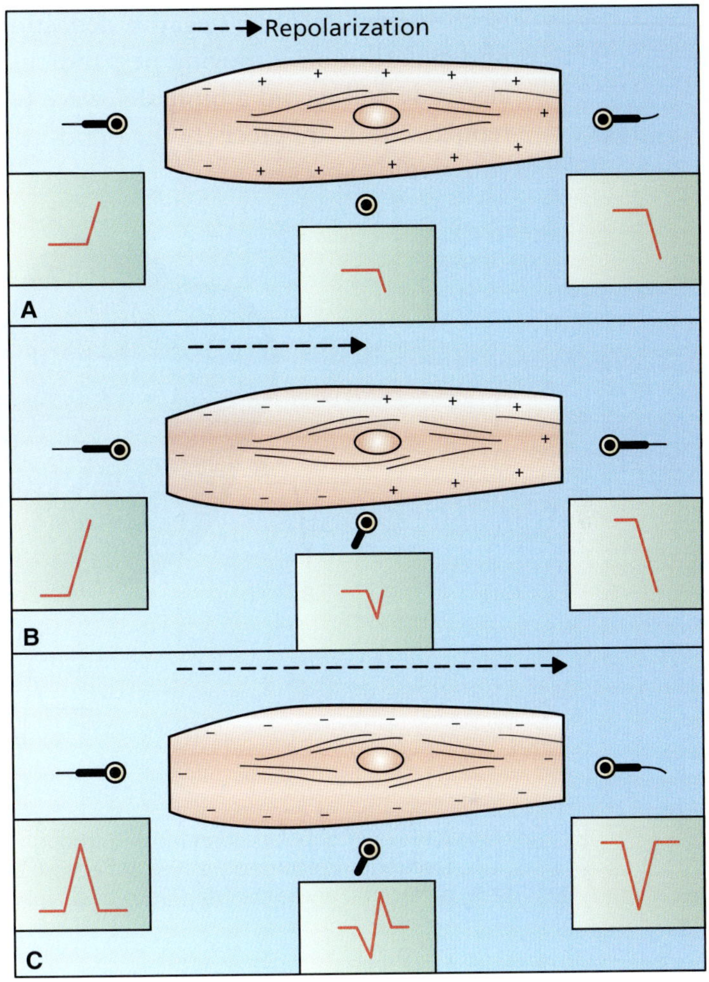

A wave of repolarization moving through muscle tissue is recorded by three different positive electrodes. (*A*) Early repolarization. (*B*) Late repolarization. (*C*) Repolarization is complete.

We can easily apply these concepts to the entire heart. Electrodes placed on the surface of the body will record waves of depolarization and repolarization as they sweep through the heart.

If a wave of depolarization passing through the heart is moving toward a surface electrode, that electrode will record a positive deflection (see the illustration on the next page—electrode *A*). If the wave of depolarization is moving away from the electrode, the electrode will record a negative deflection (electrode *B*). If the wave of depolarization is moving perpendicularly to the electrode, the electrode will record a biphasic* wave (electrode *C*). The effects of repolarization are precisely the opposite of those of depolarization, as you would expect.

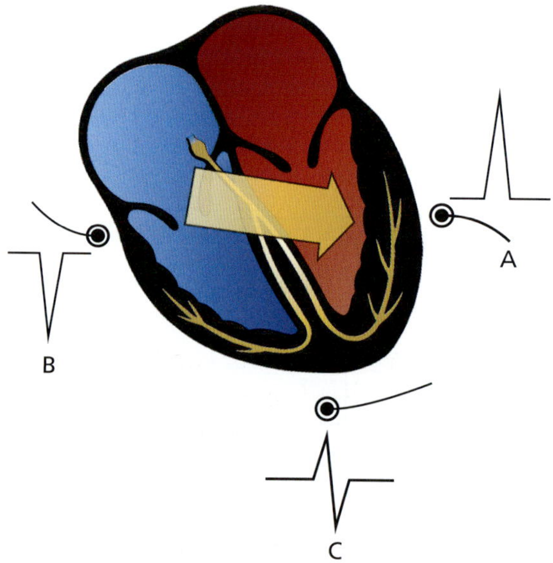

A wave of depolarization moving through the heart (*large arrow*). Electrode *A* records a positive deflection, electrode *B* records a negative deflection, and electrode *C* records a biphasic wave.

---

*Other terms used are equiphasic and isoelectric. Whatever the term, we are referring to roughly equal deflections above and below the line.

The 12 Views of the Heart

If the heart were as simple as a single myocardial cell, a couple of recording electrodes would give us all the information we need to describe its electrical activity. However, as we have already seen, the heart is *not* so simple—a burden to you, a boon to authors of EKG books.

The heart is a three-dimensional organ, and its electrical activity must be understood in three dimensions as well. A couple of electrodes are not adequate to do this, a fact that the original electrocardiographers recognized well over a century ago when they devised the first limb leads. Today, the standard EKG consists of 12 leads. Note that the definition of a *lead* is not the same as that of an *electrode.* Rather, a lead reflects the *combined* electrical activity (the actual act of combination is done inside the EKG machine by a very smart computer) of *several* electrodes or the activity of a single electrode compared to the body as a whole. Each lead is determined by the placement and orientation of 10 electrodes on the body, and each views the heart at a unique angle, enhancing its sensitivity to a particular region of the heart at the expense of others. The more views, the more the information provided.

To read an EKG and extract as much information as possible, you need to understand the 12-lead system.

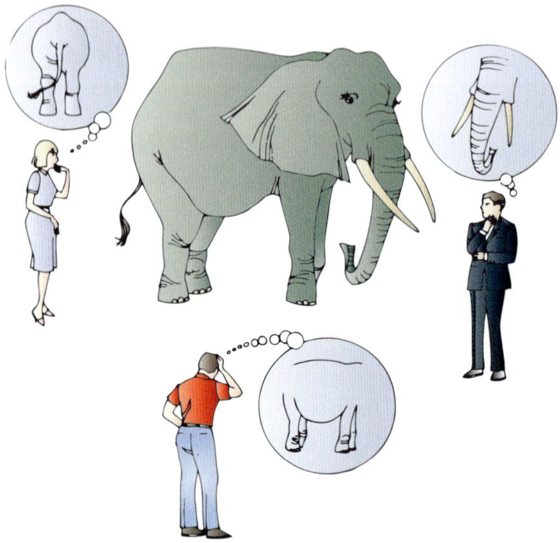

Three curious observers get three very different impressions of this consummate example of *Loxodonta africana*. One observer sees the trunk, another sees the body, and the third sees the tail. If you wanted the best description of the elephant, who would you ask? All three, of course.

To prepare a patient for a 12-lead EKG, two electrodes are placed on the arms and two on the legs. These provide the basis for the six *limb leads*, which include the three *standard leads* and the three *augmented leads* (these terms will make more sense in a moment). Six additional electrodes are also placed across the chest, forming the six *precordial leads*.

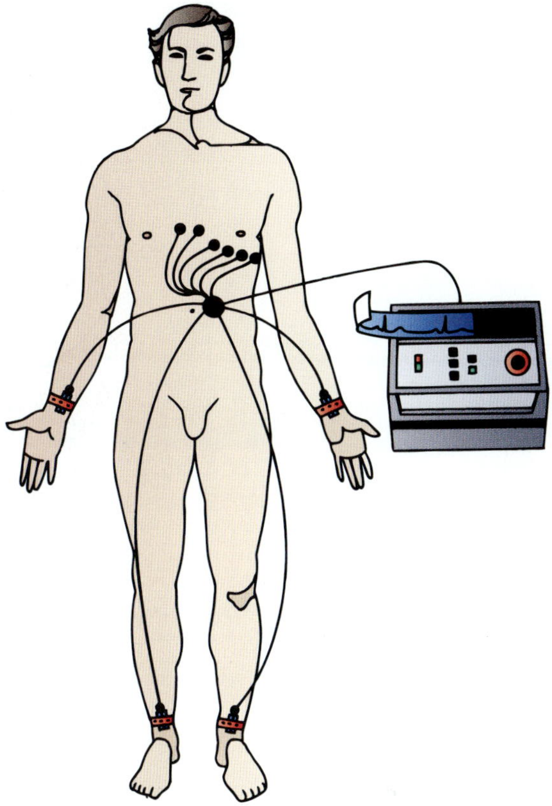

The electrical recordings will vary depending on the precise placement of the electrodes. Therefore, adherence to standard positioning protocols is very important to allow comparison between EKGs taken at different times in different settings.

The Six Limb Leads

The limb leads are created by putting electrodes on all four extremities. They view the heart in a vertical plane called the *frontal plane*. The frontal plane can be envisioned as a giant circle superimposed on the patient's body. This circle is then marked off in degrees. The limb leads view electrical forces (waves of depolarization and repolarization) moving up and down and left and right through this circle.

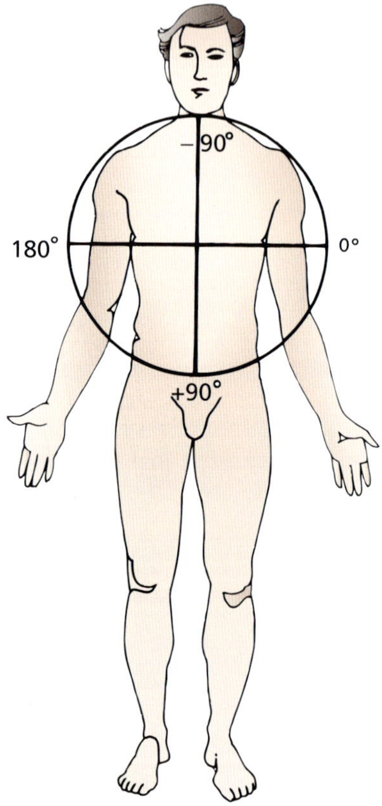

The frontal plane is a coronal plane. The limb leads view electrical forces moving up and down and left and right on the frontal plane.

To produce the six leads of the frontal plane, each of the electrodes is variably designated as positive or negative (this is done automatically by circuitry inside the EKG machine).

Each lead has its own specific view of the heart, or *angle of orientation*. The angle of each lead can be determined by drawing a line from the negative electrode(s) to the positive electrode(s). The resultant angle is then expressed in degrees by superimposing it on the 360° circle of the frontal plane. This is far less complicated than it sounds and is more easily illustrated than explained. So let's look at each limb lead individually.

The three standard limb leads are defined as follows:

1. Lead I is created by making the left arm positive and the right arm negative. Its angle of orientation is 0°.

2. Lead II is created by making the legs positive and the right arm negative. Its angle of orientation is 60°.
3. Lead III is created by making the legs positive and the left arm negative. Its angle of orientation is 120°.

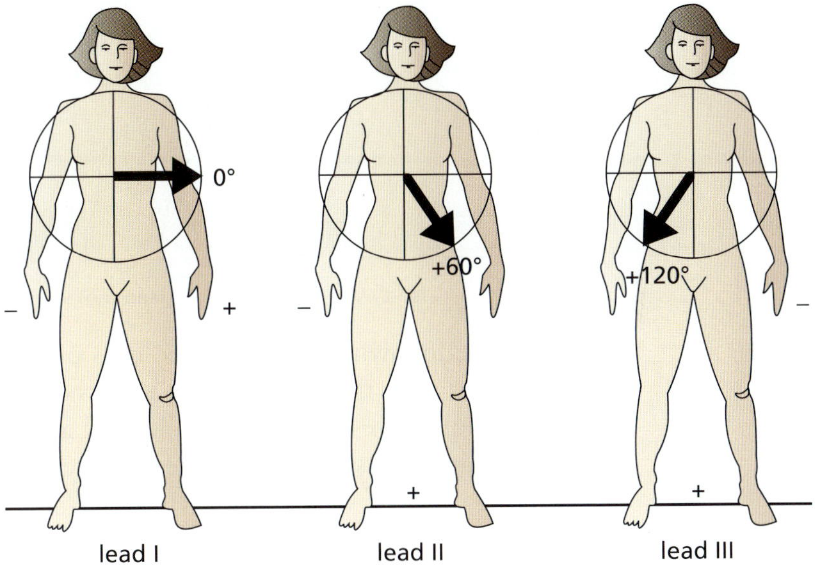

The three augmented limb leads are created somewhat differently. One or two leads are chosen to be positive, and all the others are made negative, with their average essentially serving as the negative electrode (common ground). They are called *augmented leads* because the EKG machinery must amplify the tracings to get an adequate recording.

1. Lead aVL is created by making the *left arm* positive and the other limbs negative. Its angle of orientation is −30°.
2. Lead aVR is created by making the *right arm* positive and the other limbs negative. Its angle of orientation is −150°.
3. Lead aVF is created by making the legs positive and the arms negative. Its angle of orientation is +90°, that is, toward the feet.

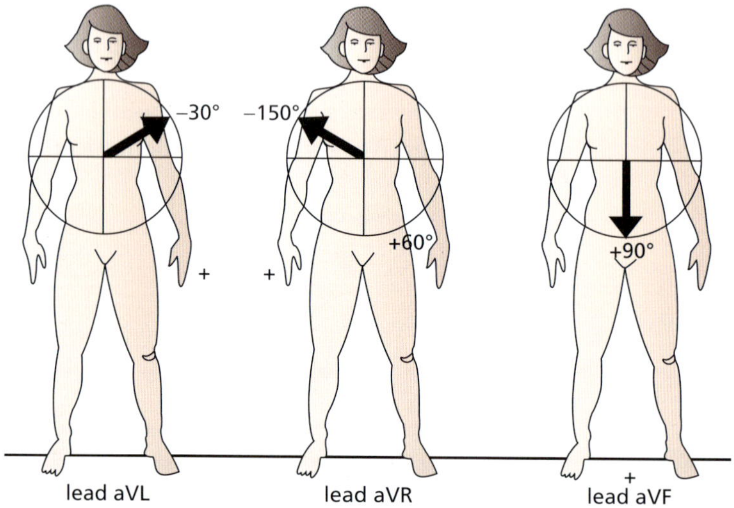

In the following figure, all six leads of the frontal plane are indicated with their appropriate angles of orientation. Just as our three inquisitive observers each looked at the elephant from their own unique perspective, each lead perceives the heart from its own unique point of view.*

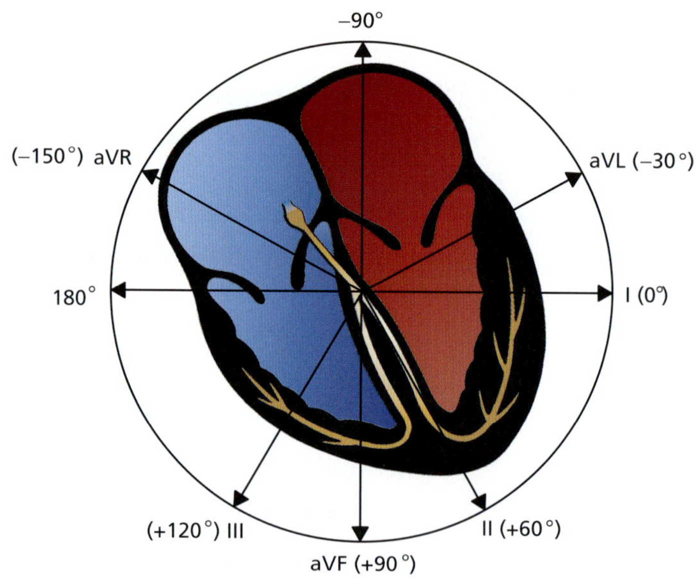

*You have no doubt noted, perhaps with some misgiving, that the circle of the frontal plane is designed such that the top half is negative and the bottom positive. Thus, the angle of the leads on the top half of the circle, aVR and aVL, are negative, whereas those below are positive (and lead I, of course, is 0°). This may not be the way we would have designed things, but it's what we are stuck with and there is simply no way around it.

Leads II, III, and aVF are called the *inferior leads* because they most effectively view the inferior surface of the heart. The inferior surface, or wall, of the heart is an anatomic term for the bottom of the heart, the portion that rests on the diaphragm.

Leads I and aVL are often called the *left lateral leads* because they have the best view of the left lateral wall of the heart.

aVR is a loner among the limb leads. It is the only true *right-sided limb lead*.

Now is as good a time as any to memorize these six leads and their angles.

Lead	Angle	
Inferior Leads		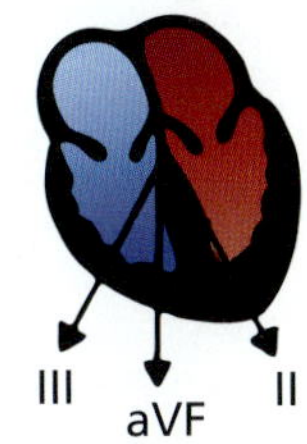
Lead II	+60°	
Lead III	+120°	
Lead aVF	+90°	
Left Lateral Leads		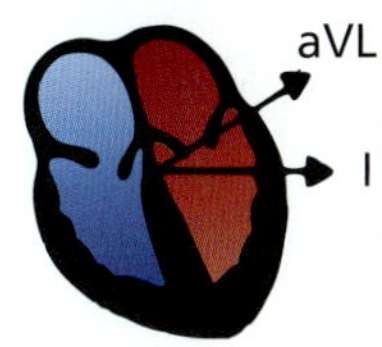
Lead I	+0°	
Lead aVL	−30°	
Right-sided Lead		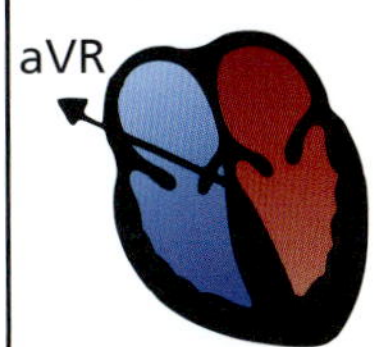
Lead aVR	−150°	

Of the six limb leads, three are standard (I, II, and III), and three are augmented (aVR, aVL, and aVF). Each lead views the heart from its own particular angle of orientation.

The Six Precordial Leads

The six precordial leads, or chest leads, are easier to understand. They are arranged across the chest in a *horizontal plane* as illustrated below. Whereas the leads of the frontal plane view electrical forces moving up and down and left and right, the precordial leads record forces moving anteriorly and posteriorly.

To create the six precordial leads, each chest electrode is made positive in turn, and the whole body is taken as the common ground. The six positive electrodes, creating the precordial leads V1 through V6, are positioned as follows:

- V1 is placed in the fourth intercostal space to the right of the sternum.
- V2 is placed in the fourth intercostal space to the left of the sternum.
- V3 is placed between V2 and V4.
- V4 is placed in the fifth intercostal space in the midclavicular line.
- V5 is placed between V4 and V6.
- V6 is placed in the fifth intercostal space in the midaxillary line.

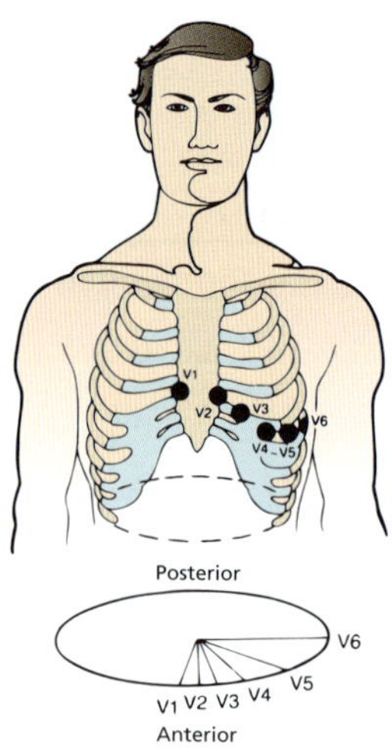

The precordial leads define a horizontal or transverse plane and view electrical forces moving anteriorly and posteriorly.

Just like the limb leads, each precordial lead has its own particular line of sight and region of the heart that it views best.

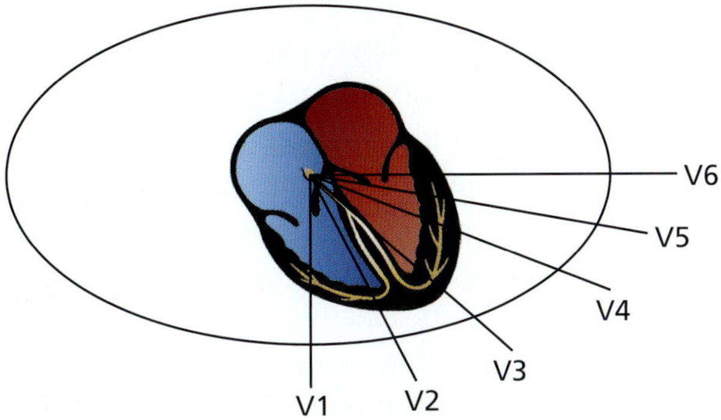

The right ventricle lies anteriorly and medially within the body cavity, and the left ventricle lies posteriorly and laterally. Lead V1 lies directly over the right ventricle, V2 and V3 over the interventricular septum, V4 over the apex of the left ventricle, and V5 and V6 over the lateral left ventricle.

Leads V2 through V4 are often referred to as the *anterior leads*, V5 and V6 join I and aVL as *left lateral leads*, and lead V1, along with aVR, comprise the *right ventricular leads*.

Leads	Group
V2, V3, V4	Anterior
I, aVL, V5, V6	Left lateral
II, III, aVF	Inferior
aVR, V1	Right ventricular

What Happens If You Misplace the Electrodes?

Perhaps you can already guess the answer to this question. If you reverse the limb electrodes—the most common mistake is to reverse the electrodes on the right and left arms—the EKG machine has no way of knowing that you have messed up. It can't adjust and correct your error.* Therefore, current moving left to right or right to left

*The artificial intelligence baked into many of the current EKG systems may be able to give an interpretation of possible limb lead reversal, but the EKG tracing on the page will still be reversed.

will have its electrical recording reversed 180°. In other words, a lead that would normally show a tall, positive wave will now show a deep negative one, and vice versa. Your interpretation of the EKG will be seriously flawed, and you may think that a perfectly healthy patient has a serious heart condition.

You must also be careful to place the precordial leads, V1 through V6, as precisely as possible on the chest wall. Even a slight misplacement can lead to a mistaken interpretation, indicating, for example, that a previous heart attack has taken place where none has occurred. Placing these precordial leads on the chest can be particularly challenging in an obese patient or in someone with large, pendulous breasts. You may also be tempted from time to time to move some of the chest wall electrodes just a smidgeon to avoid patches of thick hair on a hirsute patient; those sticky EKG electrode pads we typically use today do not adhere well when there is a thick clump of hair between the pads and the chest wall. Do not take the easy way out and give in to temptation and move the electrode pad out of position to a more congenial location. Ask your patient if it is okay to remove some of the hair and, if permission is granted, shave off the little spot of skin that you need. The hair will grow back quickly.

As many as 4% of all EKGs are run with incorrect lead placement by well-intentioned health care providers who are simply not being careful or who are understandably in a hurry (the emergency department and cardiac intensive care unit can be very stimulating and distracting environments!).

Does My Patient Have to Be Lying Down?

Yes, and as flat as possible. Some patients won't be able to lie perfectly flat—perhaps they have congestive heart failure and lying down makes them short of breath (orthopnea), or perhaps they have cervical arthritis and lying flat causes neck pain. Well, we are not tyrants—give your patient a pillow or elevate the head of the bed or examining table. But don't raise them up more than is necessary. Why does it matter? Changes in body posture affect the position of the heart within the body, and this in turn affects the voltage measurements on the EKG. Among the subtle changes that can occur are variations in the ST segments and the appearance of new Q waves, both of which, as we will discuss in Chapter 6, can be critical in diagnosing a myocardial infarction.

A Word About Vectors

It is important to recognize that each EKG electrode records only the *average* current flow at any given moment. Thus, although tiny swirls of current may simultaneously be going off in every direction, each lead records only the instantaneous average of these forces. In this way, out of chaos, some very simple patterns emerge.

This concept is really quite simple; an analogy may be helpful. During the course of a soccer match, a goalie may kick the ball many different times to various members of his team (or, if our hypothetical goalie is not very good, the other team). Some balls will go left, others right, and still others straight down the field. Now, imagine that all these kicks are made simultaneously rather than throughout the 90 minutes of a match. Once we sum up all the kicks the *average direction* of the goalie's kicks and tosses is likely to be straight ahead, toward the opposing net. This average direction can be represented by a single arrow, or *vector*.

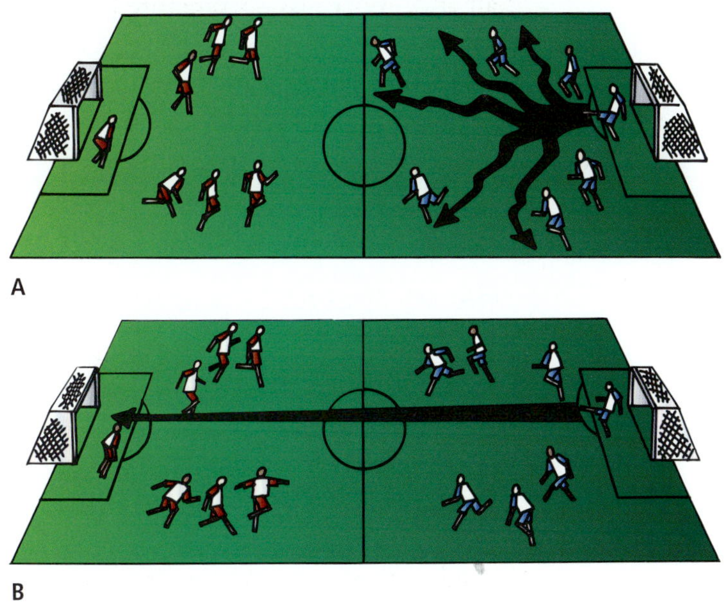

(*A*) The directions of each of the goalie's kicks during the course of the game. (*B*) A single vector represents the average direction and distance of all of these kicks.

This vector is precisely what our EKG electrodes record when measuring the electrical flow within the heart. The vector's angle of orientation represents the average *direction* of current flow, and its length represents the voltage (*amplitude*) attained.

At any given moment, the electrical forces moving within the heart can be represented by a single vector. Furthermore, over any particular period of time during the cardiac cycle (eg, atrial depolarization), these individual vectors can be summed into a kind of *vector of vectors*, which describes the average direction and magnitude of current flow during that time period (eg, during atrial depolarization, corresponding, let us say, to all the goalie's kicks over the first half of the game). Thus, any wave (in this case, the wave of atrial depolarization) can be described by a single vector with a particular direction and magnitude. You will see how this works and how it simplifies our understanding of the 12-lead EKG in the following section.

The Normal 12-Lead EKG

You now know the three things necessary to derive the normal 12-lead EKG:

1. The normal pathway of cardiac electrical activation and the names of the segments, waves, and intervals that are generated
2. The orientation of all 12 leads, 6 in the frontal plane and 6 in the horizontal plane
3. The concept that each lead records the average current flow at any given moment

All we need to do now is to take what you already know and figure out what each wave looks like in each of the 12 leads.

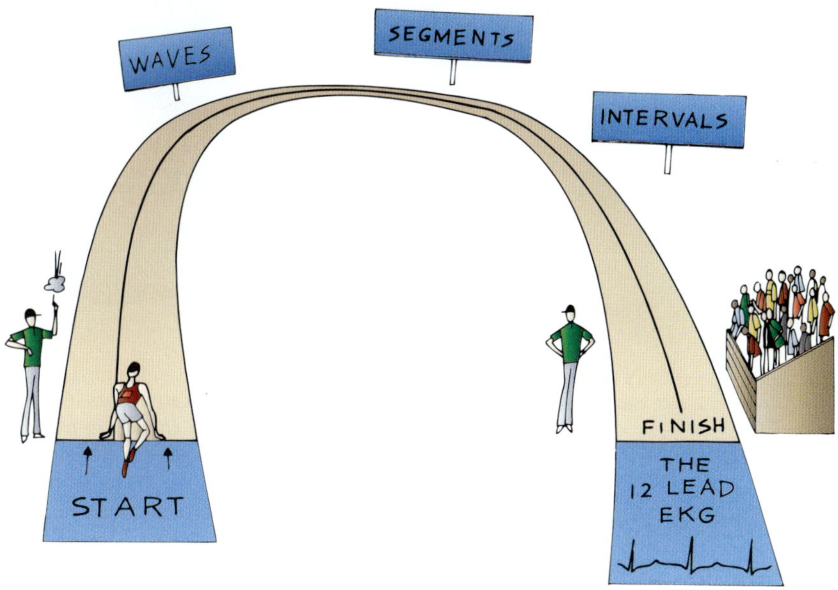

The P Wave

Atrial depolarization begins at the sinus node, high up in the right atrium. The right atrium depolarizes first and then the left atrium. The vector of current flow for atrial depolarization, therefore, points from right to left and slightly inferiorly (*large arrow shown on the next page*).

Any lead that views the wave of atrial depolarization as moving toward it will record a positive deflection on the EKG paper. The left lateral and inferior leads clearly fit this description. In the *frontal plane*, these leads include the left lateral leads I and aVL and the inferior leads II and aVF.

Lead III, which is also one of the inferior leads, is positioned a bit differently. It is the most rightward (orientation +120°) of the inferior leads and actually lies nearly perpendicular to the atrial current. Predictably, lead III frequently records a biphasic P wave.

Lead aVR, the most rightward of all the leads of the frontal plane (orientation −150°), sees the electrical current as moving away; hence, it records a purely negative deflection.

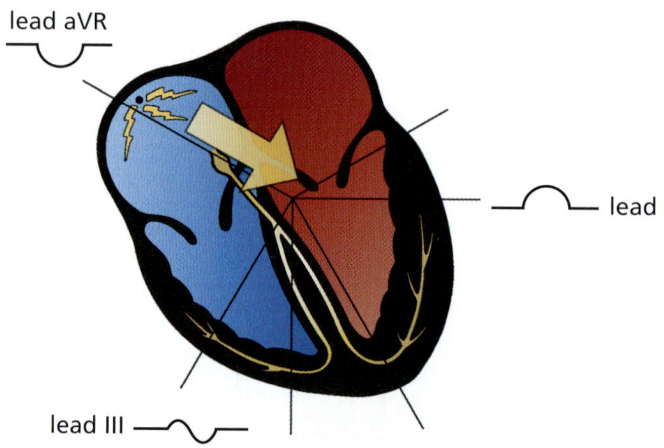

The vector of atrial depolarization points leftward and inferiorly. Therefore, lead I records a positive wave, aVR records a negative wave, and lead III records a biphasic wave.

In the *horizontal plane*, the left lateral leads V5 and V6 record a positive deflection, just as leads I and aVL did in the frontal plane. Lead V1, lying over the right heart, is oriented perpendicularly to the direction of current flow and records a biphasic wave, just like lead III. Leads V2 through V4 are variable.

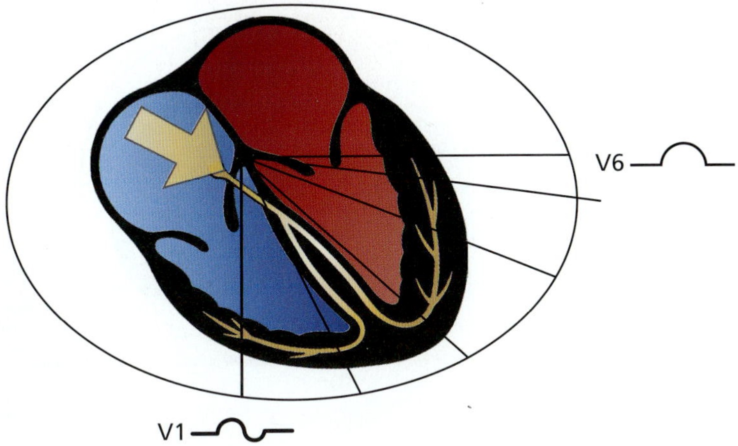

Atrial depolarization in the horizontal plane. V1 records a biphasic wave, and V6 records a positive wave.

Usually, the best leads to view atrial depolarization (the P wave) are leads II and V1.

Because the atria are small, the voltage they can generate is also small. The amplitude of the P wave does not normally exceed 0.25 mV (2.5 mm, or two and one-half small squares on the EKG paper) in any lead. The P-wave amplitude is usually most positive in lead II and most negative in lead aVR. It is less than 0.12 seconds in duration.

But People Are Individuals

A word of caution is needed. Variations in anatomy and orientation of the heart from person to person make absolute rules impossible. For example, although the P wave in lead III is usually biphasic, it is not uncommon for it to be negative in perfectly normal hearts. All it takes is a change of a few degrees in the vector of current flow to turn a biphasic wave into a negative or positive one. This can happen, for instance, if the patient's heart is angled slightly differently in the chest cavity. For this reason, the normal angle of orientation of current vectors is given in ranges, not precise numbers. For example, the normal range of the P-wave vector is 0° to +70°.

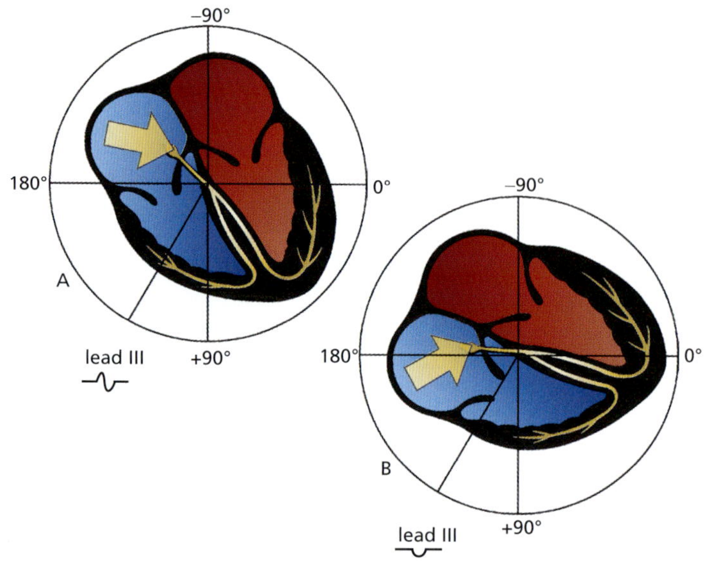

Rotation of the heart within the chest cavity redirects the perceived direction of current flow. Lead III is normally oriented perpendicularly to atrial depolarization. With the apex of the heart turned leftward, lead III will view atrial depolarization as receding and will record a wave that is largely negative.

The PR Interval

The PR interval represents the time from the start of atrial depolarization to the start of ventricular depolarization. It includes the delay in conduction that occurs at the AV node. The PR interval normally lasts from 0.12 to 0.2 seconds (3–5 mm on the EKG paper). This turns out to be convenient because if the PR interval is not longer than one big box (five small boxes) on the EKG paper, then we know it is not prolonged.

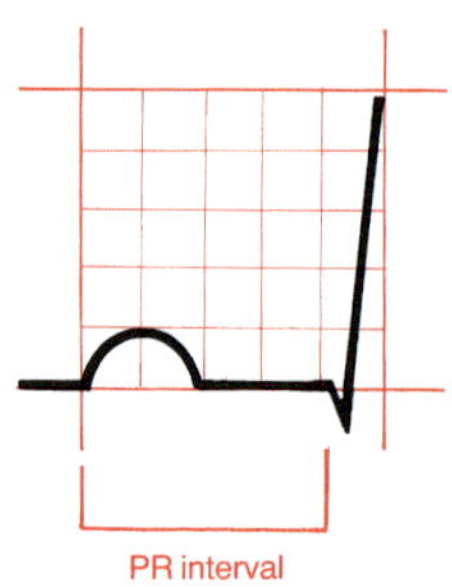

The normal PR interval lasts 0.12–0.2 seconds.

The PR Segment

The PR segment represents the time from the end of atrial depolarization to the beginning of ventricular depolarization. The PR segment is usually horizontal and runs along the same baseline as the start of the P wave.

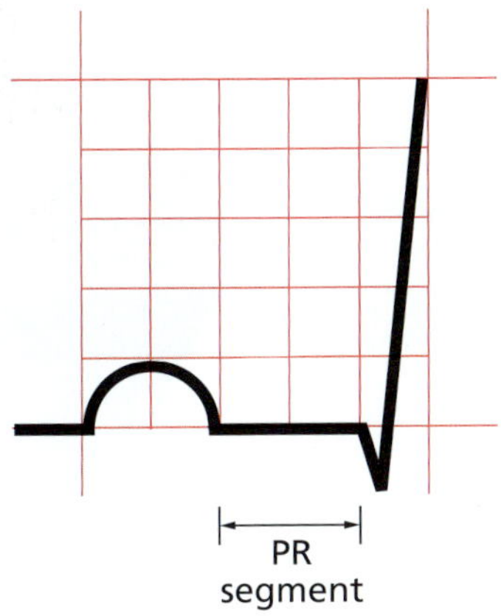

The PR segment is horizontal.

The QRS Complex Is Complex but Not Complicated

Our wave of electrical depolarization pauses at the AV node and then begins its journey into the ventricles.

Septal Q Waves

The interventricular septum, the wall of muscle separating the right and left ventricles, is the first to depolarize, and it does so in a left-to-right direction. The tiny septal fascicle of the left bundle branch is responsible for rapidly delivering the wave of depolarization to this region of the heart.

Septal depolarization is not always visible on the EKG, but when it is, this small left-to-right depolarization inscribes a tiny negative deflection in one or several of the left lateral leads. This initial negative deflection, or Q wave, may therefore be seen in leads I, aVL, V5, and V6. Sometimes, small Q waves may also be seen in the inferior leads and in V3 and V4.

Normal septal Q waves have an amplitude of not >0.1 mV.

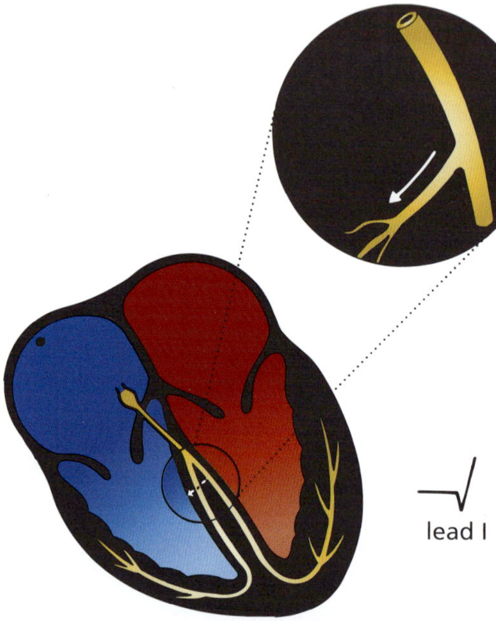

The left lateral leads view left-to-right septal depolarization as moving away; therefore, they record a small initial negative deflection, or Q wave. Small Q waves are also sometimes seen in the inferior leads; these are normal.

The Rest of the Ventricular Myocardium Depolarizes

The remainder of the ventricles, the vast bulk of the myocardium, depolarizes next. Because the left ventricle is so much more massive than the right ventricle, it dominates the QRS complex, and the average vector of current flow swings leftward. Normally, this vector points anywhere from 0° to +90°. In the frontal plane, therefore, large positive deflections (R waves) may be seen in many of the left lateral and inferior leads. Lead aVR, lying rightward, records a deep negative deflection (S wave).

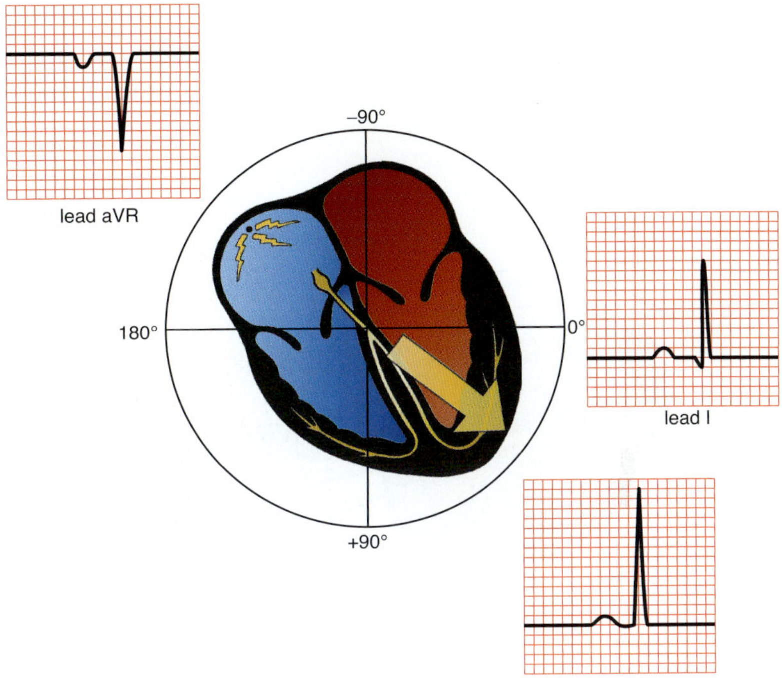

Ventricular depolarization as seen in leads I, II, and aVR. Lead I records a small Q wave due to septal depolarization followed by a tall R wave. Lead II also records a tall R wave and, less often, a small Q wave. The QRS complex in lead aVR is deeply negative, here shown as a QS wave.

In the horizontal plane, lead V1, which overlies the right ventricle, usually records a small R wave followed by a deep S wave reflecting the initial depolarization of the septum and a bit of the right ventricle and then, as both ventricles depolarize, the more robust voltage generated by the left ventricle. The current vector swings dramatically to the left. Leads V5 and V6, lying over the left ventricle, record tall positive R waves. Leads V3 and V4 represent a *transition zone*, and usually one of these leads records a biphasic wave, that is, an R wave and an S wave of nearly equal amplitude.

This pattern of progressively increasing R-wave amplitude moving right to left in the precordial leads is called *R-wave progression*. Lead V1 has the smallest R wave and lead V5 the largest (the R wave in lead V6 is normally a little smaller than that in lead V5).

The amplitude of the QRS complex is much greater than that of the P wave because the ventricles, having so much more muscle mass than the atria, can generate a much greater electrical potential.

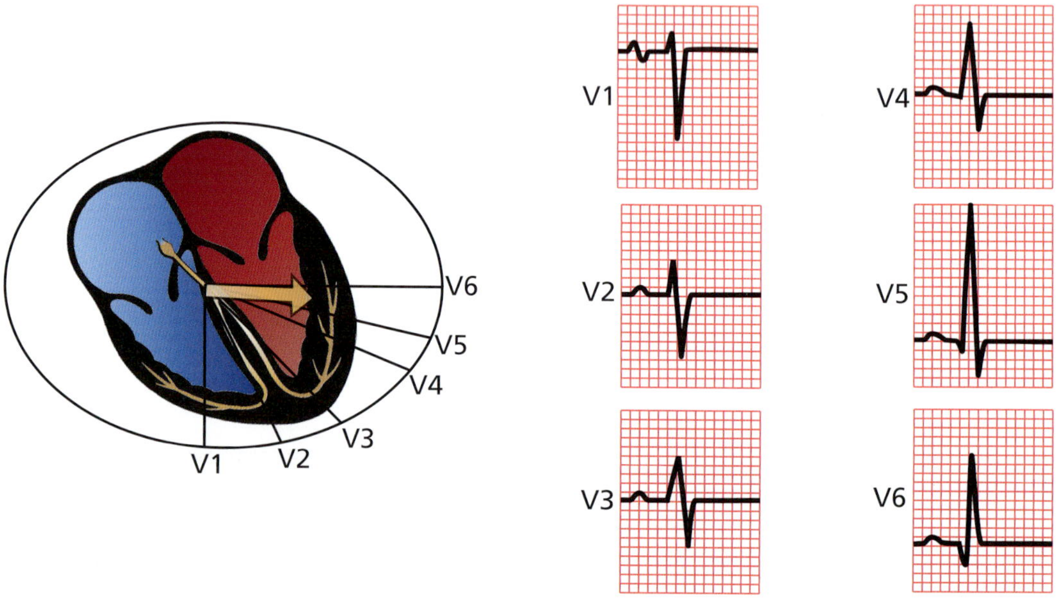

Ventricular depolarization in the precordial leads. Note the normal pattern of R-wave progression. The wave in lead V3 is biphasic.

The QRS Interval

A normal QRS interval, representing the duration of the QRS complex, is 0.06–0.1 seconds (60–100 ms) in duration.

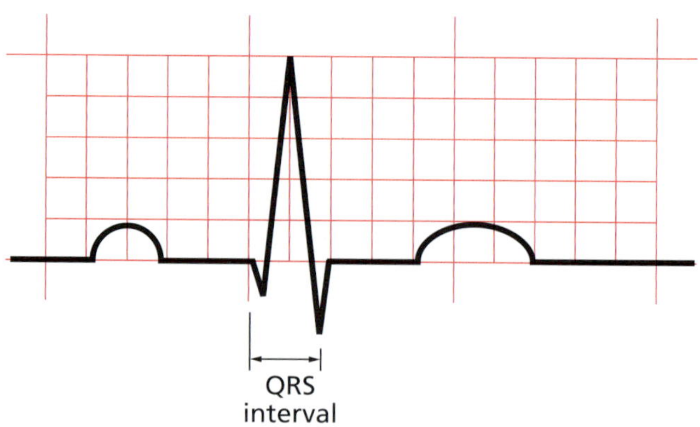

The ST Segment

The ST segment is usually horizontal or gently upsloping in all leads. It represents the time from the end of ventricular depolarization to the start of ventricular repolarization.

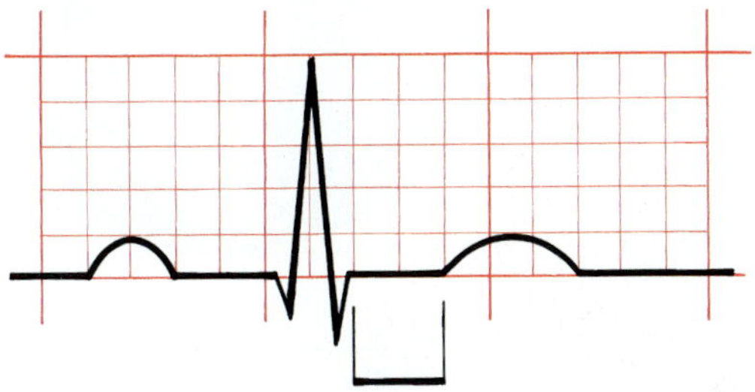

The T Wave

The T wave represents ventricular *repolarization*.

Unlike depolarization, which is largely passive, repolarization requires the expenditure of a great deal of cellular energy (remember the membrane pump?). The T wave is therefore highly susceptible to all kinds of influences, both cardiac and noncardiac (eg, hormonal, neurologic), and is therefore variable in its appearance.

Nevertheless, certain general statements can be made. In the normal heart, repolarization usually begins in the last area of the heart to have been depolarized and then travels backward, in a direction opposite to that of the wave of depolarization (see the *large arrow* on the following illustration). Because both an approaching wave of depolarization and a receding wave of repolarization generate a positive deflection on the EKG, the same electrodes that recorded a *positive* deflection during *depolarization* (appearing as a tall R wave) will also generally record a *positive* deflection during *repolarization* (appearing as a positive T wave). **It is therefore typical and normal to find positive T waves in the same leads that have tall R waves.**

The amplitude, or height, of a normal T wave is one-third to two-thirds that of the corresponding R wave.

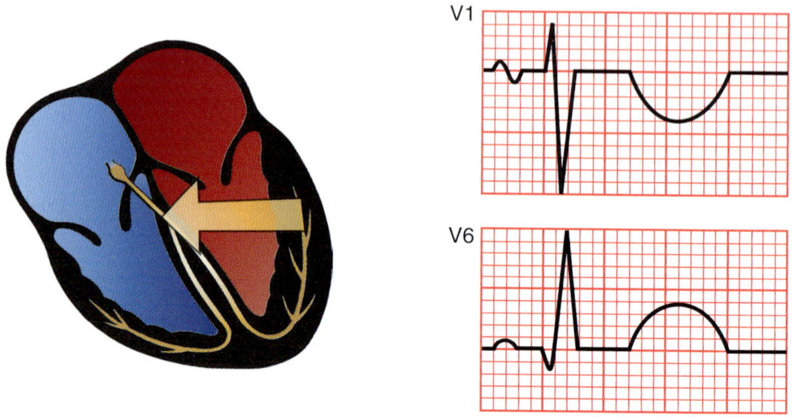

Ventricular repolarization generates a T wave on the EKG. The T wave is usually positive in leads with tall R waves.

The QT Interval

The QT interval encompasses the time from the beginning of ventricular depolarization to the end of ventricular repolarization. It therefore includes all of the electrical events that take place in the ventricles. From the standpoint of time, more of the QT interval is devoted to ventricular *repolarization* than depolarization (ie, the T wave is wider than the QRS complex).

The duration of the QT interval is proportionate to the heart rate. The faster the heart beats, the faster it must repolarize to prepare for the next contraction; thus, the shorter the QT interval. Conversely, when the heart is beating slowly, there is little urgency to repolarize, and the QT interval is long. In general, the QT interval constitutes about 40% of the normal cardiac cycle, as measured from one R wave to the next.

A quick and easy way to tell if the QT interval is prolonged is to look at the midpoint of the R-R interval (ie, the interval between two QRS complexes). The QT interval should end prior to this midpoint regardless of the heart rate.

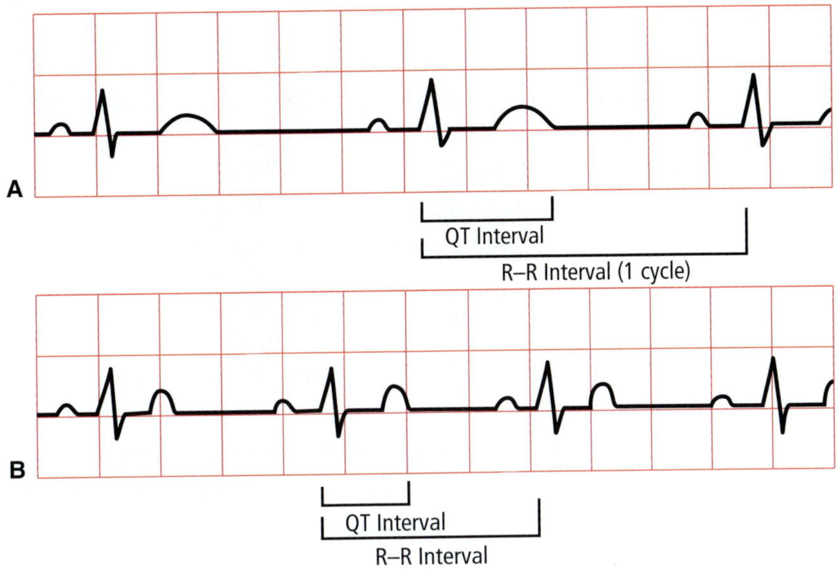

The QT interval constitutes about 40% of each cardiac cycle (R–R interval). The faster the heart beats, the shorter the QT interval. The heart rate in *B* is considerably faster than that in *A*, and the QT interval is correspondingly much shorter (less than one and one-half boxes vs. two full boxes). A simple way to determine if the QT interval is normal is to look at the R-R interval, that is, one cardiac cycle; the T wave should end prior to the midpoint.

SUMMARY

Orientation of the Waves of the Normal EKG

1. The P wave is small and usually positive in the left lateral and inferior leads. It is often biphasic in leads III and V1. It is usually most positive in lead II and most negative in lead aVR.
2. The QRS complex is large, and tall R waves (positive deflections) are usually seen in most left lateral and inferior leads. R-wave progression refers to the sequential enlargement of R waves as one proceeds across the precordial leads from V1 to V5. A small initial Q wave, representing septal depolarization, can often be seen in one or several of the left lateral leads, and sometimes in the inferior leads.
3. The T wave is variable, but it is usually positive in leads with tall R waves.

Now, take a good look at the following EKG. Does it seem familiar?

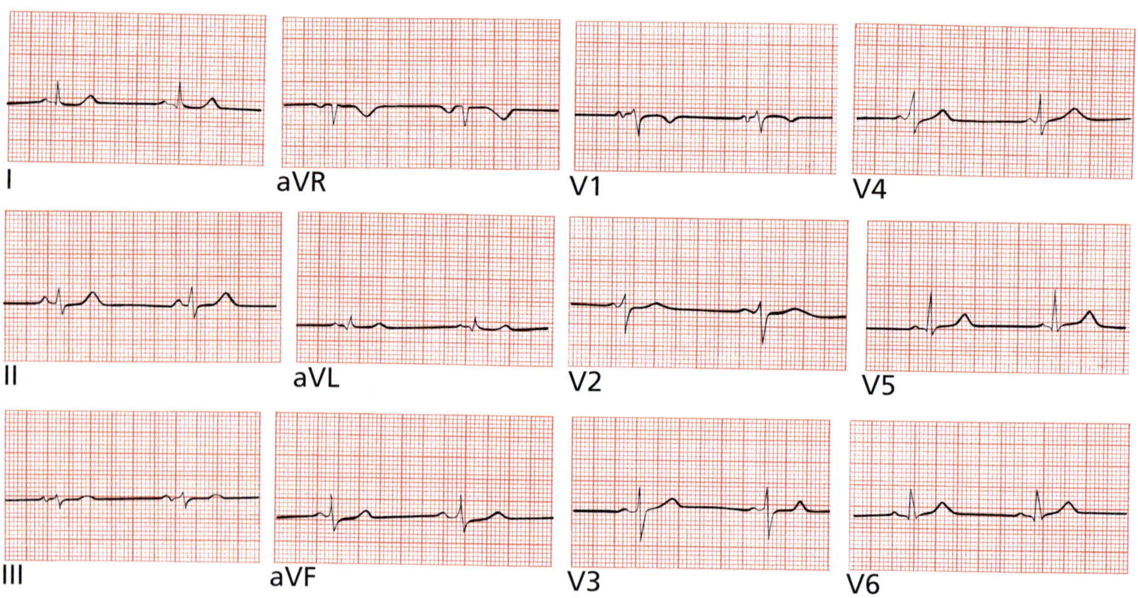

Of course, it seems familiar. It's a normal 12-lead EKG, identical to the one that began the book.

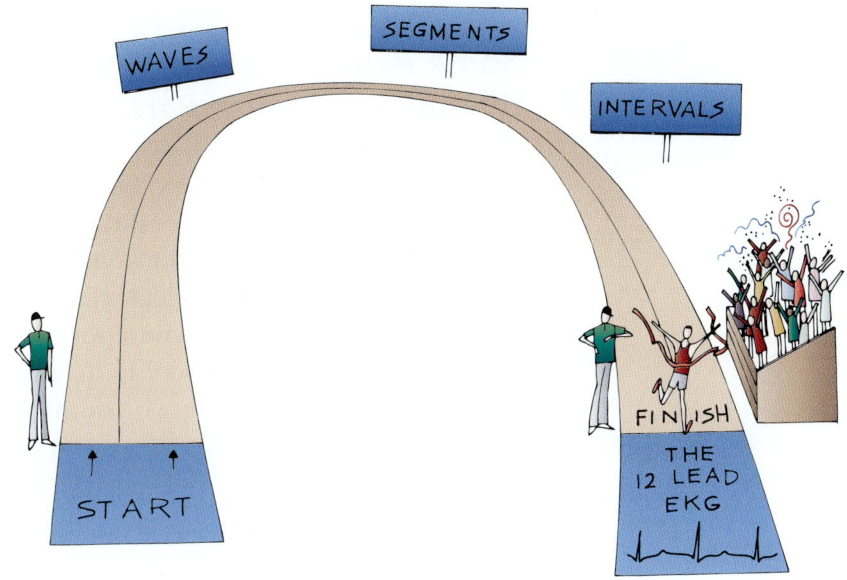

Congratulations! You have successfully traversed the most difficult terrain in this book. Everything that follows builds logically from the few basic principles you have just mastered.

Some Really Important Stuff That You May Be Wondering About: Part 1: Why Not Just Let the Computer Do It?

Before we leave the comfortable realm of the normal EKG for the more harrowing domain of the abnormal, let's squarely face an important and frequently neglected issue. When you use a modern EKG machine, you get more than just a tracing. You get an interpretation straight from the computer's, er, mouth. Since we all know how smart computers are, why bother to learn to read EKGs at all?

There are two major reasons:

1. The computer, even with the advent of artificial intelligence (AI), often—surprisingly often—doesn't get it right. It does certain things very well, such as measuring intervals and identifying obvious deviations from the norm. But frequently, it will overcall subtle but normal findings, sending you and your patient into a tizzy. Or, conversely, it will miss slight abnormalities that may actually have important consequences for your patient. And—this is the one that will really drive you crazy—sometimes it will just waffle, calling something a *possible* abnormality, which doesn't help you at all.

2. You have one important thing going for you that the computer lacks—clinical context. You know your patients, how they look and feel, their past medical and medication history, their risk for cardiac disease, and so on. You also should know for certain whether the electrodes have been placed correctly. The best EKG interpretation will always be one that takes the actual patient into consideration. Borderline findings are common on EKGs, and only by considering the EKG as just one tool among many in your overall assessment are you likely to avoid unnecessary panic and start ordering needless additional tests or calling 911 to get your patient to the emergency department. On the other hand, a finding on the EKG that the machine just yawns at and dismisses as "nonspecific" may strike you quite

differently when patients are right in front of you clutching their chest in pain, complaining of shortness of breath, and too light-headed to stand up.

To quote (in English translation) the ancient Greek playwright, Euripides: "*Much effort, much prosperity.*" In the chapters that follow, you will learn how to outsmart even the most sophisticated EKG machine.

Some Really Important Stuff That You May Be Wondering About: Part 2: How Do I Get the Goop Off My Patient's Chest Once the EKG Is Finished?

Most EKG electrodes are attached to the body with special pads impregnated with adhesive. Pulling them off can be painful, especially if hairs are caught between the pads and the skin. Usually, a quick yank (with apologies to your patient) is your best bet to minimize discomfort. However, there may still be some adhesive residue left behind where the pads were placed. Happily, there are all sorts of ways to remove it—alcohol pads, petroleum jelly, baby oil, and mineral oil can all get the job done. Even after the goop has been removed, some patients may still be left with red marks where the electrode pads were placed. Assure your patient that these will resolve quickly, often within hours, sometimes days. If they find these spots intolerably itchy, a mild over-the-counter hydrocortisone cream will quickly set things right.

Coming Attractions

You are now ready to use the EKG to diagnose an extraordinary variety of cardiac and noncardiac disorders. We will group these disorders into five categories.

Hypertrophy and Enlargement (Chapter 2). The EKG can reveal whether a particular atrial or ventricular chamber is enlarged or hypertrophied. Valvular diseases, sustained hypertension, and both inherited and acquired cardiac muscle disorders can affect the heart in this way, and the EKG can therefore help to recognize and evaluate these disorders.

Abnormalities of Rhythm (Chapter 3). The heart can beat too fast or too slow, fibrillate chaotically, or come to a sudden standstill. The EKG remains—and will probably always remain—the best means to assess such rhythm disturbances, which, at their most severe, can lead to sudden death.

Abnormalities of Conduction (Chapters 4 and 5). If the normal pathways of cardiac electrical conduction become blocked, the heart rate can fall precipitously. The result can be syncope, a faint caused by a sudden decrease in cardiac output. Syncope is one of the leading causes of hospital admission. Conduction can also be *accelerated* along short circuits that bypass the normal delay in the AV node; we will look at these, too.

Myocardial Ischemia and Infarction (Chapter 6). The diagnosis of myocardial ischemia and infarction is one of the most important roles for the EKG. There are many reasons why a patient may have chest discomfort, and the EKG can help sort these out.

Electrolyte Disturbances, Drug Effects, and Miscellaneous Disorders (Chapter 7). Because all of the electrical events of the heart are dependent on electrolytes, it stands to reason that various electrolyte disorders can affect cardiac conduction and even lead to sudden death if untreated. Medications such as digitalis, antidepressants, antiarrhythmic agents, and even antibiotics can profoundly alter the EKG. A number of cardiac and noncardiac diseases can also cause dramatic shifts in the EKG. In each of these instances, a timely glance at an EKG may be diagnostic and sometimes lifesaving. We will also look at the controversial roles of the EKG in screening young athletes before sports participation and in evaluating a patient's risks before going for surgery.

2 Hypertrophy and Enlargement of the Heart

In this chapter, you will learn:

1 | what happens to a wave on the EKG when an atrium enlarges or a ventricle hypertrophies

2 | the meaning of electrical axis and its importance in diagnosing hypertrophy and enlargement

3 | how to use the EKG to diagnose right and left atrial enlargement

4 | how to use the EKG to diagnose right and left ventricular hypertrophy

5 | about your patients Mildred W. and Tom L., cases which will test your ability to recognize what happens to the EKG with hypertrophy and enlargement, and why these diagnoses matter

A Few Introductory Remarks

The EKG can diagnose many important and urgent problems—things that can really get your heart pumping. Hypertrophy and enlargement, alas, are—with a few exceptions—not among them. Don't misunderstand—recognizing atrial enlargement or ventricular hypertrophy can have important clinical implications for your patients. For example, the diagnosis of left ventricular hypertrophy on the EKG is associated with a substantially increased risk of adverse cardiovascular events (eg, stroke and myocardial infarction). But for genuine soul-stirring excitement, it does not compare to diagnosing an evolving heart attack or a potentially lethal rhythm disturbance.

So why start here? First, because hypertrophy and enlargement are easy to understand. Second, their EKG manifestations build logically from what we have discussed so far. And third, any good book should have an appealing narrative arc, building relentlessly to an exciting climax. Starting high and finishing low would not leave you at the end with that shiver down the spine, that feeling that you can't wait to get out there into the real world and save some lives.

So, here we go—our initial foray into how we can use the EKG to diagnose abnormalities of the heart.

Definitions

The terms *hypertrophy* and *enlargement* are often used interchangeably, but they are not really the same thing.

Hypertrophy refers to an *increase in muscle mass*. The wall of a hypertrophied ventricle is thick and powerful. Most hypertrophy is caused by *pressure overload*, in which the heart is forced to pump blood against an increased resistance, as can occur in patients with systemic hypertension or aortic stenosis. Just as weightlifters develop powerful pectoral muscles as they bench press progressively heavier and heavier weights, so the heart muscle grows thicker and stronger (at least for a while) as it is called on to eject blood against increasing resistance.

Enlargement refers to *dilation* of a particular chamber. An enlarged ventricle can hold more blood than a normal ventricle. Enlargement is typically caused by *volume overload*; the chamber dilates to accommodate an increased amount of blood. Enlargement is most often seen with certain valvular diseases. Aortic insufficiency, for example, may cause left ventricular enlargement, and mitral insufficiency may result in left atrial enlargement.

Enlargement and hypertrophy frequently coexist. This is not surprising because both represent ways in which the heart tries to increase its cardiac output or maintain normal stress on the walls of its chambers. In both instances, the cardiac myocytes and their extracellular milieu undergo changes that can include inflammation and fibrosis that can affect the way the heart conducts electricity and therefore, are often detectable on the EKG.

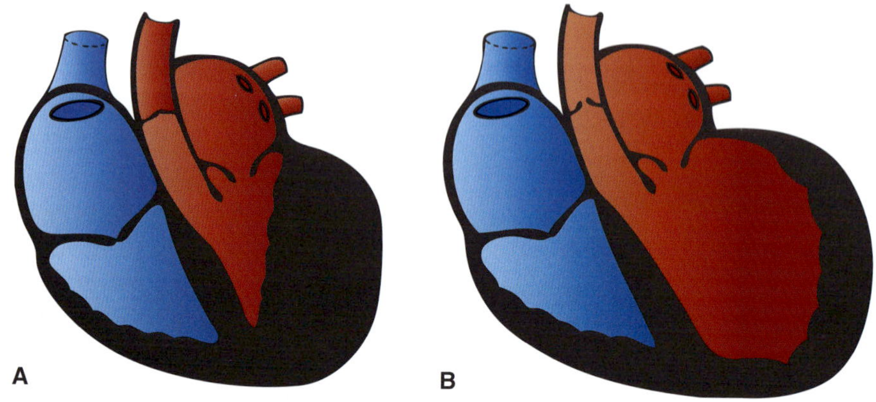

(*A*) A hypertrophied left ventricle caused by aortic stenosis. The wall is so thick that the chamber size is significantly diminished. (*B*) An enlarged left ventricle. The chamber is bigger, but the wall thickness is normal.

The EKG is not very good at distinguishing between hypertrophy and enlargement. However, it is traditional to speak of *atrial enlargement* and *ventricular hypertrophy* when reading EKGs.

The term atrial enlargement has been supplanted in the minds of some by the term *atrial abnormalities*. This change in terminology reflects the recognition that a variety of electrical abnormalities can cause the changes on the EKG that are characteristically associated with atrial enlargement. However, we will continue to use the term atrial enlargement in this book, both because the term is more rooted in tradition (and traditional values still matter as we race headlong through the 21st century) and because the vast majority of cases of P-wave changes are due to enlargement of the atria.

Because the P wave represents atrial depolarization, we look at the P wave to assess atrial enlargement. Similarly, we examine the QRS complex to determine whether there is ventricular hypertrophy.

Hypertrophy and enlargement can represent healthy and helpful adaptations to stressful situations, but because they may also reflect serious underlying disorders affecting the heart, it is important to learn how to recognize them on the EKG. In addition, over time, the increase in muscular thickness and/or size can compromise the heart's ability to adequately pump blood to the rest of the body, causing heart failure. Hypertrophied myocardium also demands more blood supply for the overgrown heart muscle and can compress the coronary arteries, and is therefore more susceptible to ischemia than normal myocardium.

How the EKG Can Change With Hypertrophy and Enlargement

Three things can happen to a wave on the EKG when a chamber hypertrophies or enlarges:

1. The chamber can take longer to depolarize. The EKG wave may therefore *increase in duration.*
2. The chamber can generate more current and thus a larger voltage. The wave may therefore *increase in amplitude.*
3. A larger percentage of the total electrical current will move through the expanded chamber. The mean electrical vector, or what we call the *electrical axis*, of the EKG wave may therefore shift.

Because the concept of axis is so important for diagnosing hypertrophy and enlargement, we need to digress for just a moment to elaborate on this idea.

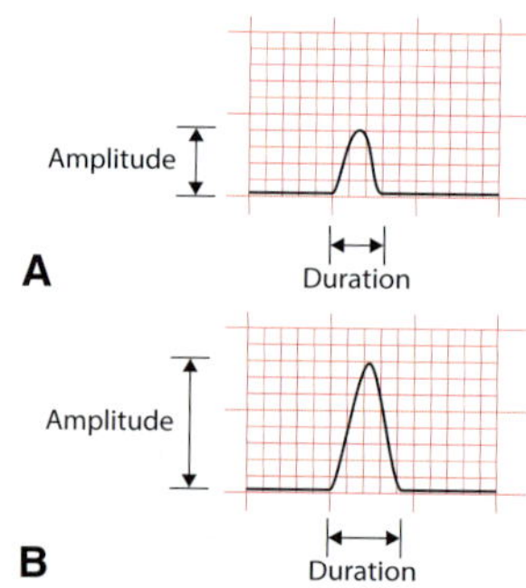

(*A*) A normal wave. (*B*) The same wave when the chamber has enlarged or hypertrophied. The amplitude and duration of the wave have increased. A third alteration, a shift in the electrical axis, is discussed in the following pages.

An increase in amplitude is the most dramatic change that occurs when a chamber enlarges and is critical to all EKG criteria for diagnosing enlargement and hypertrophy as you will shortly see. However, be aware that very thin people, particularly those with pectus excavatum, a common congenital deformity of the anterior thoracic wall, can have abnormally large EKG waves in the precordial leads simply because the chest electrodes are so much closer to the heart and not dampened by overlying tissue.

Axis

In the preceding chapter (see page 49), we discussed how the EKG records the instantaneous vector of electrical forces at any given moment. Using this idea, we can represent the complete depolarization (or repolarization) of a chamber by drawing a series of sequential vectors, each vector representing the sum of all the electrical forces at a given moment.

Because it is easier to visualize than to talk about, let's use some simple illustrations to amplify the text. We will first look at ventricular depolarization (the QRS complex) before turning to atrial depolarization (the P wave) and ventricular repolarization (the T wave).

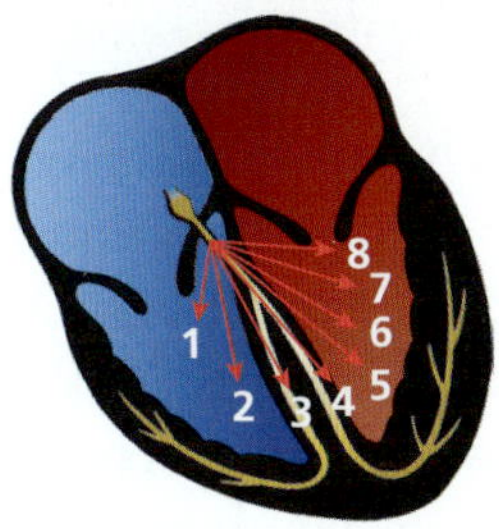

Ventricular depolarization is represented by eight sequential instantaneous vectors, illustrating how the electrical forces normally move progressively leftward. Although, for the sake of clarity, we have shown only eight instantaneous vectors, we could just as well have shown 80 or 8000.

In the illustration above, the vectors of current flow are numbered sequentially as they evolve over time. The first vectors represent septal depolarization, and each successive vector represents progressive depolarization of the remainder of the ventricles. The vectors swing progressively leftward because the electrical activity of the much larger left ventricle increasingly dominates the EKG.

Now here is the key point: We can average all of these vectors to create one summation vector, a kind of "vector to rule them all." This average vector of all of the instantaneous vectors is called the *mean vector*. And the *direction* of the mean vector is called the **mean electrical axis**.

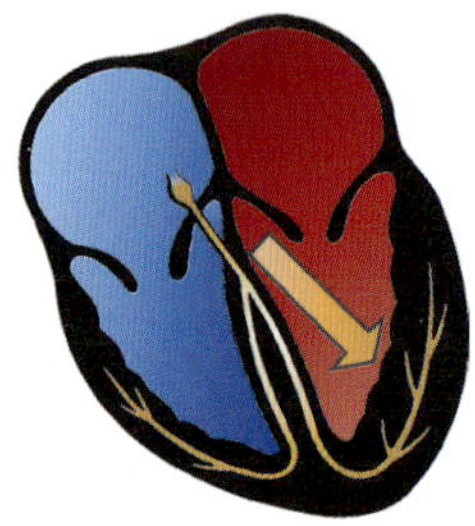

A single vector summarizes all of the instantaneous vectors. This summation vector is called the mean vector, and its direction is the axis of ventricular depolarization. Axis is defined in the frontal plane only.

The mean QRS vector points leftward and inferiorly, representing the average direction of current flow during the entirety of ventricular depolarization. The normal QRS axis—the direction of this mean vector—therefore lies between +90° and 0°. (Actually, most cardiologists extend the range of normal from +90° to −30°. In time, as you become more comfortable with the concept of axis, you should add this refinement to your electrical analysis.)

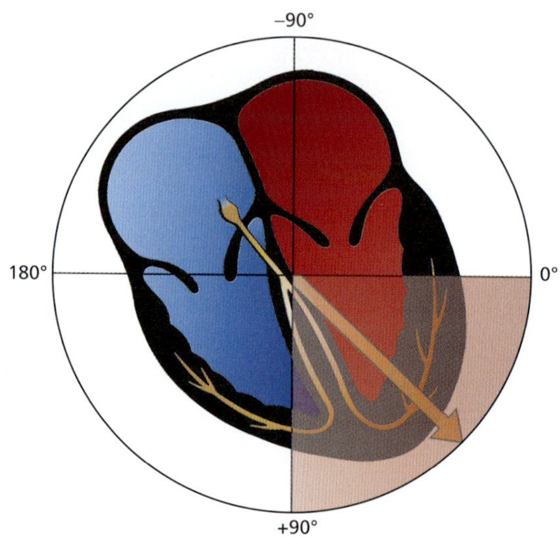

If the QRS axis lies within the *shaded quadrant*, between 0° and 90°, it is normal.

We can quickly determine whether the QRS axis on any EKG is normal by looking only at leads I and aVF which, you will recall, are oriented at 0° and +90°, respectively. **If the QRS complex is predominantly positive in both leads I and aVF, then the QRS axis must be normal** (if this sounds too simple to be true, that's because it is just a bit; as we just mentioned above, the normal QRS axis can actually lie all the way from 90° to −30°. We will expand on this idea shortly—see the box on page 80). Why is this? Let's explore.

Determining Whether the QRS Axis Is Normal

We have already discussed how any lead will record a positive deflection if the wave of depolarization is moving toward it. Lead I is oriented at 0°. Thus, if the mean QRS vector is directed anywhere between −90° and +90°, lead I will record a predominantly positive QRS complex.

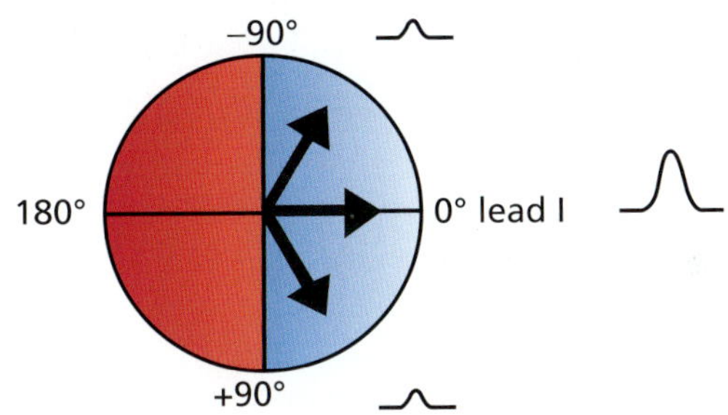

Any mean QRS vector oriented between −90° and +90° will produce a predominantly positive QRS complex in lead I. Three different QRS mean vectors are shown. All three are oriented between −90° and +90°; hence, they will all produce a predominantly positive QRS complex. The three QRS complexes depicted here illustrate what lead I would record for each of the three vectors.

Lead aVF is oriented at +90°. Therefore, if the mean QRS vector is directed anywhere between 0° and 180°, lead aVF will record a predominantly positive QRS complex.

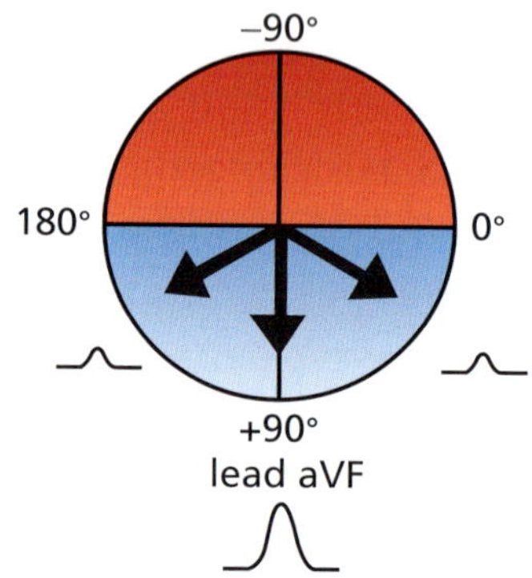

Any mean QRS vector oriented between 0° and 180° will produce a predominantly positive QRS complex in lead aVF. Three different mean QRS vectors are shown, all oriented so that lead aVF will record a predominantly positive deflection as illustrated.

You see where this is going: If the QRS complex is predominantly positive in *both* lead I and lead aVF, then the QRS axis must lie in the quadrant where *both* are positive, that is, between 0° and +90°. This is the normal QRS axis.

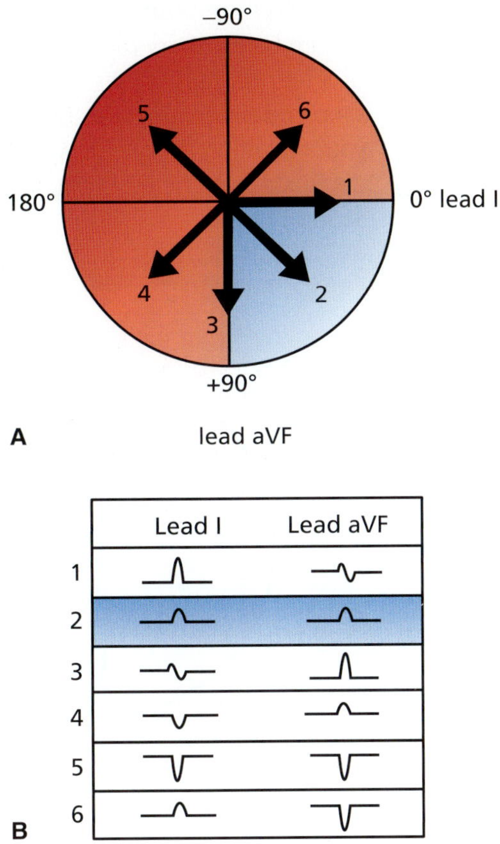

Six different QRS axes are shown (*A*). Only an axis directed between 0° and +90° (*shaded quadrant*) will produce a predominantly positive QRS complex in both lead I and lead aVF. (*B*) The QRS complexes in leads I and aVF associated with each of the six axes are shown. Only axis 2 is normal and associated with a predominantly positive QRS complex in both leads, although most cardiologists would consider axes 1 and 3 to be normal as well.

As we indicated above, many electrocardiographers believe that a normal QRS axis can extend from +90° beyond 0° all the way to −30°. Using this criterion, QRS complexes that are predominantly negative in lead aVF can still be normal if the QRS complexes in lead I *and lead II* are positive. If you can't intuitively see this, check out the picture below. Very rarely does a clinical decision turn on a variation of a few degrees of axis, so if you are more comfortable with the simpler definition, you are in good company and should not feel that you are letting anyone down. We're going to stick with the simpler definition from here on out, just to show you that we can be a good sport about it.

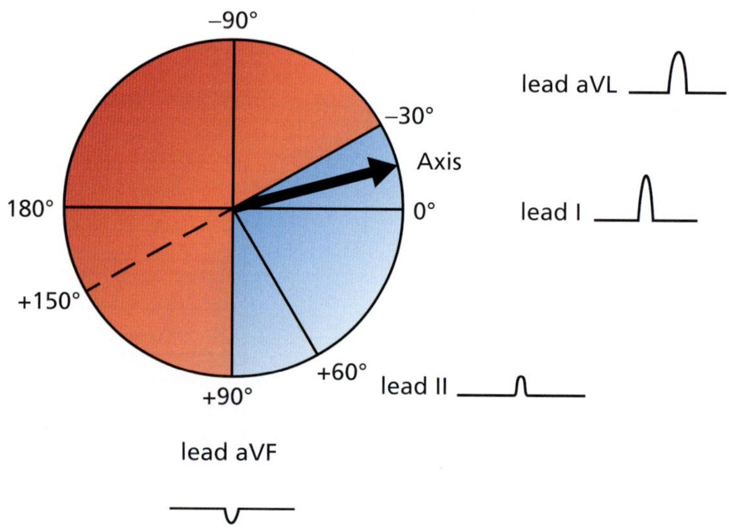

Redefining the normal axis from +90° to −30° means that the axis above is normal even though lead aVF is negative. Note that lead II, which is oriented at +60°, is positive whenever the axis lies between −30° and +150°. Therefore, when both leads I and II are positive, the axis must lie between −30° and +90°, that is, our alternative definition of "normal," as shown as the *blue area* in this picture.

Defining the Axis Precisely

Although it is usually sufficient to note whether the axis is normal or not, it is possible to be more rigorous and to define the actual angle of the axis with fair precision. All you need to do is look for the limb lead in which the QRS complex is most nearly **isoelectric**, that is, with positive and negative deflections extended equally on both sides of the baseline (sometimes, the deflections are so small that the wave appears flat). The axis must then be oriented approximately **perpendicular** to this lead because, as you already know, an electrode oriented perpendicularly to the mean direction of current flow records a biphasic wave.

Thus, for example, if the QRS complex in lead III (orientation, +120°) is biphasic, then the axis must be oriented at right angles (90°) to this lead, at either +30° or −150°. And, if we already know that the axis is normal—that is, if the QRS complex is positive in leads I and aVF—then the axis cannot be −150° but must be +30°.

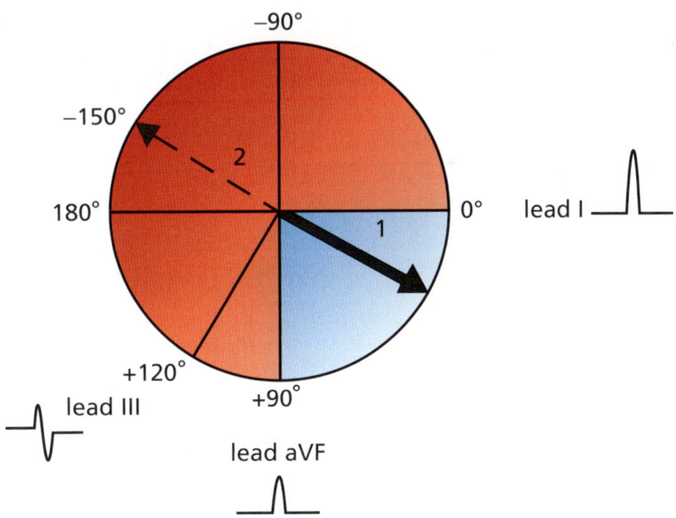

QRS complexes are shown for leads I, III, and aVF. Determining the axis is easy. The QRS complex in lead III is biphasic. The axis, therefore, must be either +30° or −150°. However, because the QRS complex is positive in both leads I and aVF, the axis must be normal; that is, it must lie within the *shaded quadrant*. The axis, therefore, can only be +30°.

Axis Deviation: Defining Abnormal Axes

The normal QRS axis lies between 0° and 90°. If the axis lies between 90° and 180°, we speak of *right axis deviation*. Will the QRS complex in leads I and aVF be positive or negative in a patient with right axis deviation?

The QRS complex in lead aVF will still be positive, but it will be negative in lead I.

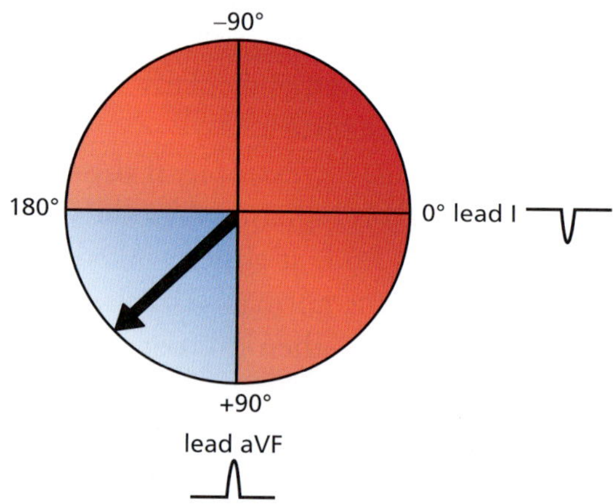

Right axis deviation. The QRS complex is negative in lead I, whereas it is positive in aVF.

If the axis lies between 0° and –90°, we speak *of left axis deviation*. In this case, the QRS complex in lead I will be positive, but it will be negative in lead aVF.

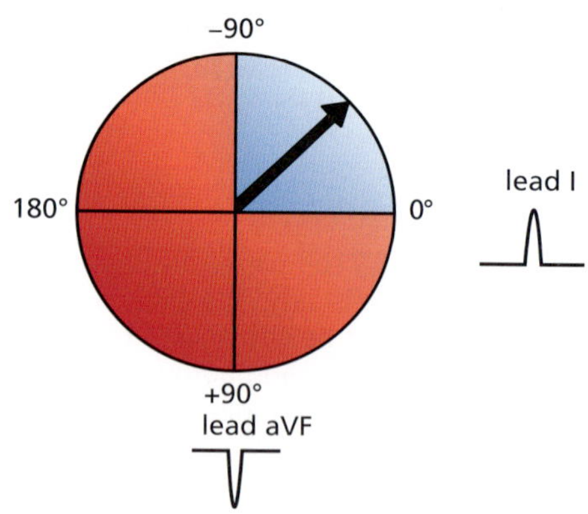

Left axis deviation.

In rare instances, the axis becomes totally disoriented and lies between −90° and 180°. This is called *extreme right axis deviation.* The QRS complex in both lead aVF and lead I will be negative.

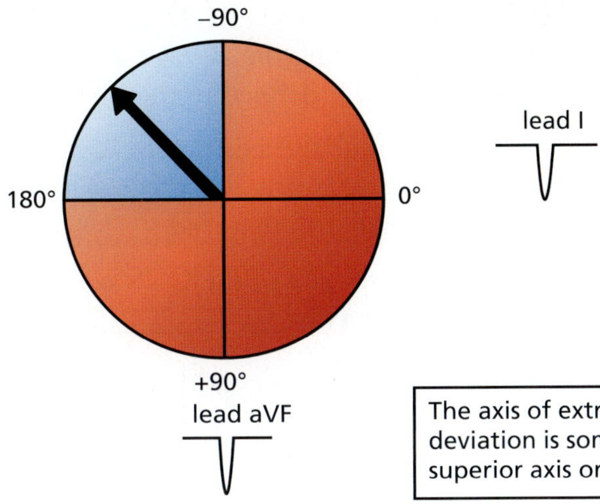

The axis of extreme right axis deviation is sometimes called a superior axis or a northwest axis.

Extreme right axis deviation.

SUMMARY

Axis

1. The term *axis* refers to the direction of the mean electrical vector, representing the average direction of current flow in a given chamber. It is defined in the frontal plane only.
2. To determine the axis of any wave, find the lead in which the wave is most nearly isoelectric. The axis must lie approximately perpendicular to that lead.
3. A quick estimate of the QRS axis can be made by looking at leads I and aVF:

Axis	Lead I	Lead aVF
Normal axis	Positive	Positive
Left axis deviation	Positive	Negative
Right axis deviation	Negative	Positive
Extreme right axis deviation	Negative	Negative

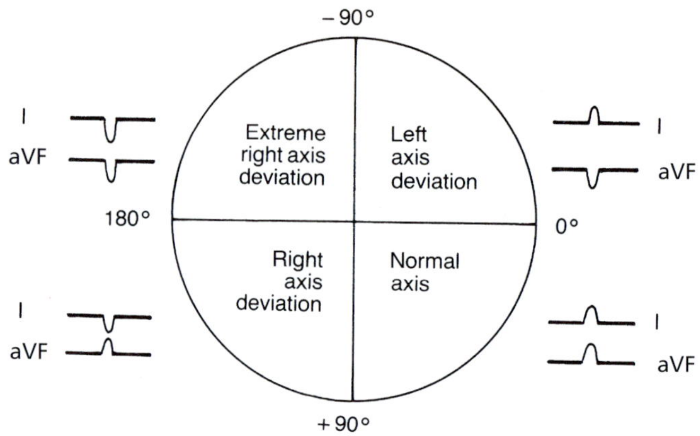

On the EKG below, the waves recorded by the six leads of the frontal plane are shown. Is the QRS axis normal or is there axis deviation?

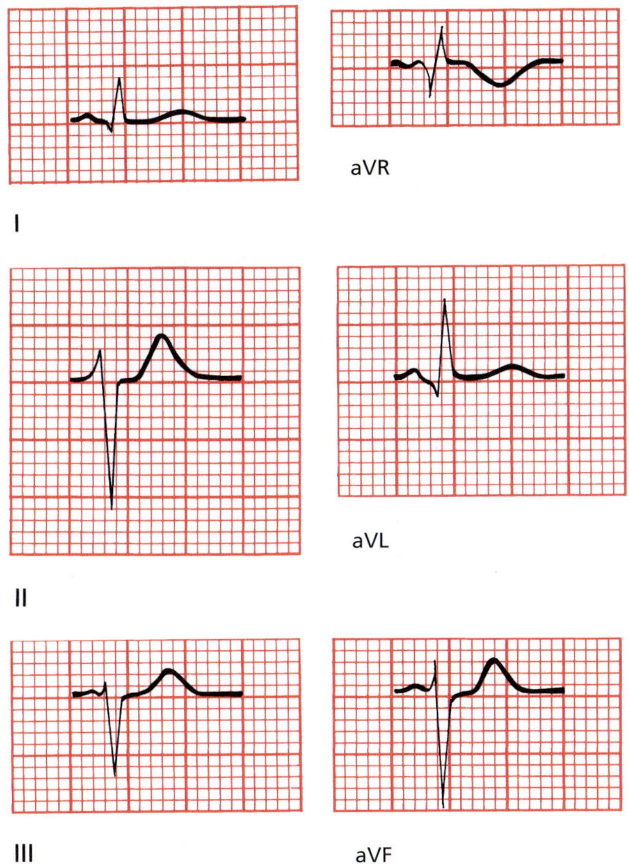

This patient has left axis deviation; the QRS complex is predominantly positive in lead I and negative in lead aVF.

Now, can you define the axis more precisely by finding the lead with a biphasic QRS complex?

The QRS complex in lead aVR is approximately biphasic; therefore, the electrical axis must lie nearly perpendicular to it. Lead aVR is oriented at −150 degrees, so the axis of the QRS complex, perpendicular to aVR, must be either −60° or +120°. Because we already know that the axis falls within the zone of left axis deviation (ie, between 0° and −90°), the correct axis must be −60°.

Just as we have done for the QRS complex, we can define an axis for the P wave and T wave on every EKG. The normal **P-wave axis** lies approximately between 0° and 70° in adults (between 0° and 90° in children). The **T-wave axis** is variable, but it should approximate that of the QRS axis, lying within 50° to 60° of the QRS axis.

Can you identify the axis of the QRS complex, P wave, and T wave on the following EKG?

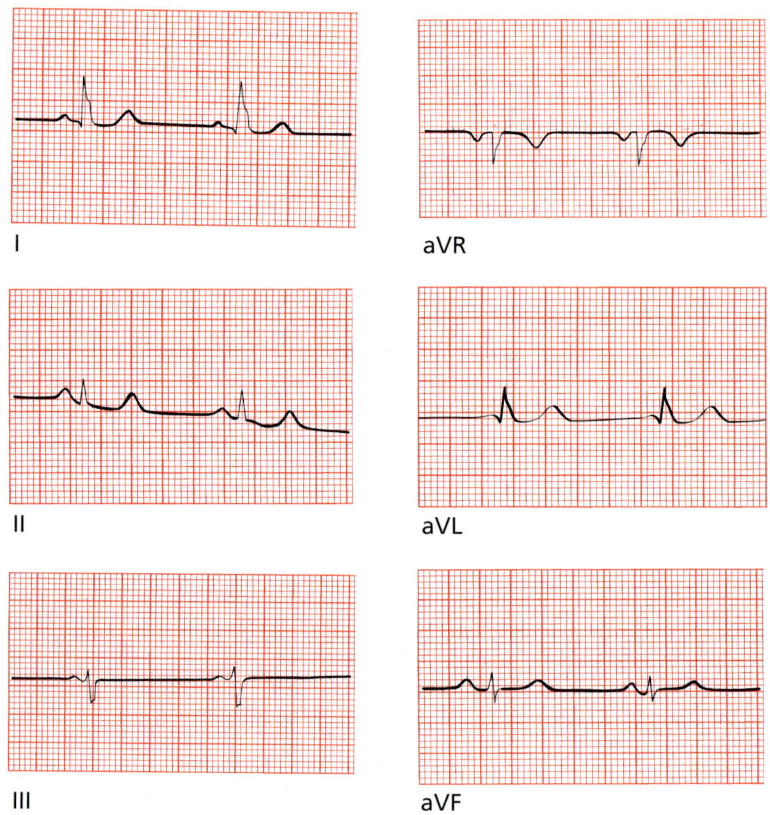

The QRS complex: the QRS axis is about 0°. It is nearly equiphasic in aVF, implying an axis of 0° or 180°. Because the QRS complex in lead I has a tall R wave, the axis must be 0°. *The P wave:* In lead aVL, the P wave is virtually invisible (isoelectric), so the P-wave axis must lie perpendicular to this lead and is either 60° or –120°. Since the P wave is positive in leads I and aVF, the axis must be 60°. *The T wave:* all of the leads with tall R waves have positive T waves. The T waves are flat in lead III, indicating an axis perpendicular to lead III (either +30° or –150°). Because there is a tall T wave in lead I, the axis must be about +30°.

Axis Deviation, Hypertrophy, and Enlargement

Now that we have beaten the concept of axis deep into the ground, you are justified in wondering why axis deviation has anything to do with hypertrophy and enlargement. Because the concept of axis deviation is most successfully applied to ventricular hypertrophy, let's consider what happens to the flow of electricity when a ventricle hypertrophies.

In the normal heart, the QRS axis lies between 0° and +90°, reflecting the electrical dominance of the much larger left ventricle over the right ventricle. Imagine a 65-year-old patient who has allowed her hypertension to go untreated for many years, and now comes to see you for headaches and shortness of breath. You discover a greatly elevated blood pressure of 190/115 mm Hg. This sustained and severe hypertension has forced the left ventricle to work too hard for too long, and as a result, it has hypertrophied. Its electrical dominance over the right ventricle has therefore become even more profound. The mean electrical vector is therefore drawn even further leftward, and the result is *left axis deviation*. The presence of left axis deviation therefore, raises the possibility of left ventricular hypertrophy.

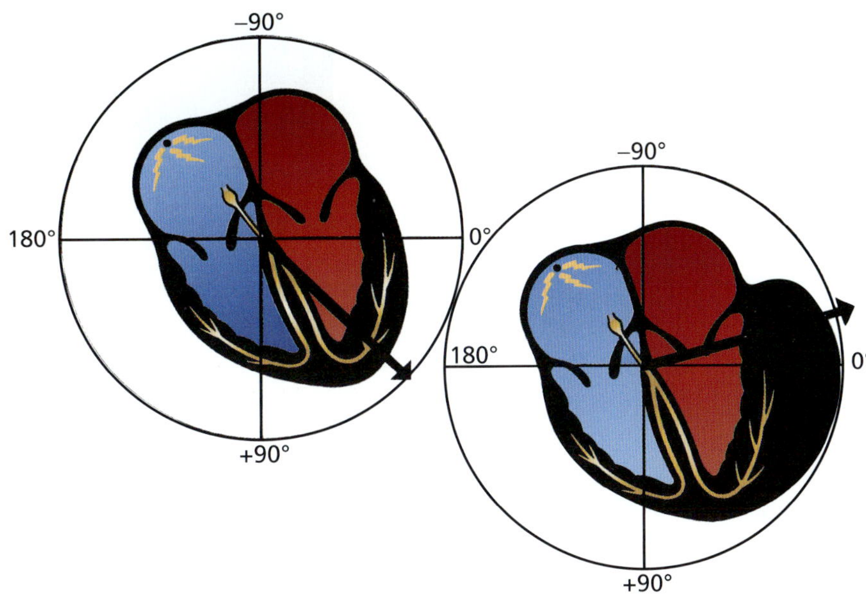

With left ventricular hypertrophy, the electrical axis moves further leftward, resulting in left axis deviation.

Right ventricular hypertrophy is far less common and requires a huge change in the proportions of the right ventricle in order to overcome the electrical forces generated by the normally dominant left ventricle. It can occur, however, in patients with chronic obstructive pulmonary disease sufficiently severe to cause pulmonary artery hypertension or in patients with uncorrected congenital heart disease associated with profound volume or pressure overload of the right ventricle. If the right ventricle greatly hypertrophies, it can be detected on the EKG as a shift in the QRS axis. The mean electrical axis of current flow is drawn rightward, and the result is *right axis deviation*. The presence of right axis deviation therefore raises the possibility of right ventricular hypertrophy.

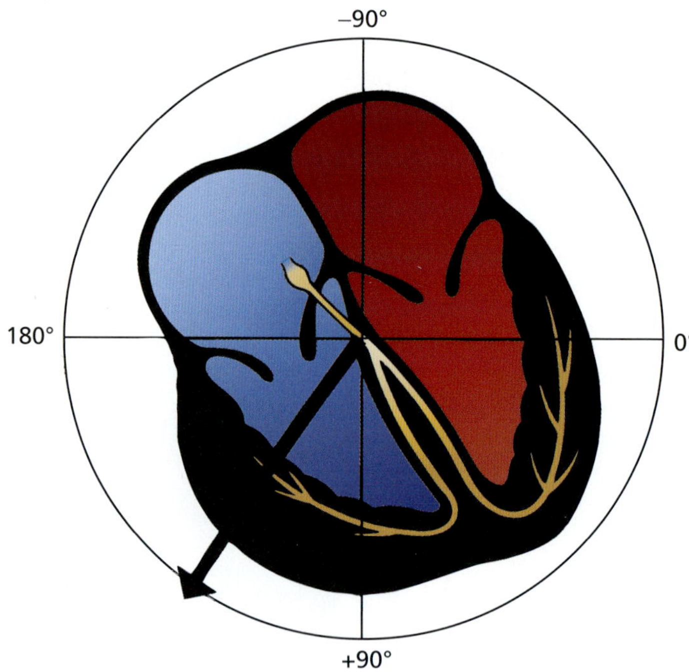

With right ventricular hypertrophy, the electrical axis moves rightward, resulting in right axis deviation.

Now is a good time to restate the three things that can happen to a wave on the EKG with enlargement or hypertrophy:

1. The wave can increase in duration.
2. The wave can increase in amplitude.
3. The electrical axis of the wave can deviate from normal.

Specific EKG criteria for the diagnosis of atrial enlargement and ventricular hypertrophy have been devised, and these are discussed in the following pages.

Atrial Enlargement

You already know (see Chapter 1, page 53) that the normal P wave is <0.12 seconds in duration, and the largest voltage, whether positive or negative, should not exceed 2.5 mm (0.25 mV) in any of the 12 leads. The first part of the P wave represents right atrial depolarization and the second part left atrial depolarization.

Virtually, all of the information you need to assess atrial enlargement can be found in leads II and V1. Lead II is useful because it is oriented nearly parallel to the flow of current through the atria (ie, parallel to the mean P-wave vector). It, therefore, typically records the largest positive deflection and is very sensitive to any perturbations in atrial depolarization. Lead V1 is useful because it is oriented perpendicularly to the flow of electricity and is therefore biphasic, allowing easy separation of the right and left atrial components.

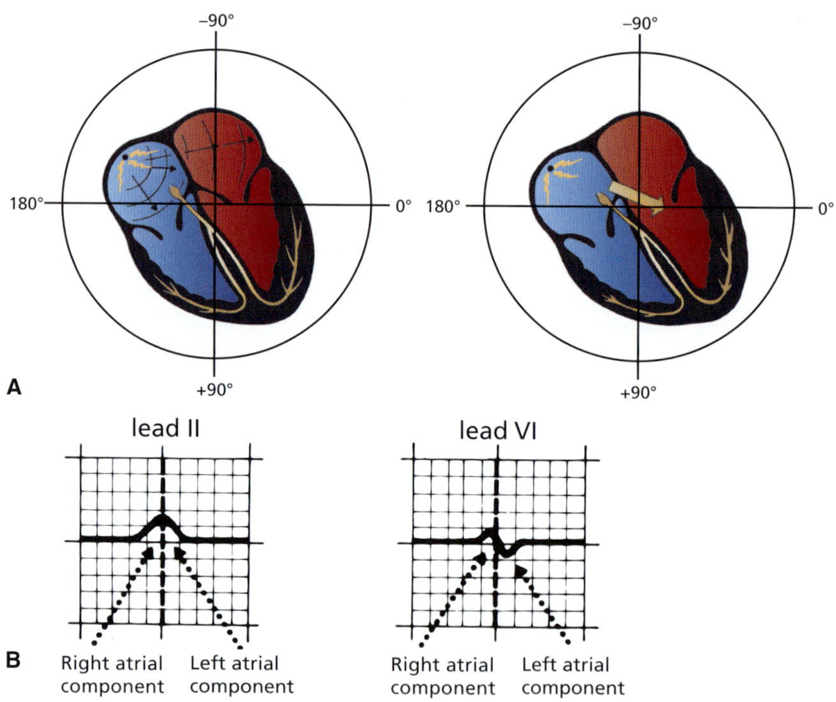

(*A*) Normal atrial depolarization; the large arrow in the second figure shows the mean electrical axis. (*B*) The normal P wave in leads II and V1. The first part of the P wave represents right atrial depolarization, and the second part represents left atrial depolarization.

Right Atrial Enlargement

With *right atrial enlargement*, the amplitude of the first portion of the P wave increases. The width does not change because the terminal component of the P wave is *left* atrial in origin, and this remains unchanged.

Enlargement of the right atrium may also cause the right atrium to dominate the left atrium electrically. The vector of atrial depolarization may swing rightward, and the P-wave axis may move rightward toward or even beyond +90°. The tallest P wave may therefore no longer appear in lead II but in lead aVF or lead III.

The classic picture of right atrial enlargement is illustrated in leads II and V1, below, and is often caused by severe lung disease (Why? Because the right side of the heart has to work harder to pump blood through the lungs. As you will shortly see, chronic lung disease is a leading cause of *right ventricular* hypertrophy as well).

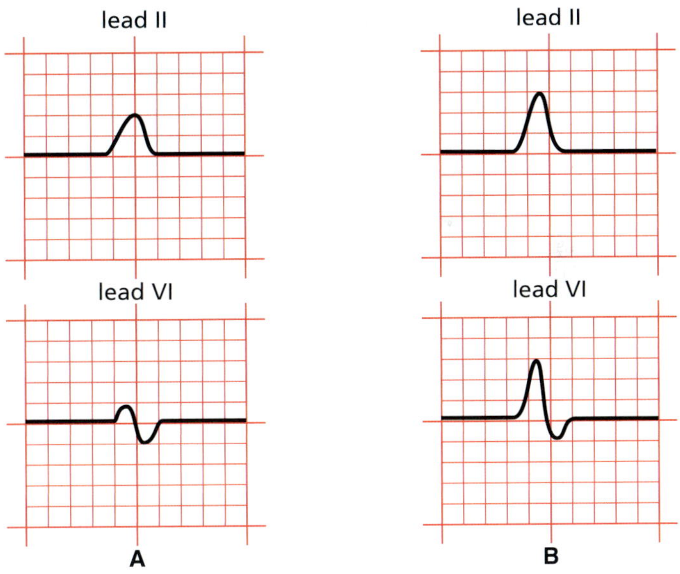

(*A*) The normal P wave in leads II and V1. (*B*) Right atrial enlargement. Note the increased amplitude of the early, right atrial component of the P wave. The terminal left atrial component, and hence the overall duration of the P wave, is essentially unchanged.

The bottom line: Right atrial enlargement can be diagnosed by the presence of P waves with an amplitude exceeding 2.5 mm in at least one of the inferior leads II, III, and aVF. A rightward P-wave axis may or may not be present.

Left Atrial Enlargement

With *left atrial enlargement*, the second portion of the P wave may increase in amplitude. The diagnosis of left atrial enlargement requires that *the terminal (left atrial) portion of the P wave should drop more than 1 mm below the isoelectric line in lead V1* (remember that lead V1 overlies the right heart, not the left, so when an enlarged left atrium depolarizes, the result will be a larger *negative* deflection in lead V1).

However, a more prominent change in the P wave is an increase in its *duration*. This occurs because left atrial depolarization represents the terminal portion of the P wave, and prolonged depolarization can be readily seen (with *right* atrial enlargement, prolonged depolarization of the right atrium is hidden by the left atrial portion of the P wave). The diagnosis of left atrial enlargement, therefore, also requires that *the terminal portion of the P wave should be at least 1 small block (0.04 second) in width.*

The electrocardiographic picture of left atrial enlargement is often seen with mitral valve disease and systemic hypertension (Why? In this case, it is the left side of the heart that has to do more work to pump blood against increased resistance. And if you guess that these disorders can also cause left ventricular hypertrophy, you have guessed correctly).

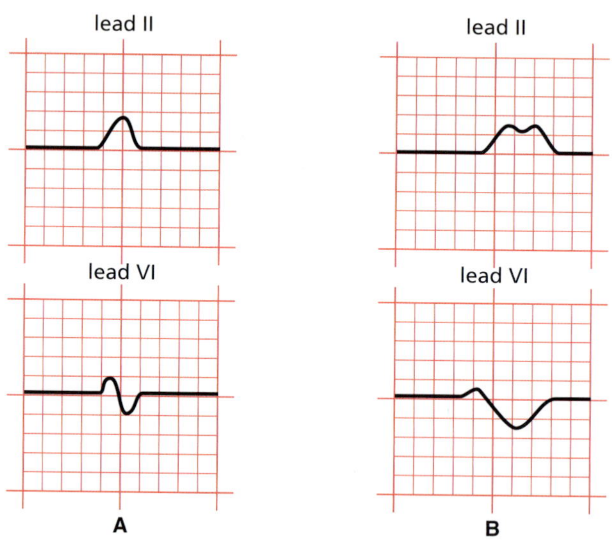

(*A*) Again, the normal P wave in leads II and V1. (*B*) Left atrial enlargement. Note the increased amplitude and duration of the terminal, left atrial component of the P wave.

SUMMARY

Atrial Enlargement

To diagnose atrial enlargement, look at leads II and V1.

Right atrial enlargement is characterized by the following:

1. P waves with an amplitude exceeding 2.5 mm in the inferior leads
2. No change in the duration of the P wave
3. Possible right axis deviation of the P wave

Left atrial enlargement is characterized by the following:

1. The amplitude of the terminal (negative) component of the P wave may be increased and must descend at least 1 mm below the isoelectric line in lead V1.
2. The duration of the P wave is increased, and the terminal (negative) portion of the P wave must be at least 1 small block (0.04 second) in width.
3. No significant axis deviation is seen because the left atrium is normally electrically dominant.

It should be stressed that electrocardiographic evidence of atrial enlargement (especially left atrial enlargement) sometimes has no obvious pathologic correlate and in these cases may merely reflect a nonspecific conduction abnormality. Abnormalities of the P-wave axis can also be seen when the heart rhythm arises from a source other than the sinus node, something we shall discuss later. Interpretation of atrial enlargement on the EKG must, therefore, be tempered by knowledge of the clinical setting (a good idea in any circumstance!).

Ventricular Hypertrophy

The diagnosis of ventricular hypertrophy requires a careful assessment of the QRS complex in multiple leads.

Right Ventricular Hypertrophy

Looking at the Limb Leads

In the limb leads, the most common feature associated with right ventricular hypertrophy is *right axis deviation*; that is, the electrical axis of the QRS complex, normally between 0° and +90°, veers off between +90° and +180°. This reflects the new electrical dominance of the usually electrically submissive right ventricle.

Many cardiologists feel that the QRS axis must exceed +100° in order to make the diagnosis of right ventricular hypertrophy. Therefore, the QRS complex in lead I (oriented at 0°) must be at least slightly more negative than positive.

Special note: In children, in whom the left ventricle has not yet achieved its full robust muscularity and power, a right axis is common and normal.

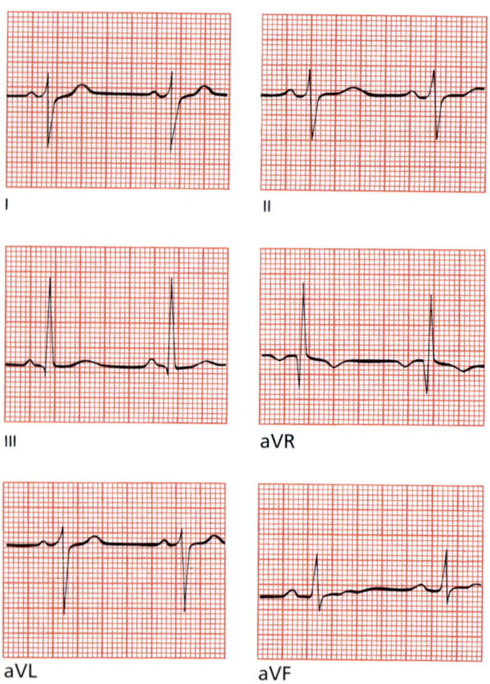

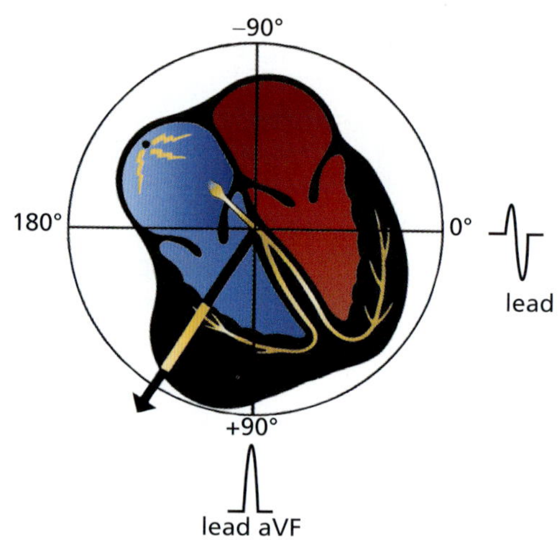

Right ventricular hypertrophy shifts the axis of the QRS complex to the right. The EKG tracings show right axis deviation. In addition, the QRS complex in lead I is slightly negative, a criterion that many believe is essential for properly establishing the diagnosis of right ventricular hypertrophy.

Looking at the Precordial Leads

The precordial leads can also be helpful in diagnosing right ventricular hypertrophy. As you might expect, the normal pattern of R-wave progression, whereby the R-wave amplitude enlarges as you proceed leftward from lead V1 to V5, is disrupted. Instead of the R-wave amplitude increasing as the leads move closer to the left ventricle, the reverse may occur. There may be a large R wave in lead V1, which lies over the hypertrophied right ventricle, and a small R wave in leads V5 and V6, which lie over the normal, but now electrically humble, left ventricle. Similarly, the S wave in lead V1 is small, whereas the S wave in lead V6 is large.

These criteria can be expressed in the simplest possible mathematics:

- In lead V1, the R wave is larger than the S wave.
- In lead V6, the S wave is larger than the R wave.

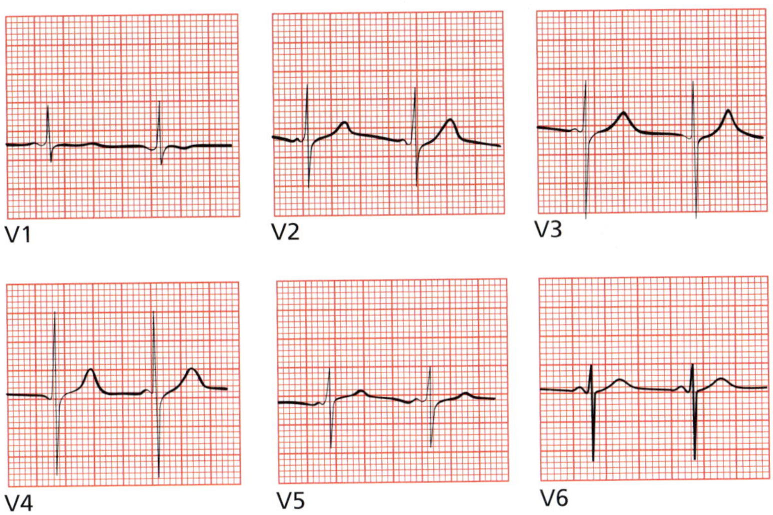

In lead V1, the R wave is larger than the S wave. In lead V6, the S wave is larger than the R wave.

The most common causes of right ventricular hypertrophy are lung disease and congenital heart disease.

Left Ventricular Hypertrophy

The diagnosis of left ventricular hypertrophy is, alas, somewhat more complicated. Left axis deviation beyond −15° is often seen, but by and large, this is not a very useful diagnostic feature. Instead, *increased R-wave amplitude in those leads overlying the left ventricle forms the basis for the EKG diagnosis of left ventricular hypertrophy.*

Unfortunately, there are almost as many criteria for diagnosing left ventricular hypertrophy on the EKG as there are books about EKGs. Nevertheless, all the criteria reflect a common theme: *There should be increased R-wave amplitude in leads overlying the left ventricle and increased S-wave amplitude in leads overlying the right ventricle.* The criteria listed here are not by any means the only ones, but they will serve at least as well as any others.

Looking at the Precordial Leads

In general, the precordial leads are more sensitive than the limb leads for the diagnosis of left ventricular hypertrophy. The most useful criteria in the precordial leads are as follows:

1. The R-wave amplitude in lead V5 or V6 *plus* the S-wave amplitude in lead V1 or V2 exceeds 35 mm.
2. The R-wave amplitude in lead V5 exceeds 26 mm.
3. The R-wave amplitude in lead V6 exceeds 20 mm.

The more criteria that are positive, the greater the likelihood that the patient has left ventricular hypertrophy.

It is, sadly, worth your while to memorize all of these criteria, but if you want to be selective, choose the first because it seems to have the best predictive value.

Note: These criteria are less valuable in individuals younger than 35 years of age, who frequently have increased voltage due, at least in some cases, to a relatively thin chest wall. They are particularly unreliable in young children. Thus, in these individuals, specificity is low.

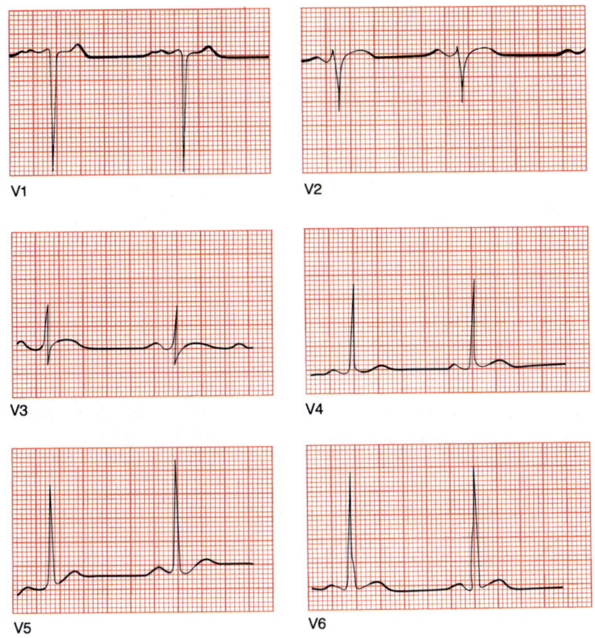

Left ventricular hypertrophy in the precordial leads. Two of the three criteria are met. The R-wave amplitude in V5 plus the S-wave amplitude in V1 exceeds 35 mm, and the R-wave amplitude in V6 exceeds 20 mm. The only criterion not met is for the R wave in lead V5 to exceed 26 mm.

Looking at the Limb Leads

The most useful criteria in the limb leads are as follows:

1. The R-wave amplitude in lead aVL exceeds 11 mm.
2. The R-wave amplitude in lead aVF exceeds 20 mm.
3. The R-wave amplitude in lead I exceeds 13 mm.
4. The R-wave amplitude in lead I *plus* the S-wave amplitude in lead III exceeds 25 mm.

Again, if you aspire to electrocardiographic nirvana, learn them all. If you must pick one, pick the first; it is the most specific for left ventricular hypertrophy.

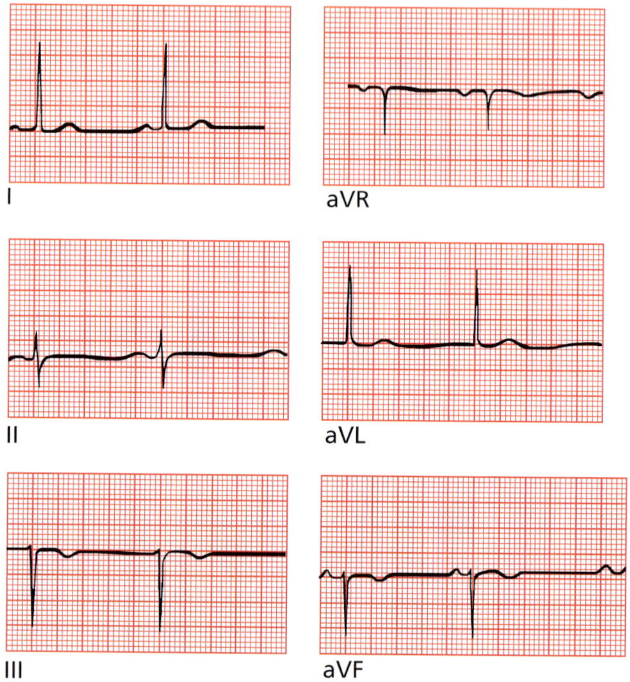

Left ventricular hypertrophy in the limb leads. Criteria 1, 3, and 4 are met; only criterion 2, regarding the R-wave amplitude in lead aVF, is not met.

There is one other criterion that is regarded by some experts as the most accurate of all (but again, far from perfect), and it combines one limb lead and one precordial lead:

The R-wave amplitude in aVL plus the S-wave amplitude in V3 exceeds 20 mm in women and 28 mm in men.

You may have noticed that, in our discussion of ventricular hypertrophy, unlike atrial enlargement, no comment has been made about the *duration* of the QRS complex. Both right and left ventricular hypertrophy often slightly prolong the QRS complex (current takes longer to traverse the enlarged muscle), but rarely beyond 0.1 seconds. A slightly widened QRS complex can support your diagnosis of left ventricular hypertrophy if other criteria are present.

The leading causes of left ventricular hypertrophy are systemic hypertension and valvular disease.

When Both Ventricles Are Hypertrophied

What happens when *both* the right ventricle and left ventricle are hypertrophied? As you might expect, there may be a combination of features (eg, criteria for left ventricular hypertrophy in the precordial leads with right axis deviation in the limb leads), but in most cases, the effects of the usually dominant left ventricle obscure those of the right ventricle.

Now Test Yourself: Is There Ventricular Hypertrophy in the Tracing Below? The Patient Is a 50-Year-Old Female

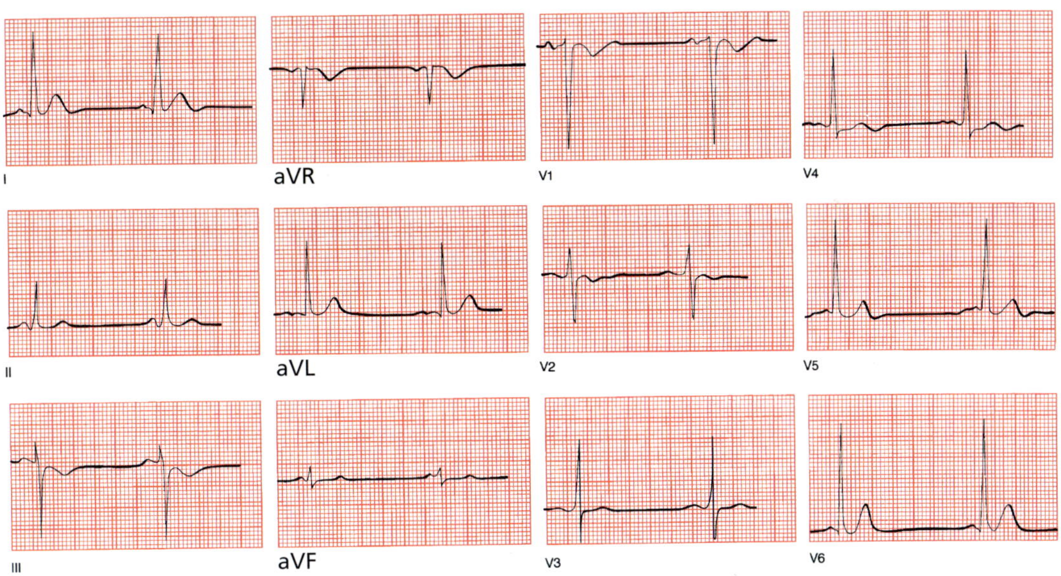

Yes. This patient has aortic stenosis and has left ventricular hypertrophy on the EKG. She meets the criteria in both the precordial and limb leads.

Secondary Repolarization Abnormalities of Ventricular Hypertrophy

We are not quite done with hypertrophy just yet. Something else may happen with hypertrophy of a ventricle that can dramatically alter the EKG, specifically the ST segment and the T wave. As we discussed in Chapter 1, the ST segment plus the T wave represent the time from the end of ventricular depolarization to the end of ventricular repolarization. Therefore, these changes are called *secondary repolarization abnormalities* and include the following:

1. Downsloping ST-segment depression
2. T-wave inversion (ie, the T wave changes its axis so that it is no longer closely aligned with the QRS axis)

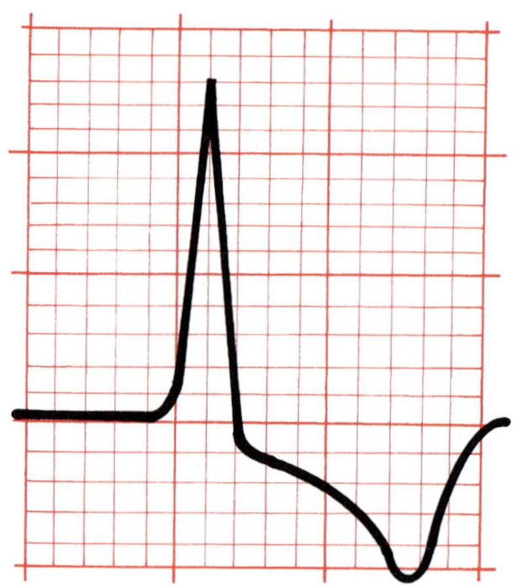

Note how the depressed ST segment and the inverted T wave appear to blend together to form a single asymmetric wave. The downward slope is gradual; the upward slope is abrupt.

A Word on Why

Several theories have been advanced to explain the cause of these repolarization abnormalities, ranging from inadequate blood flow in the capillary beds of the subendocardium (the inner layer of the myocardium lying just beneath the endocardial lining of the ventricle) to an overlapping of depolarization and repolarization forces in the region of thickened muscle. No one knows for sure. These changes were once referred to as *strain*, but the implication that these changes necessarily reflect the *straining* of an overworked and hypoxic muscle has proven to be more simplistic than true, and the term should be discarded.

Repolarization abnormalities are common. They are most evident in those leads with tall R waves (reasonably so, because these leads lie over, and most directly reflect, the electrical forces of the hypertrophied ventricle). Thus, right ventricular repolarization abnormalities will be seen in leads V1 and V2, and left ventricular repolarization abnormalities will be most evident in leads I, aVL, V5, and V6. Left ventricular secondary repolarization abnormalities are far more common than right ventricular abnormalities.

The presence of repolarization abnormalities in a patient with voltage criteria for hypertrophy increases the likelihood that the patient truly has ventricular hypertrophy.

Repolarization abnormalities may be seen with significant hypertrophy and may herald the onset of further decompensation and ventricular dilatation. For example, a patient with aortic stenosis and no clinical symptoms may show a stable pattern of left ventricular hypertrophy for years. Eventually, however, the left ventricle may fail, and the patient will develop shortness of breath and other symptoms of congestive heart failure. The EKG may then show left ventricular hypertrophy with secondary repolarization abnormalities. This progression is illustrated in the two EKGs below. It is, however, important to stress that the EKG changes of left ventricular dilatation with or without repolarization abnormalities are not present in all patients with severe aortic stenosis.

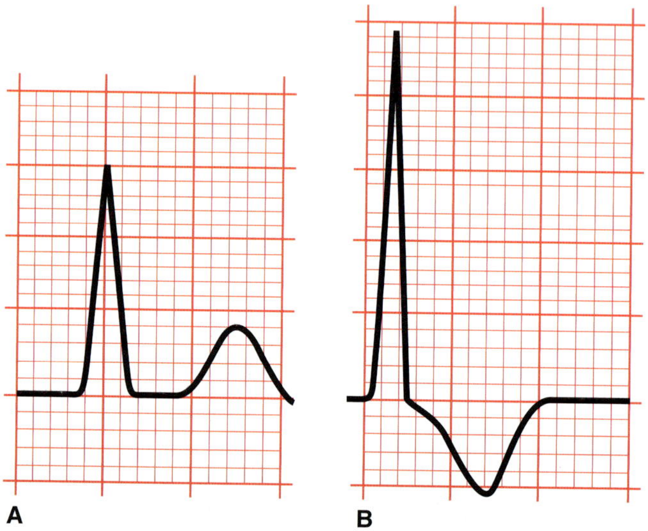

(*A*) Lead aVL in a patient with aortic stenosis and left ventricular hypertrophy. Note the tall R wave, meeting the criteria for left ventricular hypertrophy. The ST segment is flat, and the T wave is upright. (*B*) One year later, the same lead shows the development of secondary repolarization abnormalities, reflecting the onset of left ventricular failure. The ST segment is depressed, and the T wave is inverted. Note, too, that the amplitude of the R wave has increased.

It is important to recognize the asymmetric contour of the ST-segment and T-wave changes that occur with secondary repolarization abnormalities. The descent is gradual and is followed by a more abrupt ascent. In Chapter 6, we will see that ST-segment depression and T-wave inversion are also hallmarks of cardiac ischemia, and one of the key ways to tell ischemia from secondary repolarization is by their differing configurations—asymmetric with secondary repolarization abnormalities and symmetric with cardiac ischemia. However, as with all rules, this one is imperfect too, and the clinical context in which you interpret these changes in the ST segment and T wave matters a great deal.

SUMMARY

Ventricular Hypertrophy

Right ventricular hypertrophy is characterized by the following:

1. Right axis deviation is present, with the QRS axis exceeding +100°.
2. The R wave is larger than the S wave in V1, whereas the S wave is larger than the R wave in V6.

Left ventricular hypertrophy is characterized by voltage criteria and, not infrequently, secondary repolarization abnormalities. The most useful criteria are the following:

1. The R wave in V5 or V6 plus the S wave in V1 or V2 exceeds 35 mm.
2. The R wave in aVL exceeds 11 mm.
3. The R wave in aVL plus the S wave in V3 exceeds 20 mm in women and 28 mm in men.
4. Left axis deviation exceeding −15° is often present, and the QRS complex may be slightly prolonged.

Secondary repolarization abnormalities include asymmetric T-wave inversion and downsloping ST-segment depression.

A Cautionary Note About the EKG Diagnosis of Left Ventricular Hypertrophy

Although the EKG pattern of left ventricular hypertrophy is easily recognized, it is present in only about 50% of patients whose echocardiograms demonstrate a thickened left ventricle. The sensitivity of the EKG criteria for left ventricular hypertrophy is thus fairly low. In other words, many patients with left ventricular hypertrophy will have normal EKGs. Why might this be? There are many reasons, but one is that a hypertrophied left ventricle often contains diffuse fibrotic or infarcted tissue that does not conduct electricity well, disrupting the otherwise expected correlation between increased ventricular muscle mass and increased voltage. In addition, the EKG changes of left ventricular hypertrophy may be masked by coexisting obesity, prior infarction, pericardial fluid, or emphysema, among other causes. However, when the EKG pattern of left ventricular hypertrophy does appear, there is a 90% likelihood that a thickened ventricle will be seen on an echocardiogram. The specificity of the EKG criteria for left ventricular hypertrophy is thus reasonably high.

It pains the author of an EKG book to write this, but if you really need to confirm the presence of left ventricular hypertrophy in your patient, consider ordering an imaging study, typically an echocardiogram or, if the echo is inconclusive, cardiac MRI.

CASE 1

Mildred W., a 53-year-old widow (her husband succumbed to cerebral anoxia induced by his futile efforts to memorize all of the EKG criteria for left ventricular hypertrophy), comes to your office for a routine checkup. She is new to your practice and has not seen a doctor since her last child was born, which was more than 20 years ago. She has no specific complaints other than an occasional headache. Routine physical examination is unremarkable, except that you find her blood pressure is 170/110 mm Hg. She is unaware of being hypertensive. You would like to know if her hypertension is long standing or of recent onset. Her EKG is shown below. Is the EKG helpful?

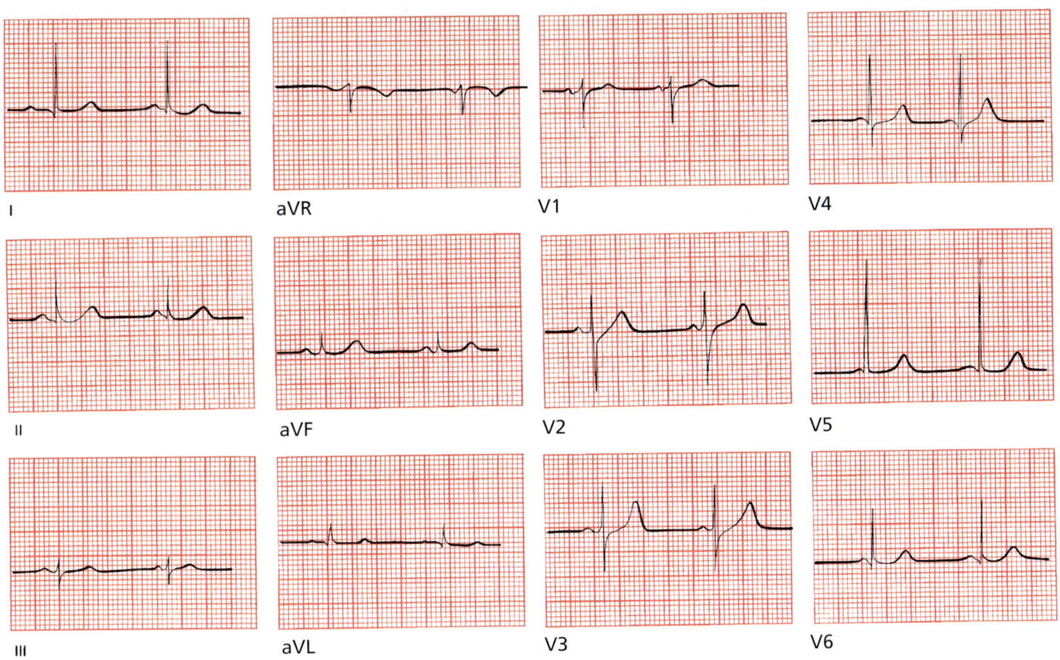

Mildred's EKG is essentially normal, which is not at all surprising. Most patients with hypertension have normal EKGs (and hopefully you recognized that this EKG is normal!). Nevertheless, had you found left ventricular hypertrophy, with or without repolarization abnormalities, you would have had at least one piece of evidence suggesting that her hypertension may be long standing. In this particular case, an imaging study could be done to exclude hypertrophy, but it is certainly not necessary for deciding that Mildred's hypertension should be treated.

CASE 2

Tom L. is a 23-year-old marathon runner. Nearing Central Park at about the 20-mile mark of the New York City Marathon, he suddenly turns pale, clutches his chest, and drops to the ground. Another runner, although on pace for a personal best, stops to help. Finding Tom pulseless and apneic, he begins cardiopulmonary resuscitation. The timely intervention proves lifesaving. Tom responds, and moments later, the following EKG is taken as he is being rushed to the nearest hospital. Why did Tom collapse?

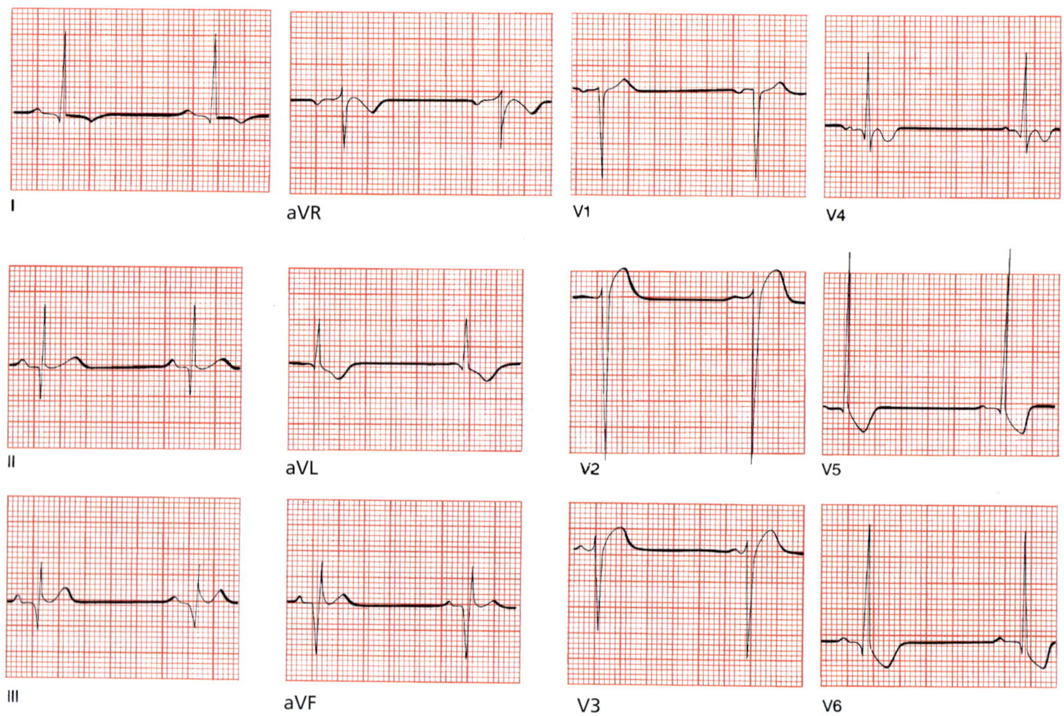

Hint: If you get this, you already know too much.

Tom L. collapsed because of a hypertrophic disease of his heart muscle. A leading cause of sudden death in young athletes is hypertrophic cardiomyopathy, of which one variant is **hypertrophic obstructive cardiomyopathy**, or HOCM (also called idiopathic hypertrophic subaortic stenosis, or IHSS). More than half of cases are familial (first-degree relatives of an affected patient should undergo genetic testing), with men affected slightly more often than women. Approximately 1 out of every 500 people is affected, and it is the leading cause of sudden cardiac death in young adults in the United States (see Chapter 7 for more about using the EKG to identify the various causes of sudden death). In this disorder, disorganized proliferation of muscle fibers in the interventricular septum can cause significant septal hypertrophy. The resultant clinical repercussions can range from severe and life threatening to virtually none. Syncope can result from (1) obstruction to left ventricular outflow by the hypertrophied muscle, and (2) an abnormal ventricular rhythm (see the next chapter).

EKG abnormalities are present in as many as 95% of patients with HOCM. The classic features on the resting EKG are the following:

1. Ventricular hypertrophy
2. Repolarization abnormalities in those leads with the tallest R waves
3. Narrow, deep spikey Q waves, of uncertain etiology, most often in the inferior and lateral leads (you can see great examples of these in leads II, III, and aVF on Tom's EKG)

Although this case was patently unfair, you may have recognized some of the features we have been talking about in this chapter, namely, the presence of criteria for left ventricular hypertrophy, especially in the precordial leads. Repolarization abnormalities are evident in all the left lateral leads (I, aVL, V5, and V6).

The timely intervention of his fellow runner saved Tom's life. It turned out that Tom had experienced similar, albeit less severe, episodes in the past, characterized by light-headedness and chest pain. Treatment has continued to evolve: pharmacotherapy now includes traditional medications to reduce both cardiac contractility and the risk of a serious arrhythmia as well as cardiac myosin inhibitors. Placement of an implantable cardioverter defibrillator (ICD) should be considered in any patient with HOCM who has recovered from an episode of sudden cardiac arrest.

3 Arrhythmias

In this chapter, you will learn:

1 | what arrhythmias are and why they matter

2 | about rhythm strips and ambulatory monitors

3 | how to determine the heart rate from the EKG

4 | the five basic types of arrhythmias

5 | how to recognize the four common sinus arrhythmias

6 | how arrhythmias develop in the first place

7 | to ask The Four Questions that will let you recognize and diagnose the common arrhythmias that originate in the sinus node, atria, atrioventricular (AV) node, and ventricles

8 | how to distinguish supraventricular arrhythmias, that is, those that arise above the ventricles, from ventricular arrhythmias, both clinically and on the EKG

9 | how programmed electrical stimulation and other techniques are used in the diagnosis and treatment of certain arrhythmias

10 | about the cases of George M. and Frederick van Z., which will leave you feeling astonished by how easily you have mastered material that has humbled even the high and mighty

The resting heart normally beats with a regular rhythm, 60–100 times per minute. Because each beat originates with depolarization of the sinus node, the usual, everyday cardiac rhythm is called *normal sinus rhythm* (or just *sinus rhythm*). Anything else is called an *arrhythmia.**

The term *arrhythmia* refers to any disturbance in the rate, regularity, site of origin, or conduction of the cardiac electrical impulse. An arrhythmia can be a single aberrant beat (or even a prolonged pause between beats) or a sustained rhythm disturbance that can persist for the lifetime of the patient.

Not every arrhythmia is abnormal or dangerous. For example, heart rates as low as 35–40 beats per minute are common and quite normal in well-trained athletes. Single aberrant beats, originating elsewhere in the heart than the sinus node, frequently occur in the majority of healthy individuals.

Some arrhythmias, however, can be dangerous and may even require immediate clinical intervention to prevent sudden death. The diagnosis of an arrhythmia is one of the most important things an EKG can do.

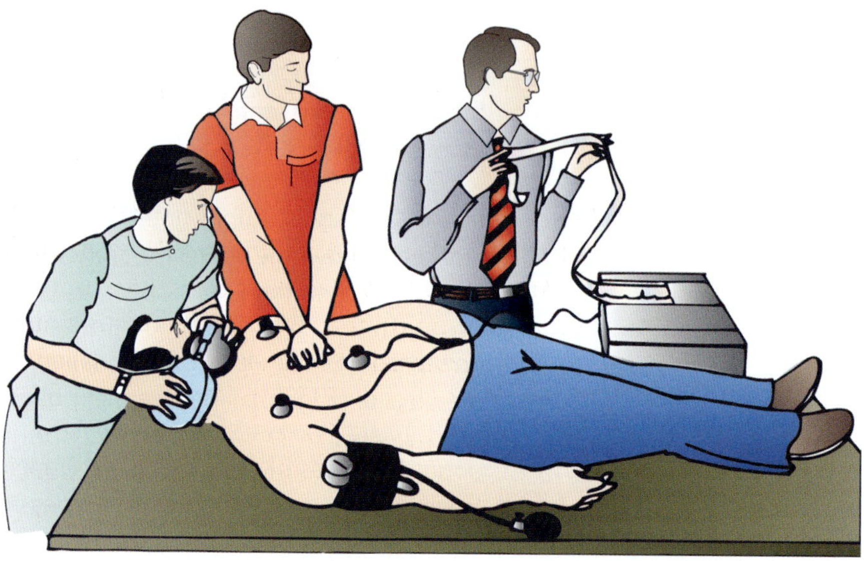

*A more accurate term might be dysrhythmia, but as this has never caught on, we will yield to social convention.

The Clinical Manifestations of Arrhythmias

When should you suspect that someone had or is having an arrhythmia?

Many arrhythmias go unnoticed by the patient and are picked up incidentally on a routine physical examination or EKG. Sometimes, however, arrhythmias elicit one of several characteristic symptoms.

First and foremost are *palpitations*, an awareness of one's own heartbeat. Patients may describe intermittent accelerations or decelerations of their heartbeat, a long pause between heartbeats, extra beats, unusually strong beats, or a sustained rapid heartbeat that may be regular or irregular. The sensation may in some cases be no more than mildly annoying, whereas in others it can be truly terrifying.

More serious are symptoms of decreased cardiac output, which can occur when the arrhythmia compromises the heart's ability to pump blood effectively. Among these are *light-headedness* and *syncope* (a sudden faint).

Rapid arrhythmias, called tachyarrhythmias, can increase the oxygen demands of the myocardium and cause *angina* (chest discomfort) or shortness of breath. The sudden onset of an arrhythmia in a patient with underlying cardiac disease can also precipitate *congestive heart failure*.

Sometimes, the first clinical manifestation of an arrhythmia is *cardiac arrest* or *sudden death*. Patients in the throes of an acute myocardial infarction are at a greatly increased risk for arrhythmic sudden death, which is why they are hospitalized in cardiac care units where their heart rate and rhythm can be continuously monitored and intervention can be performed at once and be potentially life-saving.

Increasingly, the EKG has become helpful in identifying conditions that *predispose* to serious arrhythmias and sudden death and thereby allow for clinical intervention *before* the catastrophic event.* These conditions can be inherited or acquired. We will discuss the most important of these in Chapter 7.

---

*There is exciting research using artificial intelligence to identify features on the resting 12-lead EKG that may predispose to arrhythmias and the attendant risks of syncope and sudden death. Stay tuned—this field is changing rapidly and we will be on top of all the most important developments.

Why Arrhythmias Happen

It is often impossible to identify the underlying cause of an arrhythmia, but a careful search should always be conducted for treatable precipitating factors. The mnemonic HIS BEDS should help you remember those arrhythmogenic factors that should be considered whenever you encounter a patient with an arrhythmia:

- *H—Hypoxia*: A myocardium deprived of oxygen is an irritable myocardium. Therefore, pulmonary disorders, whether severe chronic lung disease or an acute pulmonary embolus, are major precipitants of cardiac arrhythmias.
- *I—Ischemia and Irritability*: We have already mentioned that myocardial infarctions are a common setting for arrhythmias. Angina, even without the actual death of myocardial cells that occurs with infarction, is also a major precipitant. Occasionally, myocarditis, an inflammation of the heart muscle often caused by routine viral infections, can induce an arrhythmia.
- *S—Sympathetic Stimulation*: Enhanced sympathetic tone from any cause (eg, hyperthyroidism, congestive heart failure, nervousness, exercise) can elicit arrhythmias.
- *B—Bradycardia*: A very slow heart rate can predispose to arrhythmias. We can include the tachy–brady syndrome (one of a group of arrhythmias grouped under the rubric "sick sinus syndrome") in this category.
- *E—Electrolyte Disturbances*: Hypokalemia and hyperkalemia are notorious for their ability to induce arrhythmias; imbalances of calcium and magnesium can also be responsible.
- *D—Drugs*: Many drugs can cause arrhythmias. They do so by a variety of mechanisms. Ironically, the antiarrhythmic drugs are among the leading culprits.
- *S—Stretch*: Enlargement and hypertrophy of the atria and ventricles can produce arrhythmias. This is one way in which congestive heart failure, cardiomyopathies, and valvular disease can cause arrhythmias.

Rhythm Strips

In order to identify an arrhythmia correctly, it is often necessary to view the heart rhythm over a much longer period of time than the few cardiac cycles present on the standard 12-lead EKG. When an arrhythmia is suspected, either clinically or electrocardiographically, it is standard practice to run a *rhythm strip*, a long tracing of a single lead or multiple leads. Any lead can be chosen, but it obviously makes sense to choose the lead that provides you with the most information. One or more leads are preprogrammed to run automatically when you hit the Rhythm button on modern EKG machines (Lead II is the most common choice but lead V1 has its proponents as well; whereas all 12 leads can give a good sense of what is happening in the ventricles, leads II and V1 are particularly helpful in assessing atrial activity). The rhythm strip makes it much easier to identify any irregularities or intermittent bursts of unusual electrical activity.

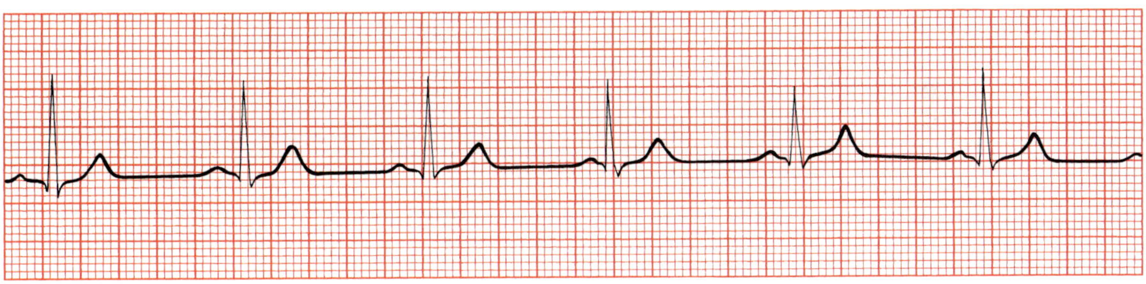

A short sample from a typical rhythm strip. You can run it as long as you need to in order to decipher the rhythm. This particular strip represents a continuous recording of lead II in a patient with normal sinus rhythm, the normal rhythm of the heart.

Ambulatory Monitors, Event Monitors, Loop Recorders, and Wearables

The ultimate rhythm strips are provided by *ambulatory monitors*. They are essentially wearable EKG recorders with memory. The original ambulatory monitor, the Holter monitor, is a small box containing the recorder that is hooked onto the patient's belt with wires running up to electrode patches attached to the chest wall. It is worn for 24–48 hours. However, far more popular today are small patches in which all the recording technology is contained within the patch. The patch is attached directly to the chest wall by an adhesive and worn for up to 2 weeks. Patients go about their normal daily activities—working, showering, exercising, sleeping—while the monitor records every single heartbeat.* A complete record of the heart rhythm is stored and later analyzed for any arrhythmic activity.

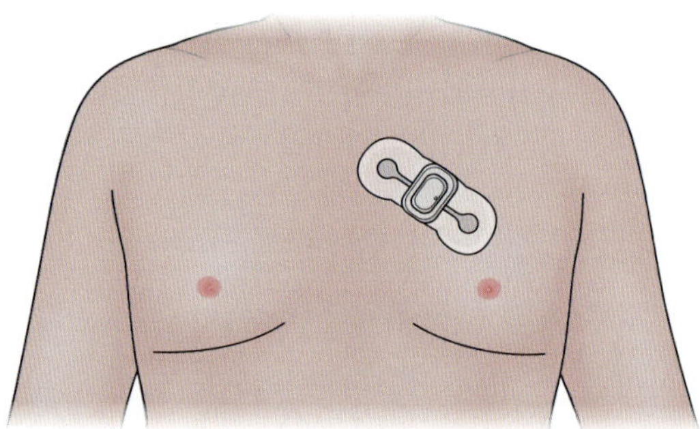

Not much larger than a typical plastic bandage, recording patches can be worn for days, even weeks, without interfering with normal daily activities.

Ambulatory monitoring is especially valuable when the suspected arrhythmia is an infrequent occurrence and unlikely to be captured on a random 12-lead EKG, which runs for only 10 seconds. Clearly, the longer one can monitor the patient, the better the chance that the arrhythmia will be detected. Patients are also instructed to write down the precise times when they experience symptoms. The

*The patches are pretty innocuous and don't interfere with whatever the patient chooses to do (even swimming is okay!). The adhesive can itch, however.

diary entries can then be compared with the ambulatory recording to determine whether there is a correlation between the patient's symptoms and any underlying cardiac arrhythmia. The patches often have a button that patients can press if they feel palpitations, thereby noting the time of their symptoms on the EKG tracing, and some devices include cell phones that allow the patients to type in their symptoms when they occur.

Some rhythm disturbances or symptoms suspicious for arrhythmias happen so infrequently that even a 2-week ambulatory monitor is likely to miss them. For these patients, an event monitor may provide a solution. An *event monitor* recording is triggered by the patient whenever he or she experiences palpitations. Some of these monitors are constantly running—they are never "off"—and they are able to go back and make a record of the rhythm from a short period before the patient activates it to several minutes after activation. The resultant EKG recording is sent out over the phone lines for evaluation. In this manner, multiple recordings can be made over the course of the several months during which the patient has rented the monitor. Other monitors are only activated by patients holding a monitor up to their chest when symptoms occur. There are also monitors that attach to a cell phone, fitness band, or other electronic device (these utilize fingertip-sized electrodes built into the device) and are used in the same way; these can be purchased by the patient and are remarkably inexpensive.

Still other abnormal rhythms are so short lived or infrequent that they are missed by any standard type of patient-activated mechanism. For these situations, an implantable loop recorder can be inserted under the skin with a small (1–2 cm) incision. These event recorders can be safely left in place for years. They automatically record and store in their memory rapid or slow heart rates (the rates that trigger the recorder are programmable). The patient can also activate the recorder whenever symptoms occur. The recorded data can be easily downloaded, typically every few months, by telemetry communication. These loop monitors are also frequently being used in patients who are asymptomatic but in whom an arrhythmia is suspected (eg, in a patient who has suffered what appears to be an embolic stroke and in whom subclinical atrial fibrillation, a potential source of embolism, must be ruled out [see page 152]).

Finally, we should mention the increasing use of consumer-oriented wearable devices, such as smartwatches, which can be purchased over the counter and can be used to monitor the heart rate and rhythm. Essentially, they are used solely to distinguish between regular (eg, sinus rhythm) and irregular (eg, atrial fibrillation) rhythms. They are easy to use and are patient activated, producing a short—usually 30 seconds—rhythm strip that can then be transmitted for expert interpretation. Although these wearable devices can be useful, there is always the risk of missing short bursts of abnormal rhythms. Just as importantly, false positives—despite increasingly sophisticated algorithms, these devices all too often lead to an incorrect diagnosis of atrial fibrillation when none is present—can cause anxiety and further needless evaluation. More subtle, perhaps, is the issue of overdiagnosis—for example, finding short runs of a supraventricular arrhythmia that may never prove clinically significant and may serve only to intensify patient anxiety and conceivably lead the patient and the health care provider to consider therapeutic interventions with all the attendant potential side effects when none may be needed.

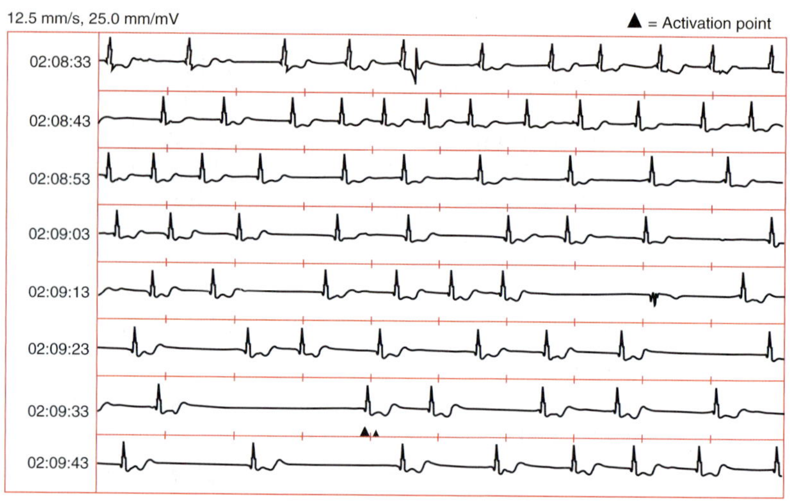

An implanted event monitor recording in a patient with syncope. The *small vertical dashes* mark off intervals of 1 second. The 3-second pause near the bottom of the strip activates the monitor, which then stores the EKG tracing from several minutes before to several minutes after the activation point. The stored recording is then downloaded and printed at a later time. In this patient, the long pause was associated with a near-syncopal episode.

How to Determine the Heart Rate From the EKG

The first step in figuring out the heart rhythm—whether we are talking about normal sinus rhythm or anything else—is to determine the heart rate, so let's start here. And it turns out that the heart rate is one of the easiest things to calculate from a standard EKG.

The horizontal axis on an EKG represents time. Recall that the distance between each light line (one small square or 1 mm) equals 0.04 seconds (40 milliseconds), and the distance between each heavy line (one large square or 5 mm) equals 0.2 seconds (200 milliseconds). Five large squares therefore constitute 1 second. Thus, a cycle that repeats itself every five large squares represents 1 beat per second, or a heart rate of 60 beats per minute.

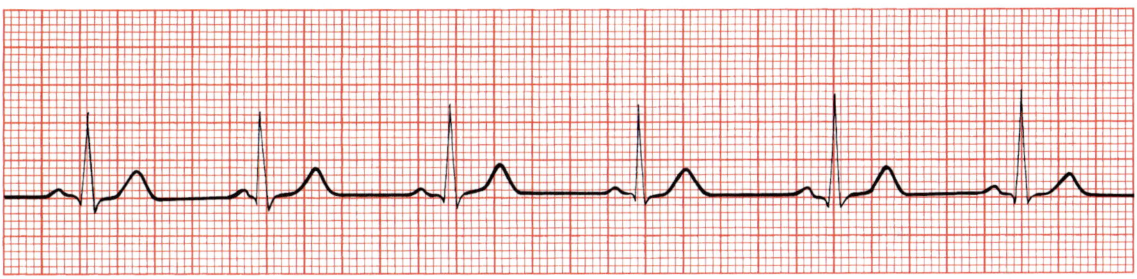

Every QRS complex is separated by five large squares (1 second). A rhythm occurring once every second occurs 60 times every minute.

Of course, not everyone's heart beats at precisely 60 beats per minute. Fortunately, whatever the heart rate, calculating it is easy.

A Simple Three-Step Method for Calculating the Heart Rate

1. Find an R wave that falls on, or nearly on, one of the heavy lines.
2. Count the number of large squares until the next R wave.
3. Determine the rate in beats per minute as follows:
   - If there is one large square between successive R waves, then each R wave is separated by 0.2 seconds. Therefore, over the course of 1 full second, there will be five cycles of cardiac activity (1 second divided by 0.2 seconds), and over 1 minute, 300 cycles (5×60 seconds). The heart rate is therefore 300 beats per minute.
   - If there are two large squares between successive R waves, then each R wave is separated by 0.4 seconds. Therefore, over the course of 1 full second, there will be 2.5 cycles of cardiac activity (1 second divided by 0.4 seconds), and over 1 minute, 150 cycles (2.5×60 seconds). The heart rate is therefore 150 beats per minute.

   By similar logic:

   - Three large squares = 100 beats per minute
   - Four large squares = 75 beats per minute
   - Five large squares = 60 beats per minute
   - Six large squares = 50 beats per minute

Notice that you can get the answer by dividing 300 by the number of large squares between R waves (eg, 300 divided by 4 squares = 75). Even greater accuracy can be achieved by counting the total number *of small* squares between R waves and dividing 1500 by this total.

What is the heart rate of the following strips?

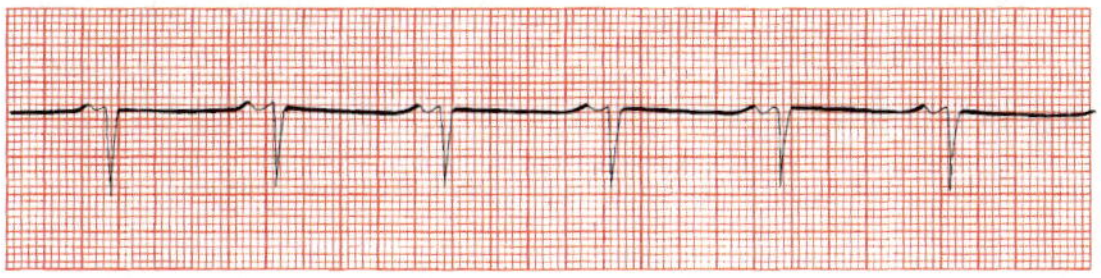

A

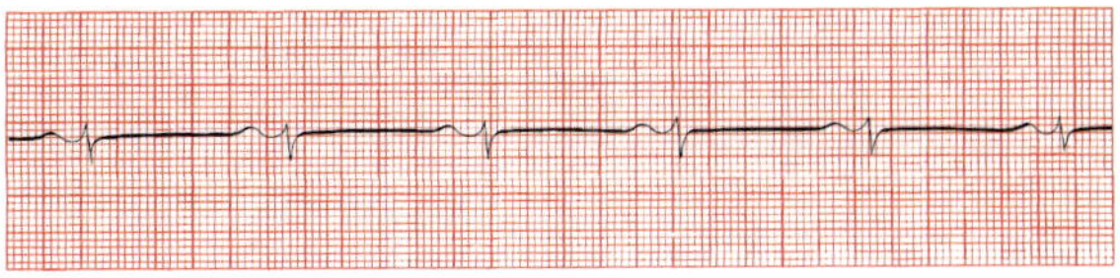

B

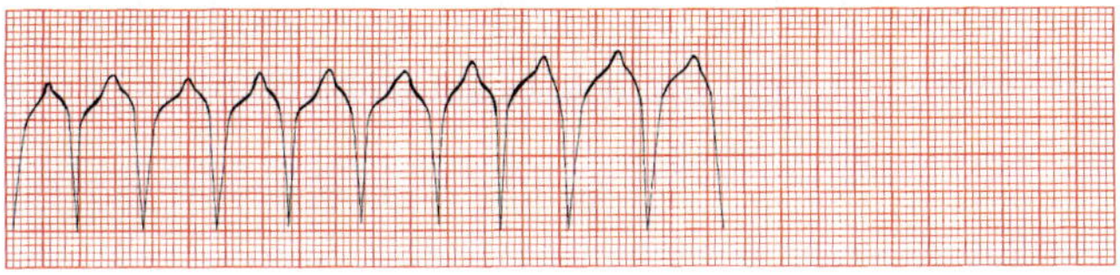

C

(*A*) About 75 beats per minute. (*B*) About 60 beats per minute. (*C*) About 150 beats per minute.

However, what if the second R wave falls *between* heavy lines, that is, if the R waves from each cycle don't conveniently fall a precise whole number of large boxes from each other? In that case, you can estimate that the rate lies between the two extremes on either side.

What is the rate of the following strip?

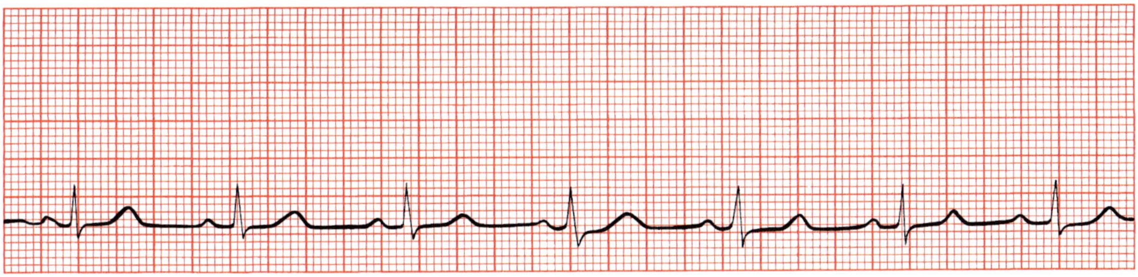

The R waves are slightly more than four squares apart—let's say four and one-quarter. The rate must therefore be between 60 and 75 beats per minute. If you guess 70, you'll be close. Alternatively, divide 300 by four and one-quarter and get 70.6 beats per minute.

If the heart rate is very slow, you can still use this system; simply divide 300 by the number of large squares between complexes to get your answer.

However, we've saved the best for last—there is an even easier way to determine the heart rate. The typical 12-lead EKG records for precisely 10 seconds from start to finish. Simply count the number of cycles, that is, R-R intervals, on the EKG (use the uninterrupted rhythm strip that runs along the bottom), and then multiply by 6 (10 seconds × 6 = 60 seconds) to get the heart rate in beats per minute. Try it both ways on the example below:

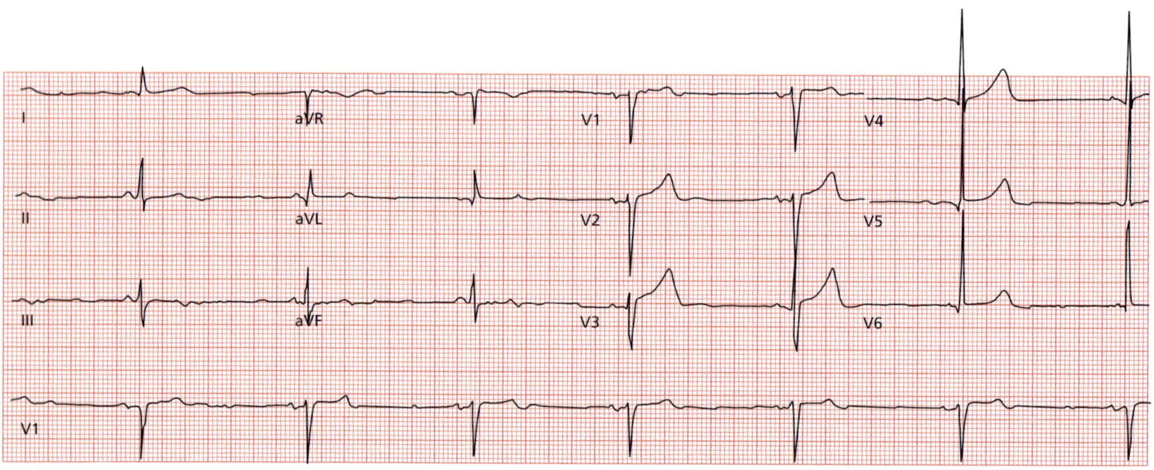

There are ~7 cardiac cycles on this ECG. Multiply by 6 and you get 42 beats per minute.

The Five Basic Types of Arrhythmias

Of all of the subjects in electrocardiography, none is guaranteed to cause more anxiety (and palpitations) than the study of arrhythmias. There is no reason for this. First, once you have learned to recognize the basic patterns, nothing is easier than recognizing a classic arrhythmia. Second, the difficult arrhythmias are difficult for everyone, including expert electrocardiographers. Nothing gladdens one's heart more than the sight of two venerable cardiologists going at it over a baffling rhythm disturbance.

The heart is capable of five basic types of rhythm disturbances:

- The electrical activity follows the usual conduction pathways we have already outlined, starting with depolarization of the sinus node, but the rhythm is too fast, too slow, or irregular. These are *arrhythmias of sinus origin*.
- The electrical activity originates from a focus other than the sinus node. These are called *ectopic rhythms*.
- The electrical activity is trapped within an electrical racetrack whose shape and boundaries are determined by various anatomic or electrical myocardial configurations. These are called *reentrant arrhythmias*. They can occur anywhere in the heart. If this sounds hard to understand, don't worry, we will walk you through it.
- The electrical activity originates in the sinus node and follows the usual pathways but encounters unexpected blocks and delays. These *conduction blocks* are discussed in Chapter 4.
- The electrical activity follows anomalous accessory conduction pathways that bypass the normal ones, providing an electrical shortcut, or short circuit. These arrhythmias are termed *preexcitation syndromes*, and they are discussed in Chapter 5.

Arrhythmias of Sinus Origin

Sinus Tachycardia and Sinus Bradycardia

Normal sinus rhythm is the normal rhythm of the heart. Depolarization originates spontaneously within the sinus node. The rate is regular and between 60 and 100 beats per minute. If the rhythm speeds up beyond 100, it is called *sinus tachycardia*; if it slows down below 60, it is called *sinus bradycardia*.

Sinus tachycardia and sinus bradycardia can be normal or pathologic. Strenuous exercise, for example, can accelerate the heart rate well over 100 beats per minute, whereas resting heart rates below 60 beats per minute are typical in well-conditioned athletes or during sleep.

On the other hand, alterations in the rate at which the sinus node fires can accompany significant heart disease. Sinus tachycardia can occur in patients with congestive heart failure or severe lung disease, or it can be the only presenting sign of an acute pulmonary embolism or hyperthyroidism in the elderly. Sinus bradycardia can be caused by opioids, many medications, and is the most common rhythm disturbance seen in the early stages of an acute myocardial infarction; in otherwise healthy individuals, it can result from enhanced vagal tone and cause fainting.

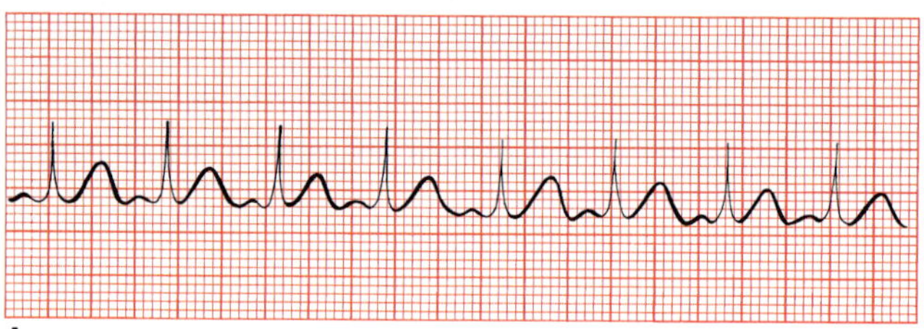

A

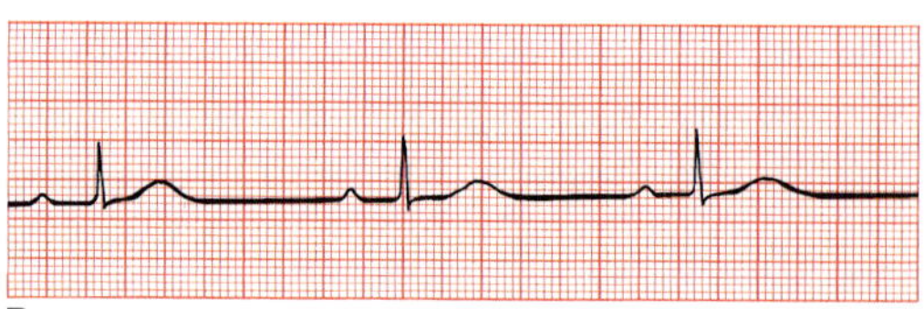

B

(*A*) Sinus tachycardia. Each beat is separated by two and one-half large squares for a rate of 120 beats per minute. (*B*) Sinus bradycardia. More than seven large squares separate each beat, and the rate is 40–45 beats per minute.

The differential diagnosis of *bradycardia* is long but worth knowing. The major causes include the following:

- Enhanced vagal tone, for example, as seen in athletes
- Medications—beta blockers, calcium channel blockers, and a long list of others
- Opioids
- Myocardial ischemia
- Hypothyroidism
- Hyperkalemia
- Hypothermia
- Stroke and other CNS catastrophes
- Obstructive sleep apnea (during the apneic periods)
- Sinus node dysfunction (see sinus arrest on page 125)
- Many—too many to list here—infectious causes

Sinus Arrhythmia

Often, the EKG will reveal a rhythm that appears in all respects to be normal sinus rhythm except that it is slightly irregular. This is called *sinus arrhythmia*. This is a *normal* phenomenon, reflecting the variation in heart rate that accompanies inspiration and expiration. The effect may be so small as to be virtually undetectable or (rarely) large enough to mimic more serious causes of an irregular heartbeat. Inspiration accelerates the heart rate, and expiration slows it down. Any variation in the R-R interval less than 15% can be attributed to sinus arrhythmia.

Sinus arrhythmia is the principle behind some yoga and meditative practices, in which you focus on slowly exhaling in order to slow the heartbeat.

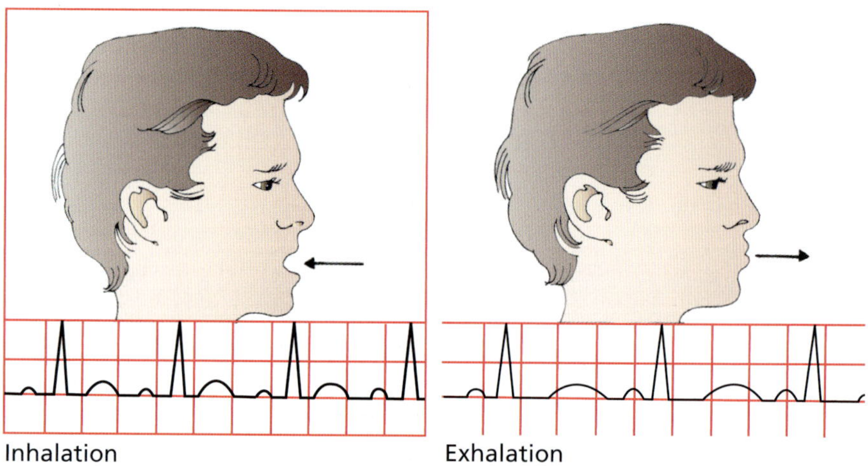

Sinus arrhythmia. The heart rate accelerates with inspiration and slows with expiration.

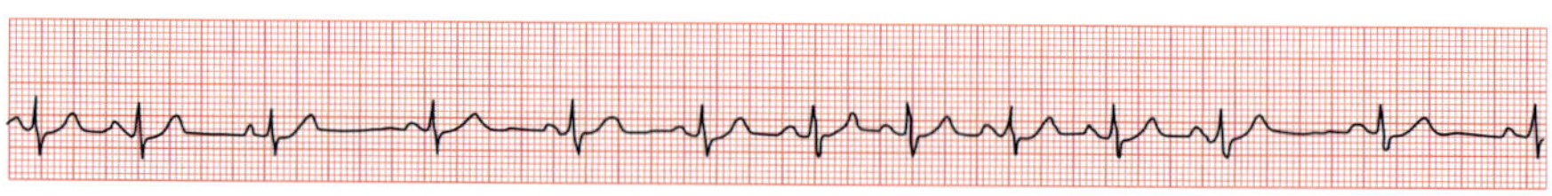

A beautiful example of sinus arrhythmia. The variation in rhythm—fast–slow–fast–slow—corresponds with inhale–exhale–inhale–exhale.

Sinus Arrhythmia Is Your Friend

Remember: sinus arrhythmia is normal. A loss of sinus arrhythmia may be caused by diminished autonomic feedback to the sinus node. It is therefore often seen in patients with diabetes mellitus who have an associated autonomic neuropathy. Sinus arrhythmia can also be diminished with aging, with obesity, and in patients with long-standing hypertension.

Have You Heard About Heart Rate Variability?

We've just pointed out that sinus arrhythmia is normal and a sign of a healthy heart. The variation in the R-R interval from beat to beat has been termed heart rate variability and is one measure of a well-functioning autonomic nervous system. Low heart rate variability is believed to reflect increased sympathetic tone and has been associated with increased mortality after a heart attack (myocardial infarction) as well as relatively poor outcomes in patients with various arrhythmias that we will be discussing in this chapter, as well as in patients with ischemic heart disease. These associations may reflect a correlation between sympathetic nervous system activity and an increased susceptibility to ventricular arrhythmias and inflammation. However, compelling data are still in short supply, and measuring heart rate variability is not currently recommended as a general screening tool. Nor has its utility in any specific high-risk situations been found to improve outcomes. Where this is all going to lead in the future is unknown, but some clinicians believe that measuring heart rate variability may eventually prove useful and allow for early therapeutic interventions for individuals at high risk of adverse cardiac outcomes.

Sinus Arrest, Asystole, and Escape Beats

Sinus arrest occurs when the sinus node stops firing. If nothing else were to happen, the EKG would show a flat line without any electrical activity, and the patient would die. Prolonged electrical inactivity is called *asystole*.

Fortunately, virtually all myocardial cells have the ability to behave as pacemakers. Ordinarily, the fastest pacemaker drives the heart, and under normal circumstances, the fastest pacemaker is the sinus node. The sinus node *overdrives* the innate pacemaker activity of the other cells in the heart by delivering its wave of depolarization throughout the myocardium before its potential competitors can complete their own, more leisurely, spontaneous depolarization. With sinus arrest, however, these other pacemakers can spring into action in a kind of rescue mission. These rescuing beats, originating outside the sinus node, are called *escape beats*.

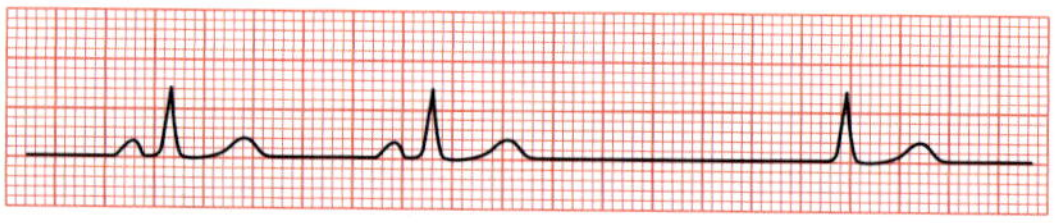

Sinus arrest occurs after the second beat—note the long pause. The third beat, restoring electrical activity, has no P wave. This beat is called a junctional escape beat, which we will explain in the very next section.

Nonsinus Pacemakers

Like the sinus node, which typically fires between 60 and 100 times each minute, the other potential pacemaker cells of the heart have their own intrinsic rate. When called upon to do so (and sometimes when not), *atrial pacemakers* usually discharge at a rate of 60–75 beats per minute. Pacemaker cells located near the AV node, called *junctional pacemakers*, typically discharge at 40–60 beats per minute. *Ventricular pacemaker* cells usually discharge at 30–45 beats per minute.

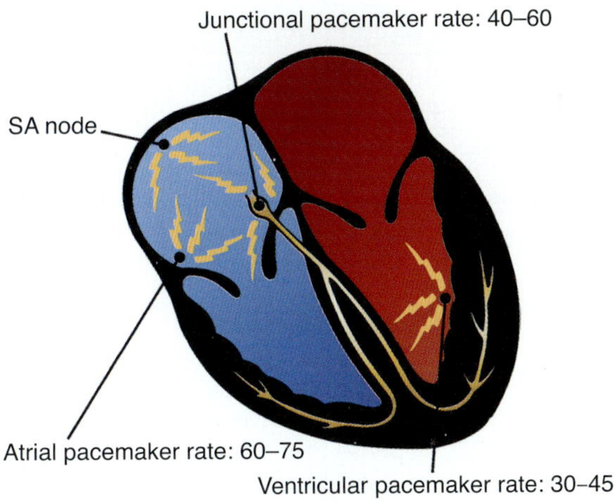

Each of these nonsinus pacemakers can rescue an inadequate sinus node by providing just one escape beat or a continual series of escape beats. Of all the available escape mechanisms, *junctional escape* is by far the most common.

With junctional escape, depolarization originates near the AV node, and the usual pattern of atrial depolarization does not occur. As a result, a normal P wave is not seen. Most often, there is no visible P wave at all. Occasionally, however, a *retrograde P wave* may be seen, representing atrial depolarization moving *upward* from the AV node back into the atria. The mean electrical axis of this *retrograde P wave* is reversed 180° from that of a normal P wave. Thus, whereas a normal P wave is upright in lead II and inverted in lead aVR, a retrograde P wave is inverted in lead II and upright in lead aVR.

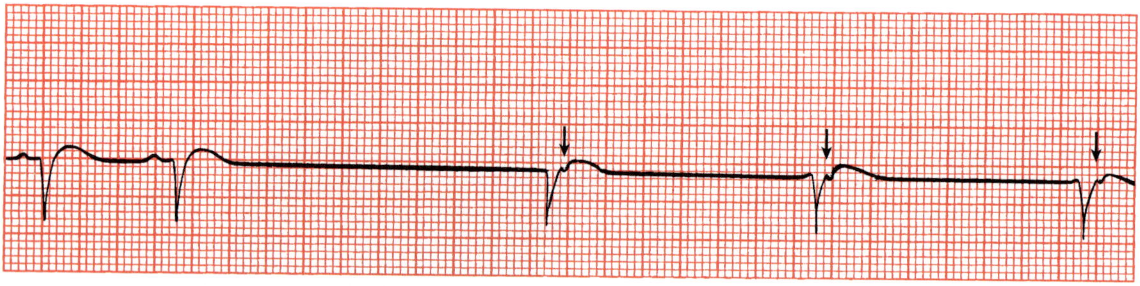

Junctional escape. The first two beats are normal sinus beats with a normal P wave preceding each QRS complex. There is then a long pause followed by a series of three junctional escape beats occurring at a rate of 40–45 beats per minute. Retrograde P waves can be seen buried in the early portion of the T waves (can you see the little downward notches where the *arrows* are pointing?). Retrograde P waves can occur before, after, or during the QRS complex, depending on the relative timing of atrial and ventricular depolarization. If atrial and ventricular depolarizations occur simultaneously, the much larger QRS complexes can completely mask the retrograde P waves.

Sinus Arrest Versus Sinus Exit Block

Because sinus node depolarization is *not* recorded on the EKG, it is almost impossible (see the Box on page 130) to determine whether a prolonged sinus pause is due to sinus arrest or to failure of a normal sinus depolarization to be transmitted out of the node and into the atria, a situation called *sinus exit block*. You may hear these different terms bandied about from time to time, but for all intents and purposes, sinus arrest and sinus exit block imply the same thing: There is a failure of the sinus mechanism to deliver its current into the surrounding tissue.

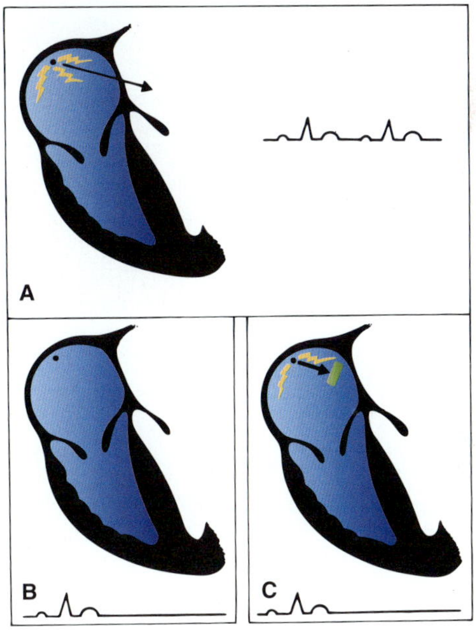

(*A*) Normal sinus rhythm. The sinus node fires repeatedly, and waves of depolarization spread out into the atria. (*B*) Sinus arrest. The sinus node falls silent. No current is generated, and the EKG shows no electrical activity. (*C*) Sinus exit block. The sinus node continues to fire, but the wave of depolarization fails to exit the sinus node into the atrial myocardium. Again, the EKG shows no electrical activity; there is not sufficient voltage to generate a detectable P wave.

Sinus exit block can be caused by many of the same medications and mechanisms that cause sinus bradycardia. Other causes include infiltrative (eg, amyloidosis) and inflammatory (eg, rheumatic fever) processes, as well as fibrosis (which can occur with aging).

More on Sinus Arrest Versus Sinus Exit Block

Special note for the electrically infatuated: There is a way in which transient sinus arrest and sinus exit block can sometimes be distinguished on the EKG. With sinus arrest, resumption of normal sinus electrical activity can occur at any random time (the sinus node simply resumes firing). However, with typical sinus exit block, the sinus node has continued to fire silently, so when the block is lifted, the sinus node resumes depolarizing the atria after a pause that is some integer multiple of the normal cycle (eg, exactly one missed P wave, or exactly two missed P waves, or more).

SUMMARY

Arrhythmias of Sinus Origin

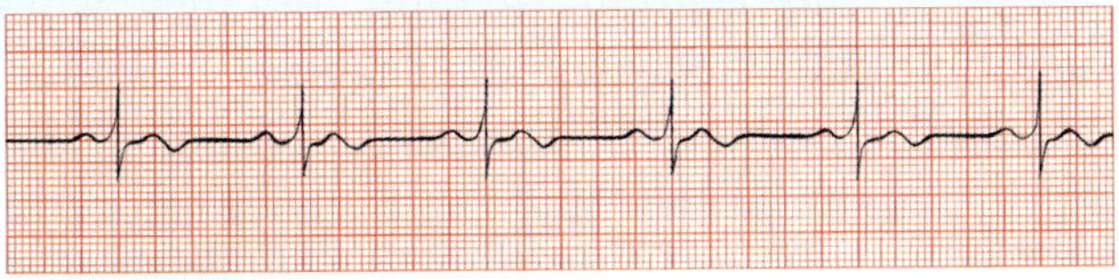

Normal sinus rhythm

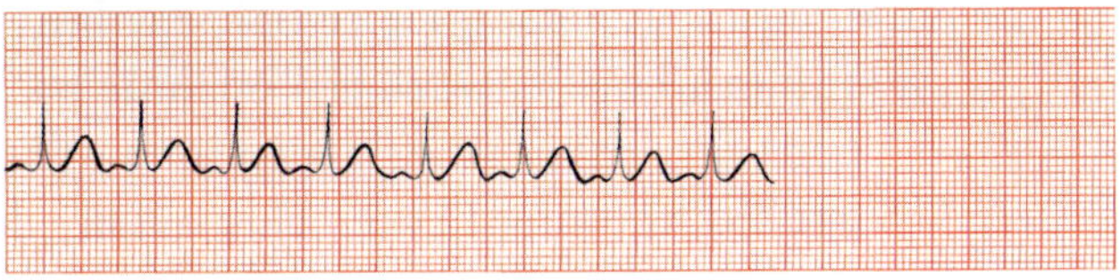

Sinus tachycardia

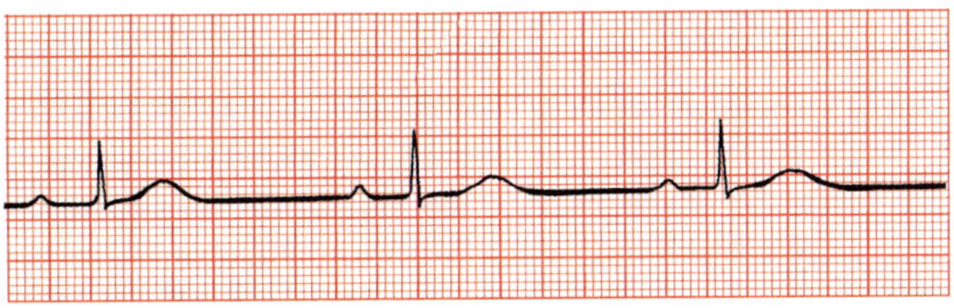

Sinus bradycardia

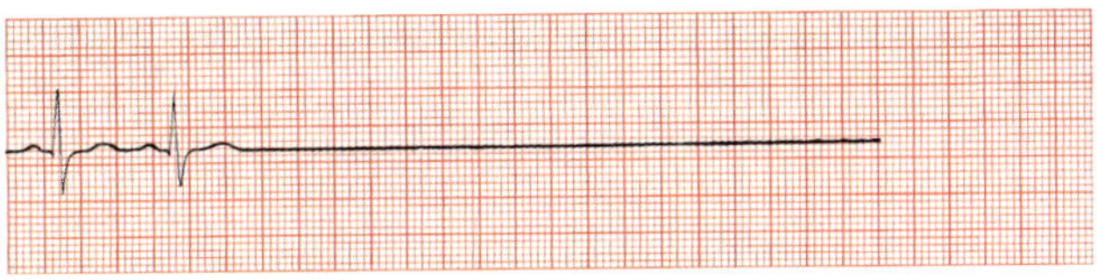

Sinus arrest or exit block

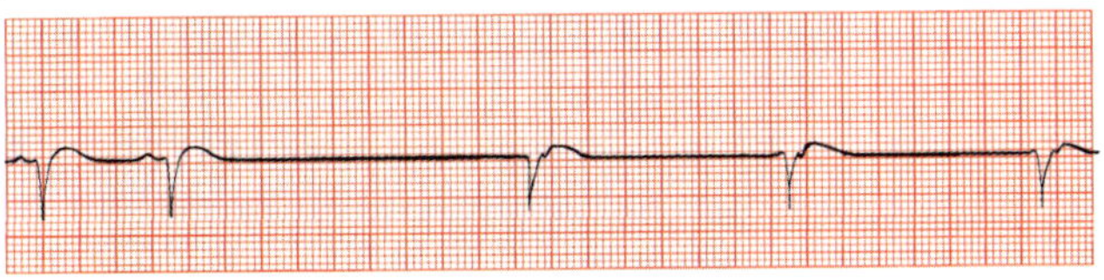

Sinus arrest or exit block with junctional escape

Ectopic Rhythms

The two major causes of nonsinus arrhythmias are ectopic rhythms and reentrant rhythms, and these will occupy the rest of this admittedly lengthy chapter.

Ectopic rhythms are abnormal rhythms that arise from regions outside the sinus node. They can consist of single, isolated beats or sustained arrhythmias. Ectopic rhythms can be caused by any of the precipitating factors described previously (see page 112).

At the cellular level, ectopic rhythms arise from enhanced automaticity (ie, enhanced intrinsic pacemaker activity) of a nonsinus node site, either a single focus or a roving one. As we have already stressed, the fastest pacemaker usually drives the heart, and under normal circumstances, the fastest pacemaker is the sinus node. Under *abnormal* circumstances, however, any of the other pacemakers scattered throughout the heart can be accelerated, that is, *stimulated to depolarize faster and faster* until they can overdrive the normal sinus mechanism and establish their own transient or sustained ectopic rhythm. Among the common causes of enhanced automaticity are digitalis toxicity, beta adrenergic stimulation from inhaler therapies used to treat asthma and chronic obstructive lung disease, caffeine, alcohol, stimulant drugs such as cocaine and amphetamines, and psychological stress. We will see examples of ectopic rhythms in the pages to come.

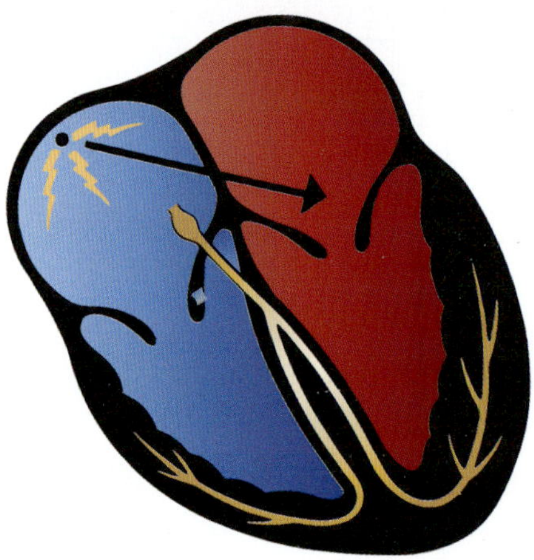

A

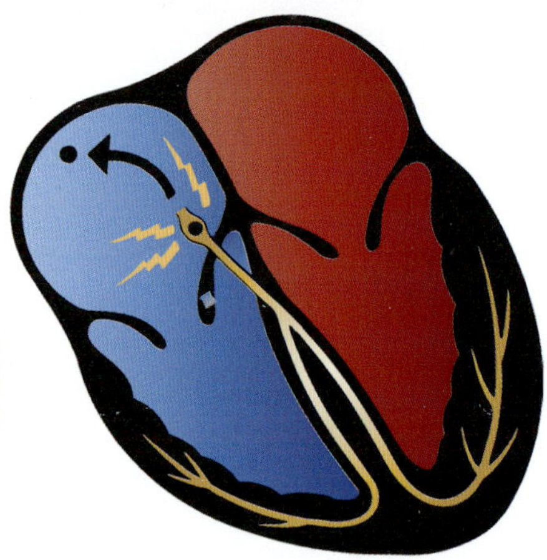

B

(*A*) Normally, the sinus node drives the heart. (*B*) If another potential pacemaker (eg, the AV junction) is accelerated, it can take over the heart and overdrive the sinus node.

Reentrant Rhythms

The second major cause of nonsinus arrhythmias is called *reentry*. Whereas enhanced automaticity represents a disorder of *impulse formation* (ie, new impulses that are formed outside the sinus node take over the heart), reentry represents a disorder of *impulse transmission*. The results, however, are similar: creation of a focus of abnormal electrical activity. In the case of reentry, we refer to the focus as a reentry loop. Because reentry is such an important driver of many important arrhythmias, we need to spend a few moments explaining how this occurs.

A reentry loop can develop in several ways. Let's look at the most common mechanism. Picture a wave of depolarization arriving at two adjacent regions of myocardium, A and B. With each normal sinus beat, current travels down both pathways to wherever it may be going. This is how things usually operate.

Suppose, however, that a premature atrial beat occurs (we will describe these types of beats shortly, but for now all you need to understand is that an early, premature beat, originating outside the sinus node, suddenly comes along and interrupts the orderly flow of normal sinus beats). Let's further assume that pathway A normally conducts faster and repolarizes more quickly than pathway B. Under normal circumstances, this doesn't matter, since both pathways have plenty of time to repolarize between beats and can continue conducting any and all subsequent beats. But this new atrial beat comes early, that is, it is premature, and pathway B, slow to repolarize, is simply not ready for it. The premature beat will therefore preferentially travel down pathway A. In doing so, however, it now renders pathway A refractory to the next sinus beat that comes along; it simply doesn't have time to repolarize and resume conducting. The ensuing sinus beat is thus forced to travel down the slower pathway B, which finally has recovered and is no longer refractory. The current can then circle back up through pathway A, at last fully recovered, and a reentry loop is established; in this case, the current circles clockwise down pathway B and up pathway A, around and around, forming a new locus of electrical activity that sends current out into the surrounding myocardium.

Sometimes pictures say much more than words, so if all this seems confusing, the following illustration should help.

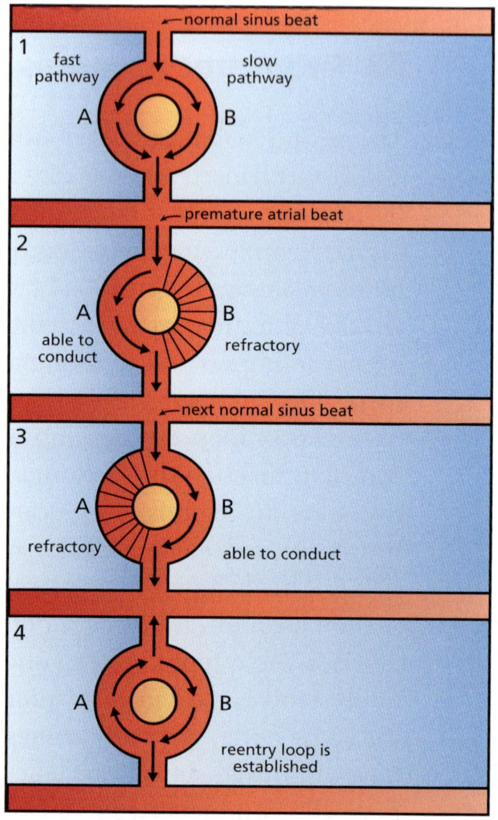

In *Figure 1*, a normal beat travels down both pathways *A* and *B*. Even though pathway A conducts more rapidly and recovers more quickly than pathway B, both have plenty of time to recover between beats and are able to conduct freely. *Figure 2* shows the arrival of a premature atrial beat, which must travel down faster pathway *A*, which recovers more quickly than pathway B (remember, normally the speed of recovery doesn't matter since there is plenty of time before the next sinus beat, but this new atrial beat arrives early, before pathway *B* can repolarize). *Figure 3* shows what happens with the arrival of the next normal sinus beat. Pathway *A* is still refractory, having just conducted the premature atrial beat, and is unable to conduct the sinus beat, which therefore is forced to travel down pathway *B*. *Figure 4* shows the normal sinus beat circling back up through pathway *A*, now recovered, and the reentry loop is off and running.

A reentry loop can vary greatly in size. It can be limited to a small loop within a single anatomic site (eg, the AV node), it can loop through an entire chamber (either an atrium or a ventricle), or it can even involve both an atrium and ventricle if there is an accessory pathway of conduction connecting the two chambers (this last point will be made more obvious in Chapter 5).

The Four Questions

As you will see in just a moment, all of the clinically important nonsinus arrhythmias—the ones you have probably heard of—are either ectopic or reentrant in origin. It is therefore critical to be able to identify them, and you will spend the rest of this chapter learning exactly how to do that. This may sound like a tall order, but to assess any rhythm disturbance on the EKG, you only need to answer four questions:

- **Are Normal P Waves Present?** The emphasis here is on the word *normal*. If the answer is yes, if there are *normal*-appearing P waves with a *normal* P-wave axis (positive in lead II and negative in lead aVR), then the origin of the arrhythmia is almost certainly within the atria, probably at or near the sinus node. If no P waves are present, then the rhythm must have originated below the atria, in the AV node or the ventricles. The presence of P waves with an *abnormal axis* and *abnormal configuration* may reflect (1) activation of the atria from impulses originating from an atrial focus other than the sinus node or (2) retrograde activation from a site within the AV node or the ventricles, that is, from current flowing backward into the atria through the AV node or through an accessory pathway connecting the atria and ventricles (more on all of this later).
- **Are the QRS Complexes Narrow (<0.12 Seconds in Duration) or Wide (>0.12 Seconds in Duration)?** A narrow normal QRS complex implies that ventricular depolarization is proceeding along the usual pathways (AV node to His bundle to bundle branches to Purkinje cells). This is the most efficient means of conduction, requiring the least amount of time, so the resulting QRS complex is of short duration (narrow). A narrow QRS complex, therefore, indicates that the origin of the rhythm must be at or above the AV node. On the other hand, a wide QRS complex usually implies that the depolarization has instead been initiated within the ventricular myocardium, not the conduction system, and therefore spreads much more slowly. Conduction does

not follow the most efficient pathway, and the QRS complex is of long duration (wide). (The distinction between wide and narrow QRS complexes, although very useful, cannot, unfortunately, be fully relied on to assess the origin of an arrhythmia. We'll see why shortly.)

Questions 1 and 2 help to make the important distinction as to whether an arrhythmia is ventricular or supraventricular (atrial or junctional) in origin.

- **What Is the Relationship Between the P Waves and the QRS Complexes?** If the P waves and QRS complexes correlate in the usual one-to-one fashion, with a single P wave preceding each QRS complex, then the rhythm almost certainly has a sinus or other atrial origin. Sometimes, however, the atria and ventricles depolarize and contract independently of each other. This will be manifested on the EKG by a lack of correlation between the P waves and QRS complexes, a dangerous situation termed *AV dissociation*.
- **Is the Rhythm Regular or Irregular?** This is often the most immediately obvious characteristic of a particular rhythm and is sometimes the most critical.

Whenever you look at an EKG, you will need to assess the rhythm. These four questions should become an intrinsic part of your thinking:

1. Are normal P waves present?
2. Are the QRS complexes narrow or wide?
3. What is the relationship between the P waves and the QRS complexes?
4. Is the rhythm regular or irregular (remember, though, that sinus arrhythmia is normal)?

For the normal EKG, the answers are easy:

1. Yes, there are normal P waves.
2. The QRS complexes are narrow.
3. There is one P wave for every QRS complex.
4. The rhythm is essentially regular.

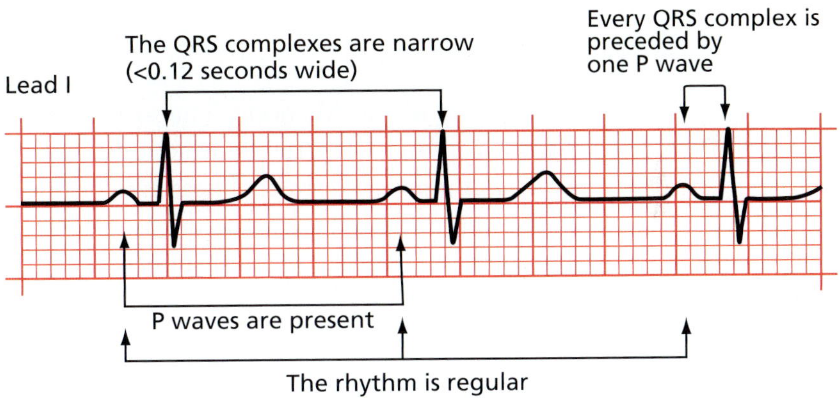

Normal sinus rhythm and "The Four Questions" answered.

We will now see what happens when the answers are different.

Supraventricular Arrhythmias

Let us look first at the arrhythmias that originate in the atria or the AV node, the **supraventricular (supra = above) arrhythmias.**

These arrhythmias can consist of a single beat or a sustained rhythm disturbance lasting for a few seconds or many years.

Atrial and Junctional Premature Beats

Single ectopic supraventricular beats can originate in the atria or in the vicinity of the AV node. The former are called *atrial premature beats* (or premature atrial contractions, PACs) and the latter, *junctional premature beats*. These are common phenomena, neither indicating underlying cardiac disease nor requiring treatment. They can, however, initiate more sustained arrhythmias.

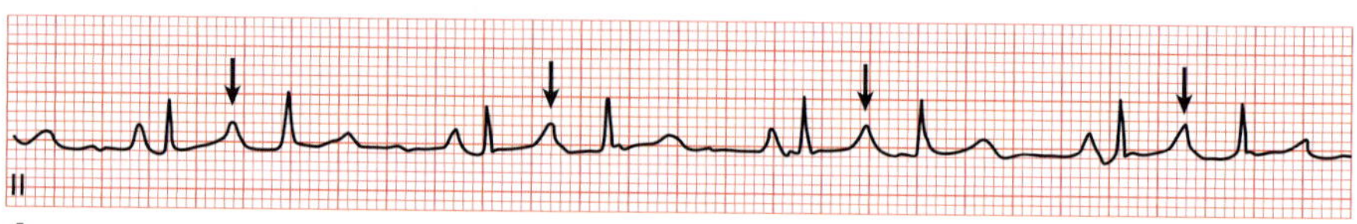

A

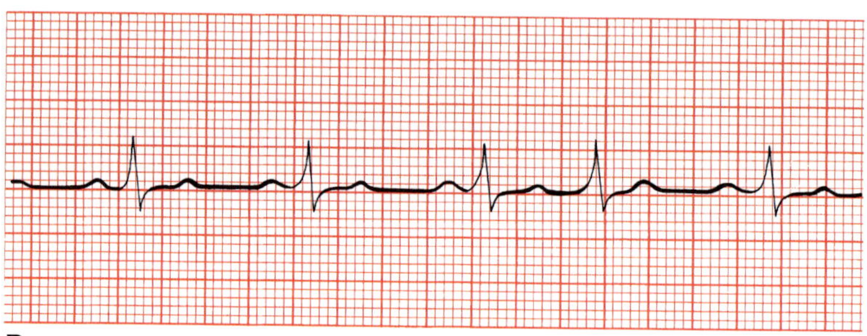

B

(*A*) Atrial premature beats alternate with normal sinus beats (this is called bigeminy). You can see that the configuration of the PACs is slightly different than the normal sinus beats (the *arrows* point to the premature atrial beats). And if you are really perceptive, you will have noticed that the interval between the premature atrial beats and the QRS complexes is different than that of the normal sinus beats and their QRS complexes; this would be expected from beats arising outside the sinus node, which have a different distance to cover before reaching the AV node and the ventricles. (*B*) The fourth beat is a junctional premature beat. There is no P wave preceding the premature QRS complex.

An atrial premature beat can be distinguished from a normal sinus beat by the *contour* (ie, morphology) of the P wave and by the timing of the beat.

Contour. Because an atrial premature beat originates at an atrial site distant from the sinus node, atrial depolarization does not occur in the usual manner, and the configuration of the resultant P wave differs from that of the sinus P waves. If the site of origin of the atrial premature beat is far from the sinus node, the *axis* of the atrial premature beat and—as in figure A on the preceding page—the interval between the P wave and the QRS complex will also differ from that of the normal P waves.

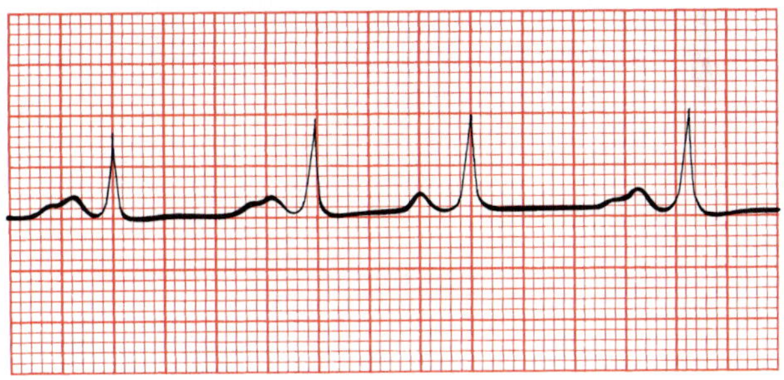

The third beat is an atrial premature beat. The P wave is shaped differently from the other, somewhat unusual-looking P waves, and the beat is clearly premature.

Timing. An atrial premature beat comes too early; that is, it intrudes itself before the next anticipated sinus wave.

With junctional premature beats, there is usually no visible P wave, but sometimes a retrograde P wave may be seen. This is just like the case with the junctional escape beats seen with sinus arrest.

What is the difference between a junctional *premature* beat and a junctional *escape* beat? They look exactly alike, but the junctional premature beat occurs *early*, prematurely, interposing itself into the normal sinus rhythm. An escape beat occurs *late*, following a pause when the sinus node has failed to fire.

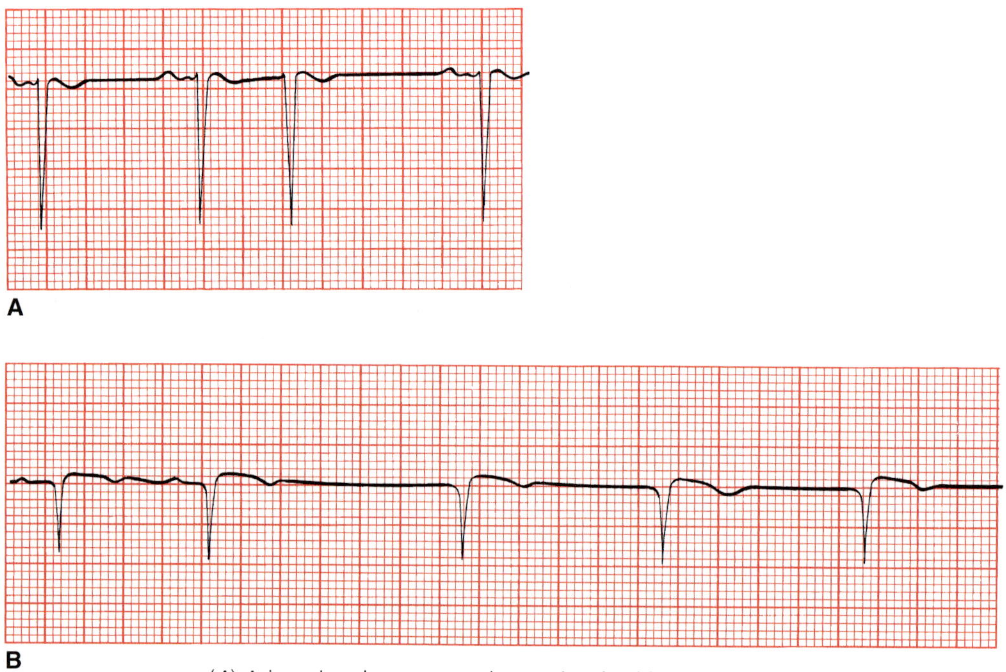

(*A*) A junctional premature beat. The third beat is obviously premature, and there is no P wave preceding the QRS complex. (*B*) The third beat is a junctional escape beat, establishing a sustained junctional rhythm. It looks just like a junctional premature beat, but it occurs late, following a prolonged pause, rather than prematurely.

Is it important to distinguish a premature beat from an escape beat? Yes, it certainly can be: a premature beat is serving no useful purpose, whereas an escape beat is essentially rescuing the heart from a prolonged pause during which the heart is effectively at a standstill. You don't want to suppress escape beats.

Both atrial and junctional premature beats are usually conducted normally to the ventricles, and the resultant QRS complex is therefore narrow.

Sometimes, an atrial premature beat may occur sufficiently early that the AV node will not have recovered (ie, repolarized) from the previous conducted beat and will therefore be unable to conduct the atrial premature beat into the ventricles. The ECG may then show only a P wave without an ensuing QRS complex. This beat is then termed a *blocked atrial premature contraction*.

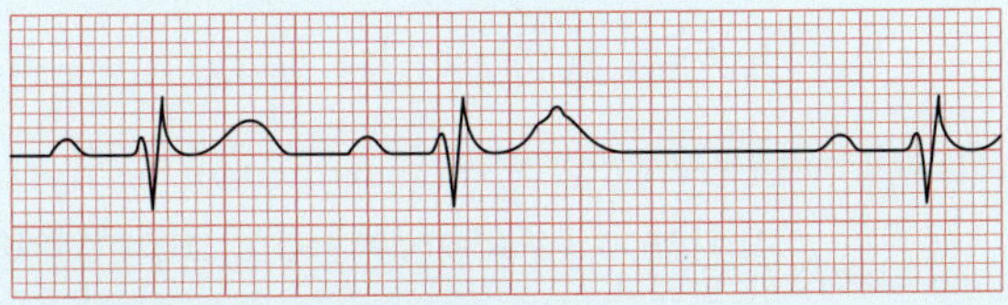

Look at the second beat. The T wave looks deformed, clearly different from the preceding T wave. Why? There is a PAC buried within it (look again and you may see a little bump near the top of the T wave—that's the PAC). At the time of the PAC, the AV node is still repolarizing and is therefore unable to conduct the PAC into the ventricles. This PAC is a blocked PAC.* It is followed by a pause—no QRS complex or T wave can be generated before the next normal P wave at last comes along and reestablishes normal conduction. Blocked PACs are the most common cause of pauses on the EKG, that is, a delay in the appearance of the next normal beat.

There are several types of *sustained* supraventricular arrhythmias that you must learn to recognize. Some of the names are a mouthful, but they are all descriptive of exactly what is going on:

1. AV nodal reentrant tachycardia (AVNRT), still referred to by some old school (and some not-so-old-school) cardiologists as paroxysmal supraventricular tachycardia
2. Atrial flutter
3. Atrial fibrillation
4. Multifocal atrial tachycardia (MAT)

---

*A PAC has three possible fates: (1) it can conduct normally; (2) it can conduct aberrantly down an atypical pathway; or (3) it can be blocked.

5. Paroxysmal atrial tachycardia (PAT), also called ectopic atrial tachycardia
6. Atrioventricular (AV) reciprocating tachycardia (we'll delay discussing this one until Chapter 5, since it is uniquely associated with a particular kind of cardiac condition called preexcitation)

AV Nodal Reentrant Tachycardia

AVNRT is a very common arrhythmia. Its onset is sudden, usually initiated by a premature supraventricular beat (atrial or junctional), and its termination is just as abrupt. It can occur in perfectly normal hearts; there may be no underlying cardiac disease at all. Persons with AVNRT typically present with palpitations, shortness of breath, dizziness, or syncope. Not uncommonly, alcohol, coffee, stimulants, or just sheer excitement can elicit this rhythm disturbance.

AVNRT is an *absolutely regular rhythm*, with a rate usually between 150 and 250 beats per minute. It is driven by a reentrant circuit looping within the AV node. Retrograde P waves may sometimes be seen in leads II or III, but your best bet would be to look in lead V1 for what is called a pseudo-*R*′, a little blip in the QRS complex that represents the superimposed retrograde P wave (check out the tracings on the next page). More often than not, however, the P waves are buried within the much larger QRS complexes and cannot be identified with any confidence. As with most supraventricular arrhythmias, the QRS complex is usually narrow.

The bottom line is if you see a rapid, narrow complex tachycardia with no clear-cut P waves that starts and stops suddenly, it's a good bet that you are dealing with AVNRT.

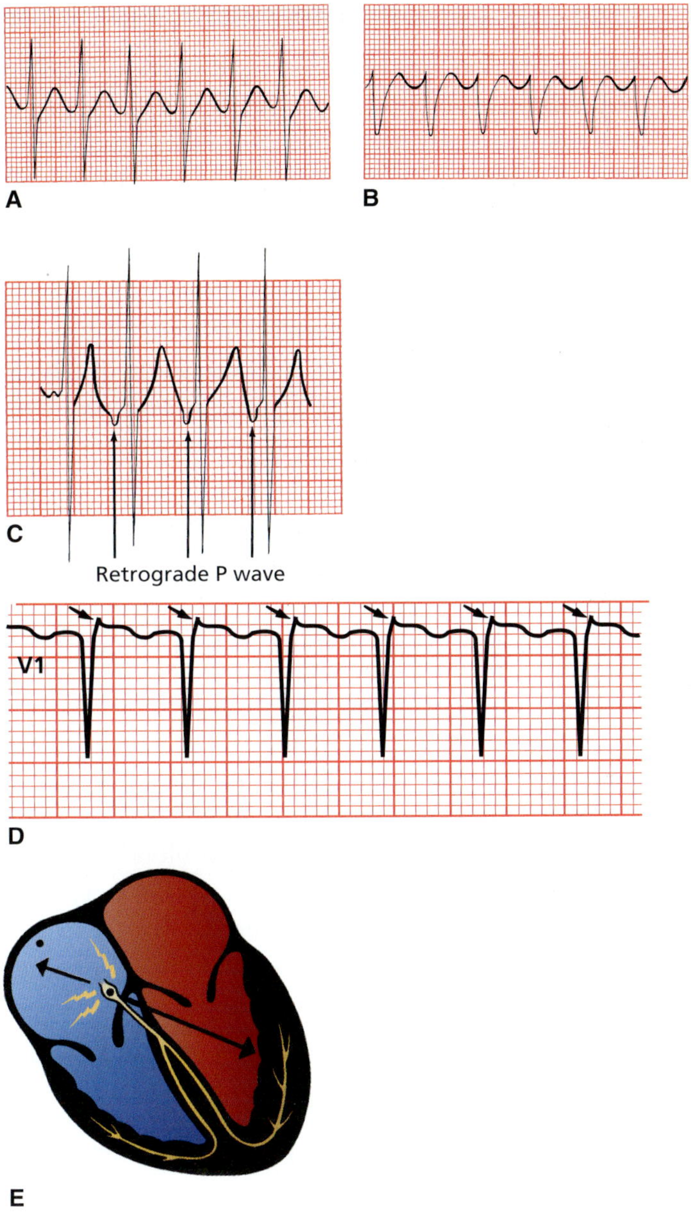

(*A–C*) AVNRT in four different patients. (*A*) Shows simultaneous activation of the atria and ventricles; therefore, the retrograde P waves are lost in the QRS complexes. (*B*) Shows a supraventricular tachycardia mimicking a more serious rhythm called ventricular tachycardia (see page 173 for a discussion of how this happens, or better yet don't—you'll get there shortly). In (*C*), retrograde P waves can be seen. (*D*) This is a good example of the pseudo-*R′* configuration in lead V1 representing the retrograde P waves (*arrows*) of AVNRT. (*E*) The AV node is usually the site of the reentrant circuit that causes the arrhythmia. Atrial depolarization therefore occurs in reverse, and if P waves can be seen, their axis will be shifted nearly 180° from normal (that is why these are called retrograde P waves).

Carotid Massage and Other Valsalva Maneuvers

Maneuvers that stimulate the vagal nerve can help to both *diagnose* and *terminate* an episode of AVNRT. Vagal input decreases the rate at which the sinus node fires and, more importantly in this setting, slows conduction through the AV node. Because AVNRT is usually caused by a reentry loop within the AV node, vagal stimulation can disrupt the loop and restore normal sinus rhythm. There are many ways to enhance vagal output that you can perform right on the spot without any fancy equipment. The most common is carotid massage, but any Valsalva maneuver* will do, some of which may be more effective than carotid massage (see Box on page 147). All of these interventions have a high success rate, so they are worth becoming comfortable with them.

Let's look first at how carotid massage works as a way to understand the underlying physiology of how these Valsalva maneuvers affect the heart. Baroreceptors that sense changes in the blood pressure are located at the angle of the jaw where the common carotid artery bifurcates. When the blood pressure rises, these baroreceptors cause reflex responses from the brain to be sent along the vagus nerve to the heart. Vagal input decreases the rate at which the sinus node fires and, more importantly, *slows conduction through the AV node*.

These carotid baroreceptors are not particularly shrewd, and they can be fooled into thinking that the blood pressure is rising by gentle pressure applied *externally* to the carotid artery. (Anything that raises the blood pressure, such as a Valsalva maneuver or squatting, will stimulate vagal input to the heart.) Carotid massage may therefore accomplish the following:

- Interrupt the reentrant circuit and terminate the arrhythmia.
- At the very least, slow the arrhythmia so that the presence or absence of P waves can be more easily determined and the arrhythmia diagnosed.

---

*A Valsalva maneuver refers to forced expiration against a closed airway; if you have ever tried to pop your ears open on an airplane by exhaling against a closed mouth and pinched nose, you have performed a Valsalva maneuver. And just to give credit where credit is due, the maneuver was named after the famous Italian anatomist and surgeon, Antonia Maria Valsalva, born 1666—yes, the same year the apocryphal apple fell on Issac Newton's head—who brilliantly delineated the structure and function of the ear and eustachain tube.

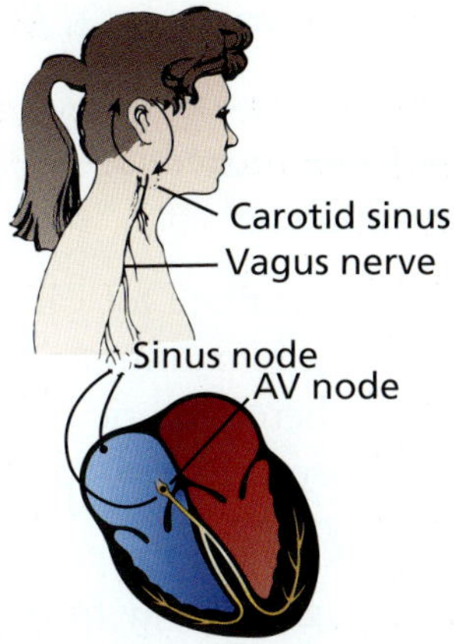

The carotid sinus contains baroreceptors that influence vagal input to the heart, primarily affecting the sinus node and AV node. Stimulation of the right carotid baroreceptors primarily stimulates sinus node vagal input, whereas stimulation of the left carotid baroreceptors is more likely to affect the vagal input to the AV node.

How to Do Carotid Massage

Carotid massage must be done with great care. Someone experienced with the procedure should be at the bedside along with resuscitation equipment.

1. Auscultate for carotid bruits. You do *not* want to cut off the last remaining trickle of blood to the brain, nor dislodge an atherosclerotic plaque. If there is evidence of significant carotid disease, do *not* perform carotid massage.
2. With the patient lying flat, extend the neck and rotate the head slightly away from you.
3. Palpate the carotid artery at the angle of the jaw and apply gentle pressure for 10–15 seconds. Press as firmly as would be required to compress a tennis ball.
4. *Never* compress both carotid arteries simultaneously!
5. Try the right carotid first because the rate of success is somewhat better on this side. If it fails, however, go ahead and try the left carotid next.
6. Have a rhythm strip running during the entire procedure so that you can see what is happening. Always have equipment for resuscitation available; in very rare instances, carotid massage may induce sinus arrest.

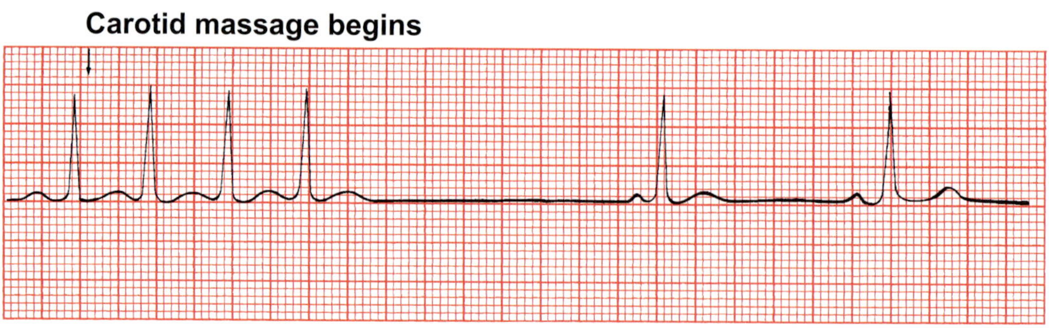

An episode of AVNRT is broken almost at once by carotid massage. The new rhythm is a sinus bradycardia with a rate of 50 beats per minute.

The modified Valsalva maneuver is becoming increasingly popular as an alternative to carotid massage. It appears to be safer and possibly more effective than carotid massage. This technique involves having patients, semirecumbent, strain for 15 seconds (you can have them blow into a syringe), then lie back in a supine position while you elevate their legs to 45° for 15 seconds.

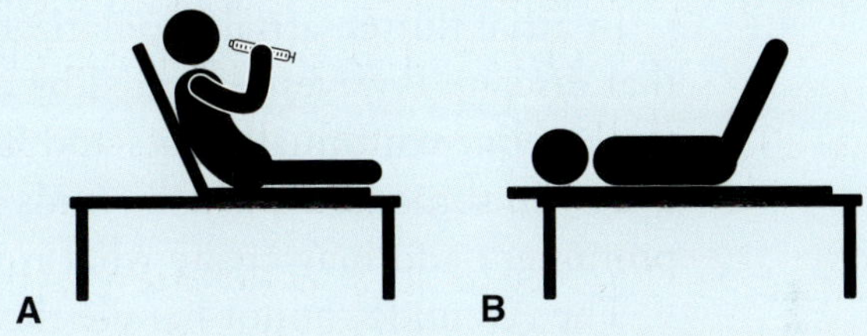

The modified Valsalva maneuver.

For patients with an acute episode of AVNRT that does not respond to carotid massage or other vagal maneuvers, pharmacologic intervention will usually terminate the arrhythmia. A bolus injection of adenosine, a short-acting AV nodal blocking agent, is almost always effective (but avoid this drug in patients with bronchospastic lung disease). Second-line therapies include beta blockers, calcium channel blockers, and, rarely, electrical cardioversion.

Atrial Flutter

Atrial flutter is less common than AVNRT. It can occur in normal hearts or, more often, in patients with underlying cardiac pathology. The atrial activation in atrial flutter, as in AVNRT, is absolutely regular but is even more rapid. Flutter waves appear at a rate of 250–350 beats per minute. In its most common form, it is generated by a reentrant circuit that runs along the annulus of the tricuspid valve.

In atrial flutter, atrial depolarization occurs at such a rapid rate that discrete P waves separated by a flat baseline are not seen. Instead, the baseline continually rises and falls, producing so-called *flutter waves*. In some leads, usually leads II and III, these may be quite prominent and may create what is referred to as a *saw-toothed pattern*.

The AV node cannot handle the extraordinary number of atrial impulses bombarding it—it simply doesn't have time to repolarize in time for each ensuing wave—and therefore not all of the atrial impulses pass through the AV node to generate QRS complexes. Some will, therefore, bump into a refractory node, and that is as far as they get. This phenomenon is called *AV block*. The typical ventricular rate averages around 150 beats per minute (Let's stress this point: although the atria are firing at 250–350 impulses per minute, thanks to the AV node you will see only approximately 150 QRS complexes per minute). A 2:1 AV block is most common. This means that for every two visible flutter waves, one passes through the AV node to generate a QRS complex, and one does not.

The bottom line here is that if you see a narrow complex tachycardia with a ventricular rate of 150 and a sawtooth baseline pattern, strongly consider the possibility of atrial flutter with 2:1 conduction.

Blocks of 3:1 and 4:1 are also frequently seen. Carotid massage may increase the degree of block (eg, changing a 2:1 block to a 4:1 block), making it easier to identify the saw-toothed pattern. Because atrial flutter originates above the AV node, carotid massage will not result in termination of the rhythm.

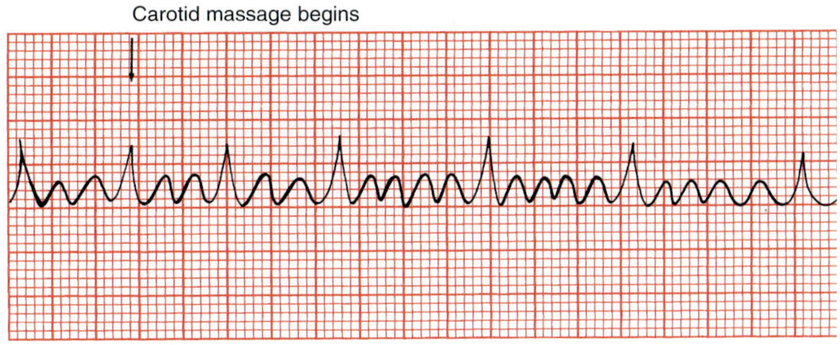

Atrial flutter. Carotid massage increases the block from 3:1 to 5:1. Why don't we call this 2:1 and 4:1? Because one P wave is invisible, hidden within the large QRS complexes.

The axis of the P waves (flutter waves) in atrial flutter depends upon whether the reentrant circuit rotates counterclockwise (the more common form, producing negative saw-toothed deflections in the inferior leads) or clockwise (positive deflections in the inferior leads) around the tricuspid valve. It can be difficult to identify flutter waves when their axis is negative; for some reason, the human eye prefers a positive wave to a negative one. Here's a pro tip: if you suspect atrial flutter (eg, in a patient with a regular, narrow QRS tachycardia with a ventricular rate in the neighborhood of 150 beats per minute), just turn the EKG upside down—miraculously, flutter waves may suddenly become apparent!

Flutter waves can also be missed when there is 2:1 AV block. This can occur because every other flutter wave may be hidden inside the much larger T waves and/or QRS complexes. If you check all 12 leads, you will probably find what you are looking for in at least one lead, often tiny bumps in the T waves that represent the hidden flutter waves.

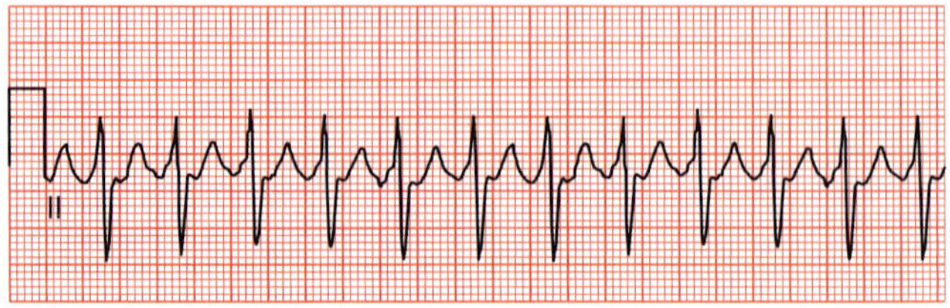

Would you ever suspect this is atrial flutter? No atrial activity at all can be seen, and this looks very much like AVNRT. However, because this is a regular narrow QRS complex tachycardia with a rate around 150 beats per minute, atrial flutter has to be in the differential diagnosis. And sure enough, this turns out to be a case of atrial flutter with 2:1 block in which the flutter waves are hidden within each QRS complex and T wave. There is no way to be sure just by looking at the rhythm strip. You can try a vagal maneuver; in AVNRT the rhythm might convert to normal sinus rhythm, whereas in the case of atrial flutter, the degree of AV block will increase, allowing the flutter waves to become visible.

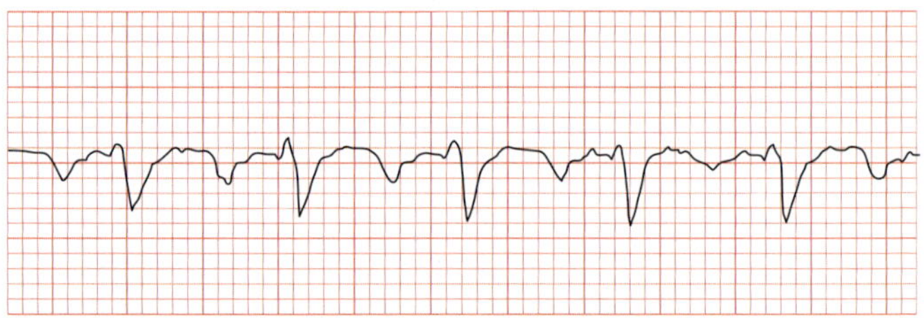

Atrial flutter. Lead II shows classic negative deflections.

Approximately 200,000 cases of atrial flutter are diagnosed each year in the United States. Common conditions associated with atrial flutter include the following:

- Hypertension
- Obesity
- Diabetes mellitus
- Electrolyte imbalances
- Alcohol intoxication
- Drug abuse, particularly cocaine and amphetamines
- Pulmonary disease (eg, chronic obstructive pulmonary disease and pulmonary embolism)
- Thyrotoxicosis
- Various underlying cardiac conditions, both congenital (eg, atrial septal defect) and acquired (eg, rheumatic valvular disease, coronary artery disease, and congestive heart failure)

Although atrial flutter is rarely life threatening, the rapid ventricular response may cause shortness of breath or angina or precipitate or worsen congestive heart failure, which may mandate urgent clinical intervention. Electrical cardioversion is usually effective at restoring normal sinus rhythm, although pharmacologic cardioversion is sometimes first attempted in patients who are hemodynamically stable. Long-term control with antiarrhythmic drugs can be difficult. Definitive treatment can now be accomplished in most patients with typical atrial flutter using a technique called catheter ablation, in which radiofrequency energy is delivered to the myocardium via a catheter to create small lesions that disrupt the reentry pathway.

It is also important to note that the rapid atrial rate in flutter increases the risk of clot formation in the atria, so anticoagulation is indicated to prevent thromboembolic events.

Atrial Fibrillation

In *atrial fibrillation*, atrial activity is completely chaotic, and the AV node may be bombarded with more than 500 impulses per minute! Whereas in atrial flutter, a single constant reentrant circuit is responsible for the regular saw-toothed pattern on the EKG, in atrial fibrillation multiple tiny reentrant circuits whirl around in totally unpredictable fashion. No true P waves can be seen. Instead, the baseline appears flat or undulates slightly. The AV node, faced with this extraordinary blitz of atrial impulses, allows only occasional impulses to pass through at variable intervals, generating an *irregularly irregular* ventricular rate—there is no discernible, predictable pattern to the appearance of the QRS complexes. The ventricular rate is usually between 120 and 180 beats (ie, 120–180 QRS complexes) per minute. However, slower or faster ventricular responses (see figures *A* and *B* below) can often be seen.

This irregularly irregular appearance of QRS complexes in the absence of discrete P waves is the key to identifying atrial fibrillation. The wavelike forms that may often be seen on close inspection of the undulating baseline are called *fibrillation waves*.

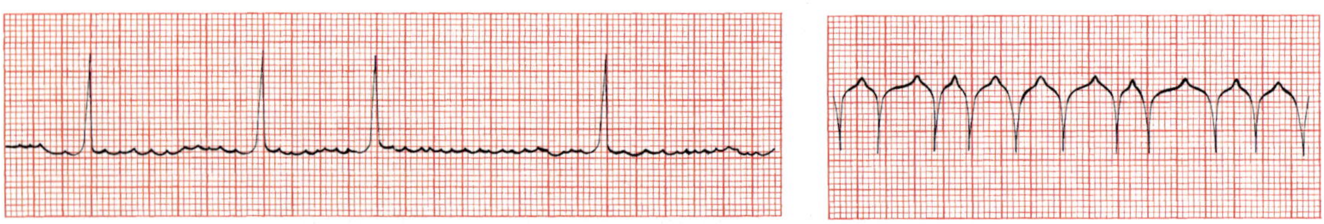

A B

(*A*) Atrial fibrillation with a slow, irregular ventricular rate. (*B*) Another example of atrial fibrillation. In the absence of a clearly fibrillating baseline, the only clue that this rhythm is atrial fibrillation is the irregularly irregular appearance of the QRS complexes.

Atrial fibrillation is not the only tachyarrhythmia that can cause an irregular rhythm, but it is by far the most common. Other possibilities include atrial flutter with variable block (although the appearance of the QRS complexes will appear irregular, they are not truly chaotic since they will occur at multiples of the flutter rate), and an arrhythmia we will be discussing shortly, multifocal atrial tachycardia (MAT). In addition, perfectly healthy people with normal hearts can have a marked sinus arrhythmia (see page 124) as they inhale and exhale; if you check their pulse, it may appear irregular. In the vast majority of cases, however, an irregular rapid rhythm means the patient has atrial fibrillation.

Carotid massage may slow the ventricular rate in atrial fibrillation, but it is rarely used in this setting because the diagnosis is usually obvious.

Atrial Fibrillation: Clinical Stuff You Should Know

Atrial fibrillation is the most common and clinically significant sustained arrhythmia in the general population. Its prevalence in the general population is estimated at 4%, and it increases with age. Atrial fibrillation can be persistent or intermittent, with episodes lasting minutes to hours to days or persist indefinitely.

Underlying causes are similar to those for atrial flutter, but there is an especially high incidence of underlying cardiovascular disorders, notably hypertension, metabolic syndrome, mitral valve disease, and coronary artery disease. Other common risk factors include obesity and alcoholism. An important cause that should not be overlooked, particularly in patients with nocturnal atrial fibrillation, is obstructive sleep apnea. In a significant minority of patients, particularly younger patients, no underlying risk factors or cardiac pathology will be found. You often won't be able to identify an *acute* precipitant in patients with atrial fibrillation, but keep in mind the possibility of a pulmonary embolism, thyrotoxicosis, and pericarditis.

Atrial fibrillation can cause palpitations, chest pain, shortness of breath, or dizziness. However, a significant number of patients, particularly the elderly, may have no symptoms at all and may not even be aware they are in atrial fibrillation until you feel their pulse and give them the news.

Atrial fibrillation can precipitate congestive heart failure and increase the risk of developing ventricular tachycardia, a potentially lethal arrhythmia (see page 165), but the major cause for concern in patients with atrial fibrillation is an increased risk of stroke. The fibrillating atria (the chambers actually quiver rather than contract and have been compared in appearance to a bag of worms) provide an excellent substrate for blood clots to form. Pieces of these clots can break off—embolize—and travel through the systemic circulation and cause a central nervous system stroke or vascular occlusion elsewhere in the body. This risk of embolization is present in patients with new-onset, recurrent, or persistent atrial fibrillation, whether symptomatic or asymptomatic.

Whereas some patients can be managed initially with a strategy of anticoagulation (to prevent clot formation and embolization) plus *rate control*, in which the atrial fibrillation is allowed to persist but the heart rate (ie, the rate at which QRS complexes appear) is limited by medications, current data make it clear that early *rhythm control*—that is, returning the patient to normal sinus rhythm—is the superior approach, greatly reducing the risk of serious complications such as stroke and congestive heart failure. Medications can be tried and may prove effective, but the preferred approach in most patients is cardioversion or an invasive technique called *catheter ablation*. The latter is becoming increasingly popular. In most patients, atrial fibrillation is triggered by electrical activity in and around the pulmonary veins where they enter the left atrium. The cornerstone of ablative therapy is to electrically isolate the pulmonary veins from the rest of the heart by essentially burning a firewall around the source of the problem, thereby preventing the abnormal electrical impulses from spreading into the heart. Whereas catheter ablation is often curative, in many patients it reduces but does not eliminate the risk of further episodes of recurrent atrial fibrillation, as demonstrated by subsequent monitoring of the patient's heart rate and rhythm. For these patients, ongoing anticoagulation is necessary to lower the risk of stroke. For patients at high risk of bleeding from an anticoagulant, the insertion of a left atrial appendage device can prevent clots from forming in the left atrium.

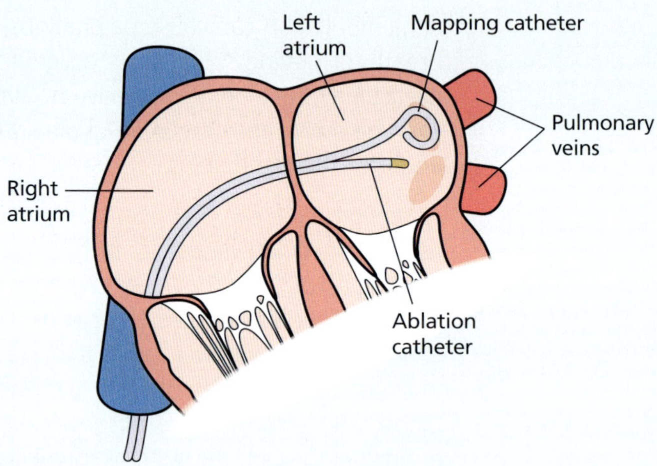

Catheter ablation therapy for atrial fibrillation. A catheter is advanced into the right atrium, through the intra-atrial septum, and into the left atrium. The site where the atrial fibrillation originates—where the pulmonary veins join the left atrium—is then electrically isolated from the rest of the heart by bursts of radiofrequency energy that create an electrical firewall.

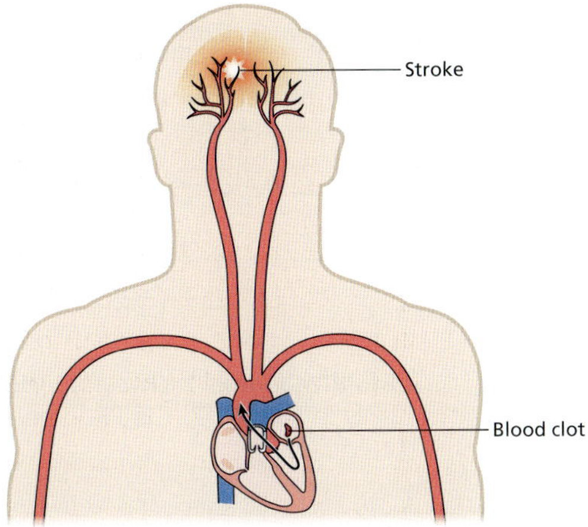

A blood clot formed in a fibrillating left atrium can come loose and travel to the brain and cause a stroke.

Multifocal Atrial Tachycardia and Wandering Atrial Pacemakers

MAT is an irregular rhythm occurring at a rate of 100–200 beats per minute. It may result from the random firing of several different ectopic atrial foci or variable conduction from a single atrial focus. In some patients, the rate is <100 beats per minute, in which case the arrhythmia is called a *wandering atrial pacemaker*.

Like atrial fibrillation, MAT is an irregular rhythm. However, it can be distinguished from atrial fibrillation by easily identifiable P waves occurring before each QRS complex, unlike the undulating baseline without clear-cut P waves seen with atrial fibrillation. The P waves vary in shape, and the interval between the different P waves and the QRS complexes varies as well. In order to make the diagnosis of MAT, you need to identify at least three different P-wave morphologies.

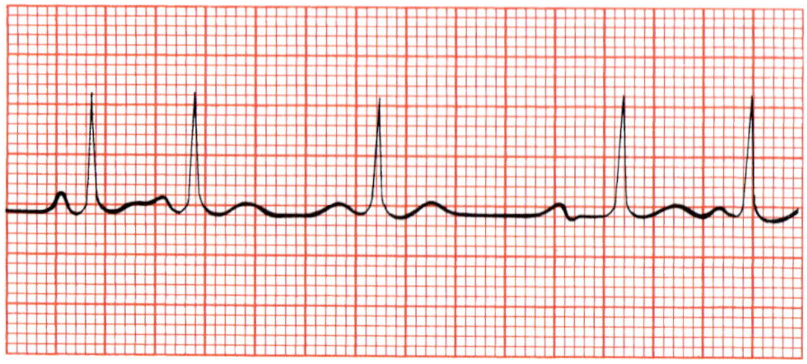

Multifocal atrial tachycardia. Note that (1) the P waves vary dramatically in shape, (2) the PR intervals vary, and (3) the ventricular rate is irregular.

In patients with a *wandering atrial pacemaker*, again at least three different P-wave morphologies can be seen. Technically, however, it is not a tachyarrhythmia because the rate is between 60 and 100 beats per minute.

MAT is generally seen in patients with lung disease. A wandering atrial pacemaker can occur in normal, healthy hearts. MAT itself rarely requires treatment. Carotid massage has no effect on MAT.

Paroxysmal Atrial Tachycardia

The last of our supraventricular arrhythmias, *PAT*, is a regular rhythm with a rate of 100–200 beats per minute. It can result either from the enhanced automaticity of an ectopic atrial focus or from a reentrant circuit within the atria. The automatic type typically displays a warm-up period when it starts, during which the rhythm appears somewhat irregular, and a similar cool-down period when it terminates. The less common reentrant form starts abruptly with an atrial premature beat. P waves are usually visible, but in some cases, may not be easily seen if the rate is fast and they are hidden within the QRS complexes or T waves.

PAT is most commonly seen in otherwise normal hearts. It can also be caused by digitalis toxicity (see Chapter 7).

How can you tell PAT from AVNRT? Most of the time it is easy, because you will see P waves before each QRS complex with PAT versus no P waves (or retrograde P waves) with AVNRT, but sometimes the P waves of PAT—especially if the rate is at the faster extremes—aren't readily apparent. One clue: if your patient is not on digitalis, AVNRT is by far the more likely diagnosis. In addition, if you see a warm-up or cool-down period on the EKG, the rhythm is likely to be PAT (remember that AVNRT starts and stops abruptly). In addition, a Valsalva maneuver can be very helpful: it will slow or terminate AVNRT, whereas it has virtually no effect on PAT (other than some mild slowing).

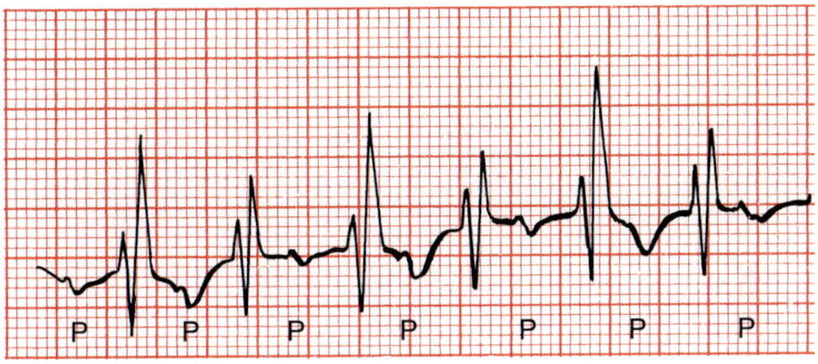

PAT. P waves are not always visible, but here they can be seen fairly easily. You may also notice the varying distance between the P waves and the ensuing QRS complexes; this reflects a varying conduction delay between the atria and ventricles that often accompanies PAT (but we are getting way ahead of ourselves; conduction delays are discussed in Chapter 4).

Test Yourself

Here are three examples of irregular supraventricular rhythms. Can you identify them?

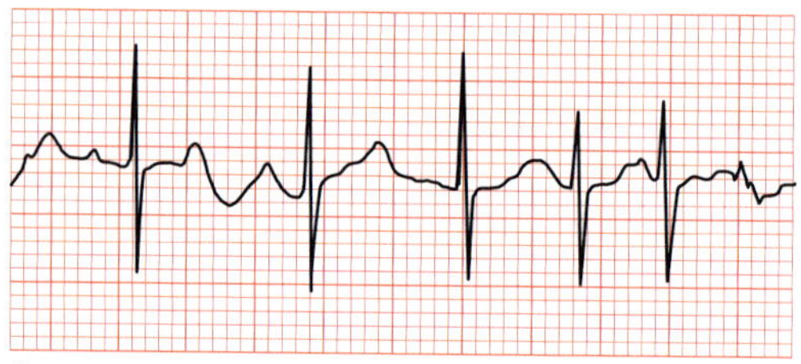

A

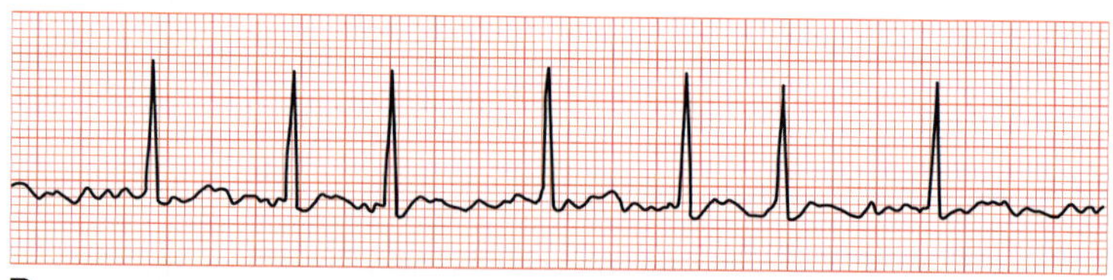

B

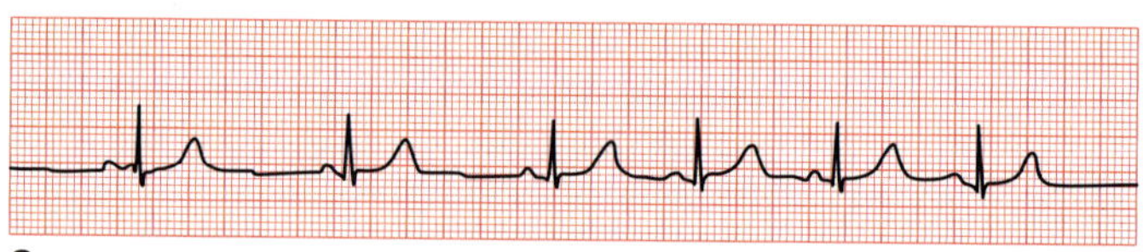

C

A. Multifocal atrial tachycardia

B. Atrial fibrillation

C. Sinus arrhythmia

Before We Move On

Here is a question to see how well you've grasped the material on supraventricular tachycardias. Suppose a patient comes to see you complaining of palpitations and feeling short of breath. You take your patient's pulse and notice two things—(1) it is very fast and (2) it is regular. Before you get an EKG, based on what you've learned so far, what is your differential diagnosis? Atrial fibrillation is off the table because it is irregularly irregular. And exclude for now the possibility of ventricular tachycardia, first because your patient would be unlikely to just come strolling in if he or she has ventricular tachycardia, and second because we will not be discussing it until the next section of this chapter.

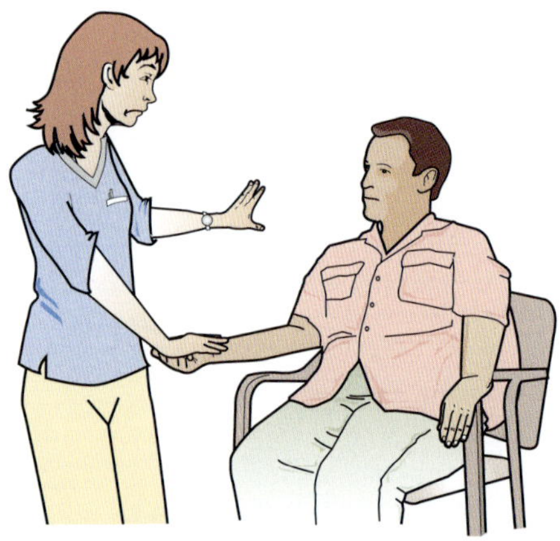

No cheating—don't look at the answer until you have thought this through. You are sorting through the differential diagnosis of regular, supraventricular tachycardias.

There are only a few possibilities, and you probably figured out that they include *sinus tachycardia, AVNRT, PAT*, and *atrial flutter with a regular block* (ie, 2:1 or 3:1 etc., without variation).

This is a handy differential diagnosis to have at your fingertips. Now, when you get your EKG on this patient, you know exactly what you are looking for:

- If you see one normal P wave for every QRS complex, your patient has sinus tachycardia.
- With atrial flutter and regular block, you should see flutter waves.
- Finally, with AVNRT or the less common PAT, the rate will usually be faster than your average sinus tachycardia, and you will see either no P waves or—particularly in the case of AVNRT—retrograde P waves.

SUMMARY

Supraventricular Arrhythmias

Arrhythmia	Characteristics	EKG
AV nodal reentrant tachycardia	Regular P waves are retrograde if visible Rate: 150–250 beats per minute Carotid massage: slows or terminates	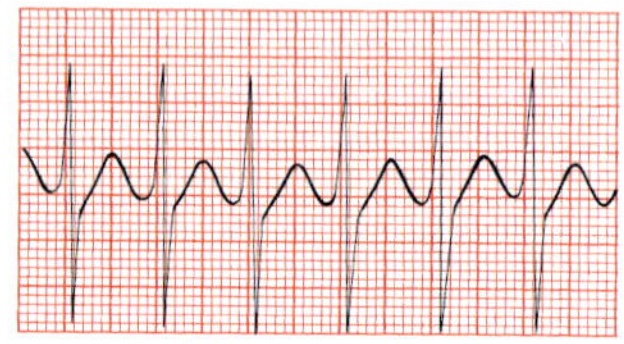
Atrial Flutter	Regular, saw-toothed 2:1, 3:1, 4:1, etc., block Atrial rate: 250–350 beats per minute Ventricular rate: one-half, one-third, one-quarter, etc., of atrial rate Carotid massage: increases block	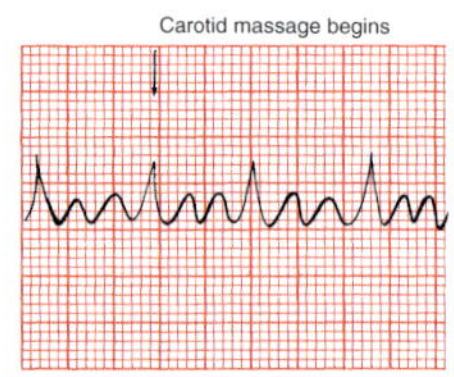
Atrial Fibrillation	Irregular Undulating baseline Atrial rate: 350–500 beats per minute Ventricular rate: variable Carotid massage: may slow ventricular rate	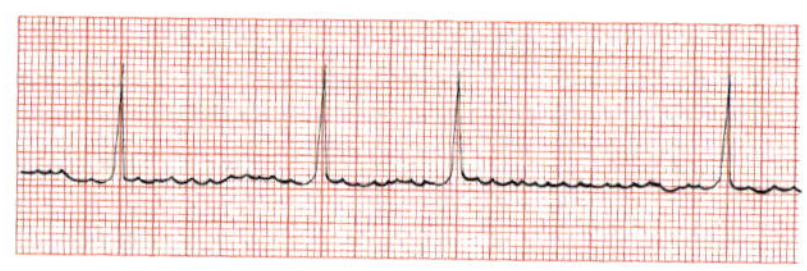
Multifocal atrial tachycardia	Irregular At least three different P-wave morphologies Rate: 100–200 beats per minute; sometimes <100 beats per minute (wandering atrial pacemaker) Carotid massage: no effect	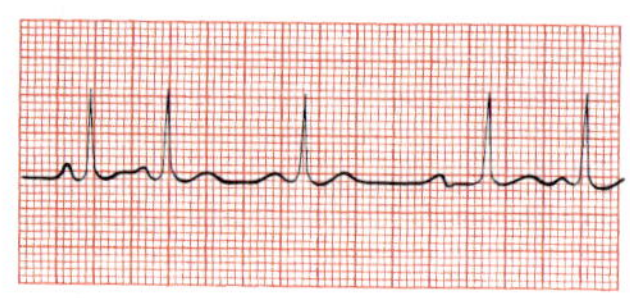
Paroxysmal atrial tachycardia	Regular Rate: 100–200 beats per minute Characteristic warm-up period in the automatic form Carotid massage: no effect, or only mild slowing	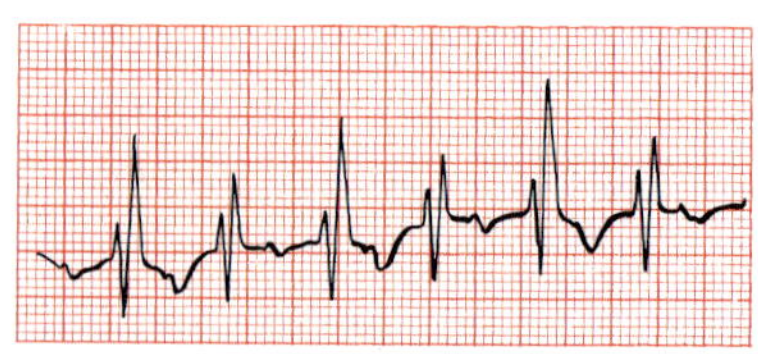

Remember: The key to diagnosing a supraventricular tachyarrhythmia is to look for P waves. They are most likely to be prominent in leads II and V1.

Ventricular Arrhythmias

Ventricular arrhythmias are rhythm disturbances arising *below* the AV node.

Premature Ventricular Contractions

Premature ventricular contractions (PVCs) are by far the most common of the ventricular arrhythmias, and can originate from either a ventricular ectopic focus or, more often, from a reentrant circuit within one of the ventricles.

The QRS complex of a PVC appears wide and bizarre because ventricular depolarization does not follow the normal ventricular conduction pathways. However, the QRS complex may not appear wide in all leads, so scan the entire 12-lead EKG before making your diagnosis. The QRS duration must be at least 0.12 seconds in most leads to make the diagnosis of a PVC. Retrograde P waves may sometimes be seen, but it is more common to see no P waves at all. A PVC is usually followed by a prolonged compensatory pause before the next beat appears. Less commonly, a PVC may occur between two normally conducted beats without a compensatory pause. These are called *interpolated PVCs*.

Isolated PVCs are common in normal hearts and rarely require treatment. An isolated PVC in the setting of an acute myocardial infarction, however, is more ominous because it can trigger ventricular tachycardia or ventricular fibrillation, both of which are life-threatening arrhythmias.

PVCs typically occur randomly, but they may alternate with normal sinus beats in a regular pattern. If the ratio is one normal sinus beat to one PVC, the rhythm—as is the case when one PAC alternates with one normal sinus beat—is called *bigeminy*. *Trigeminy* refers to two normal sinus beats for every one PVC, and quadrigeminy would be three to one.

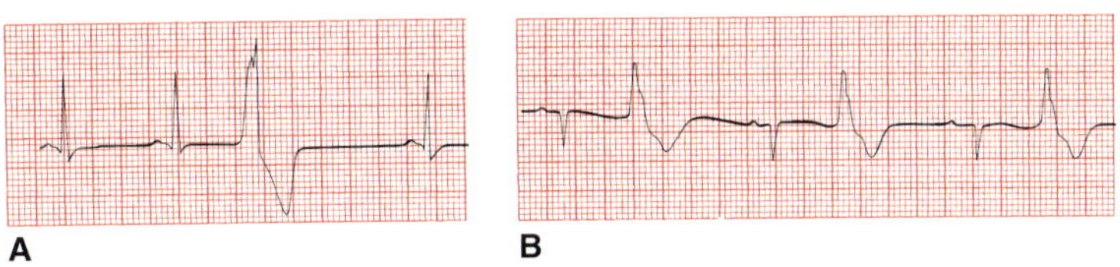

(*A*) A PVC. Note the compensatory pause before the next beat.
(*B*) Bigeminy. PVCs and sinus beats alternate in a 1:1 fashion.

When should you worry about PVCs? In most situations, you don't have to worry at all. In patients who are asymptomatic or only mildly symptomatic and have a low PVC burden, no treatment is needed. A low PVC burden is diagnosed when monitoring shows that the PVCs account for fewer than 1% of all heartbeats, or when there are fewer than 1000 PVCs per day. A high PVC burden is diagnosed when PVCs comprise 10% or more of all heartbeats. Anything in between is considered an intermediate burden. The higher the PCV burden, the greater the likelihood that the patient will develop PVC-induced cardiomyopathy due to remodeling of the myocardium. These patients can experience diminished left ventricular function and are at risk of heart failure. This condition is reversible if the PVC burden is lowered either with medications or an ablative procedure.

Treatment can be helpful in patients who are bothered by their PVCs, for example, palpitations, even if their overall burden is low. And then there are circumstances in which treatment of PVCs should be considered because they pose an increased risk for triggering ventricular tachycardia, ventricular fibrillation, and death. These include, in addition to a high PVC burden, frequent runs of consecutive PVC, especially three or more in a row; multiform PVCs which vary in their site of origin and hence in appearance; and PVCs falling on the T wave of the previous beat (called the R-on-T phenomenon; the T wave is a vulnerable period in the cardiac cycle, and a PCV falling there is more likely to set off ventricular tachycardia). The greatest risk of PVCs triggering a potentially lethal arrhythmia is when PVCs occur in the setting of active ischemia, for example, an acute myocardial infarction.

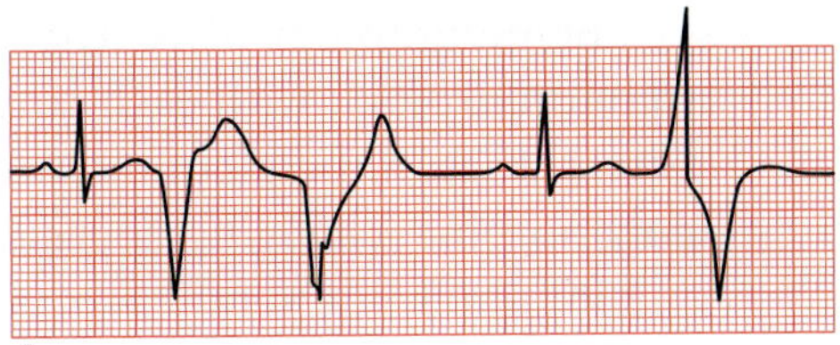
A

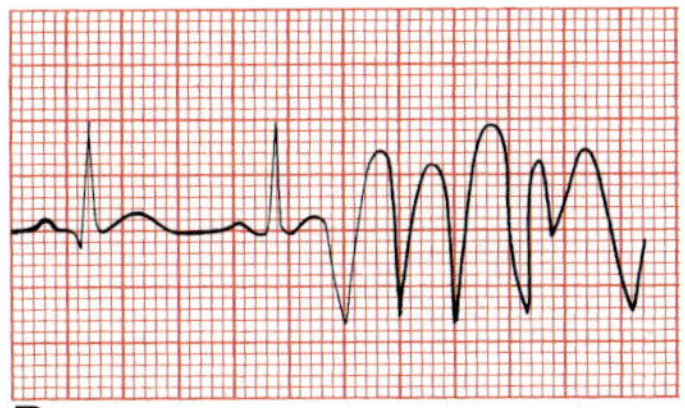
B

(*A*) Beats 1 and 4 are sinus in origin. The other three beats are PVCs. The PVCs differ from each other in shape (multiform), and two occur in a row. (*B*) A PVC falls on the T wave of the second sinus beat, initiating a run of ventricular tachycardia.

Ventricular Tachycardia

A run of three or more consecutive PVCs is called *ventricular tachycardia*. The rate is usually between 120 and 140 beats per minute, but don't make the mistake of assuming an arrhythmia can't be ventricular tachycardia if the rate is slower or faster—it can be. Unlike AVNRT, ventricular tachycardia may be slightly irregular (although it may take a very fine eye to see this). Both sustained ventricular tachycardia—defined as lasting more than 30 seconds—or ventricular tachycardia associated with hemodynamic instability are emergencies, presaging cardiac arrest, and requiring immediate treatment.

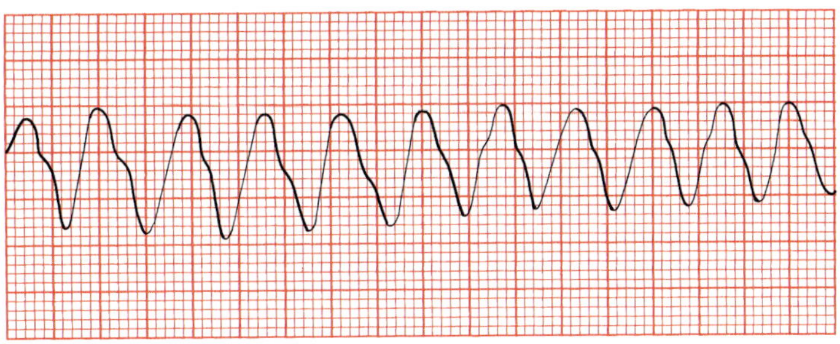

Ventricular tachycardia. The rate is about 200 beats per minute.

The morphology of ventricular tachycardia may be uniform (monomorphic), with each complex appearing similar to the one before it, as in the picture on the preceding page, or it may be polymorphic, changing appearance from beat to beat.

Monomorphic ventricular tachycardia is often seen in patients with healed infarctions; the scarred myocardium provides the substrate for the reentrant ventricular tachycardia by creating areas of slow and fast conduction (see the previous section on Reentrant Rhythms, page 133).

Polymorphic ventricular tachycardia occurs when there is more diffuse involvement of the myocardium, for example, with acute coronary ischemia, infarction, profound electrolyte disturbances, and conditions causing prolongation of the QT interval (Why a prolonged QT interval? Hang in there and you will have your answer in just a moment on page 168).

Approximately 3.5% of patients develop ventricular tachycardia after a myocardial infarction, the large majority of these within the first 48 hours. However, an increased risk of ventricular tachycardia persists for weeks beyond the myocardial infarction. The development of sustained ventricular tachycardia within the first 6 weeks postinfarction is associated with a high 1-year mortality rate.

Although ischemic heart disease is the most common cause of ventricular tachycardia, other causes include structural heart disease (eg, myocarditis or cardiomyopathy), noncardiac acute precipitants (eg, pulmonary embolism or drowning), and a variety of primary electrical disorders. A particular type of polymorphic ventricular tachycardia has numerous other causes, which we will discuss shortly (see page 168).

Take a look at the following tracing. The two leads were recorded simultaneously.

Does this represent ventricular tachycardia?

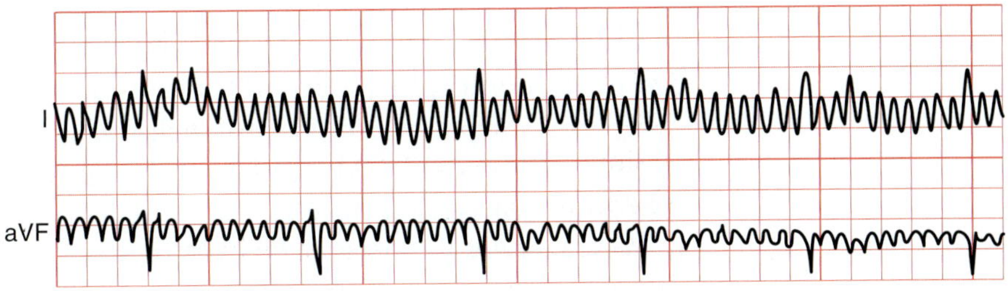

The top tracing sure looks like ventricular tachycardia. But the bottom tracing shows what are clearly regularly spaced narrow QRS complexes amidst the rest of the chaos. If you see normal QRS complexes in any lead, the rhythm can't be ventricular tachycardia. So what is going on here? This is a case of atrial flutter with a high degree of block. Now that you know that this is not ventricular tachycardia, look more closely at the top tracing. You can see taller waves among the flutter waves coinciding with the narrow QRS complexes on the bottom tracing; although it would have been almost impossible to pick these out from among the rapid, oscillating waves, these actually are normal QRS complexes, and everything else are the dramatic sawtooth waves of atrial flutter.

The lesson here is clear-cut: In patients with ventricular tachycardia, every lead must be consistent with the diagnosis. If you can find P waves or, as in this case, narrow, normal-appearing, regularly spaced QRS complexes anywhere on the tracing, even in a single lead, then it is not ventricular tachycardia.

Polymorphic Ventricular Tachycardia and Torsade de Pointes

In the previous section, we mentioned that ventricular tachycardia can be monomorphic, a progression of identical-looking QRS complexes, or polymorphic, in which the appearance of the QRS complexes is variable. The causes and treatment of the two are different, and among the latter, the one you must know is referred to as *Torsade de pointes*, meaning "twisting of the points." It is more than just the most lyrical name in cardiology. Torsade de pointes is a unique form of ventricular tachycardia that occurs in patients with a prolonged QT interval.

The QT interval, you will recall, encompasses the time from the beginning of ventricular depolarization to the end of ventricular repolarization. It normally constitutes about 40% of the complete cardiac cycle.

A prolonged QT interval can be (1) congenital in origin (resulting from mutations in genes encoding cardiac ion channels), or (2) acquired, the result of various electrolyte disturbances (notably hypocalcemia, hypomagnesemia, and hypokalemia) or the effects of a large number of pharmacologic agents (we will explore these in more detail in Chapter 7), or (3) the result of an acute myocardial infarction.

A prolonged QT interval is most often due to prolonged ventricular repolarization (ie, the T wave is lengthened), although, both hypocalcemia and hypothermia may cause a long QT interval on the basis of a prolonged ST segment. Either way, the QT interval is prolonged, and because the ventricular myocardium is susceptible to electrical stimulation during this period, a PVC falling during the QT interval can initiate torsade de pointes. Unlike ordinary, run-of-the-mill, monomorphic ventricular tachycardia, the QRS complexes in Torsade de pointes spiral around the baseline, changing their axis and amplitude (hence appearing polymorphic).

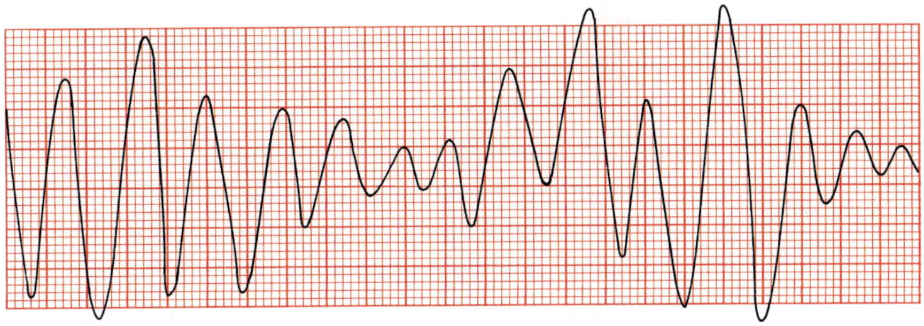

Torsade de pointes. The QRS complexes seem to spin around the baseline, changing their axis and amplitude.

Accelerated Idioventricular Rhythm

Accelerated idioventricular rhythm is a benign rhythm that is sometimes seen during an acute myocardial infarction or during the early hours following reperfusion, that is, after an occluded coronary artery has been opened in the catheterization lab. Other causes include hyperkalemia, type 1 antiarrhythmic agents, and tricyclic antidepressant overdoses.

Accelerated idioventricular rhythm is a regular rhythm occurring at 50–100 beats per minute and probably represents a ventricular escape focus that has accelerated sufficiently to drive the heart. It is rarely sustained, does not progress to ventricular fibrillation, and rarely requires treatment. In fact, the appearance of this rhythm is a favorable sign that an occluded artery has been successfully reopened, either spontaneously or via a procedure, such as angioplasty. When the rate falls below 50 beats per minute, it is then simply called an *idioventricular rhythm* (ie, the term *accelerated* is dropped).

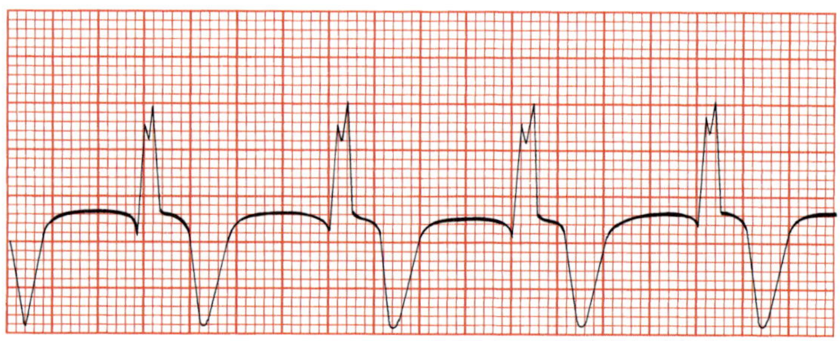

Accelerated idioventricular rhythm. There are no P waves, the QRS complexes are wide, and the rate is about 75 beats per minute.

Ventricular Fibrillation

Ventricular fibrillation is a preterminal event. It is seen almost solely in dying hearts. It is the most frequently encountered arrhythmia in adults who experience sudden death. The EKG tracing jerks about spasmodically (coarse ventricular fibrillation) or undulates gently (fine ventricular fibrillation). There are no true QRS complexes.

In ventricular fibrillation, the heart generates no cardiac output, and cardiopulmonary resuscitation and electrical defibrillation must be performed at once.

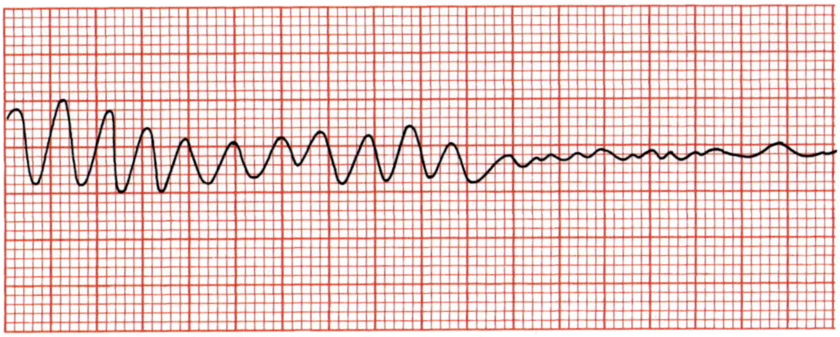

Ventricular tachycardia degenerates into ventricular fibrillation.

Common precipitants of ventricular fibrillation include the following:

- Myocardial ischemia/infarction
- Heart failure
- Hypoxemia or hypercapnia
- Hypotension or shock
- Electrolyte imbalances
- Overdoses of stimulants, especially when used in combination (eg, MDMA [eg, Ecstasy or Molly] with an amphetamine)

In many cases, ventricular fibrillation is preceded by ventricular tachycardia.

SUMMARY Ventricular Arrhythmias

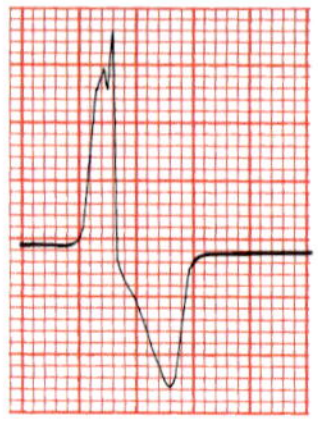

PVC

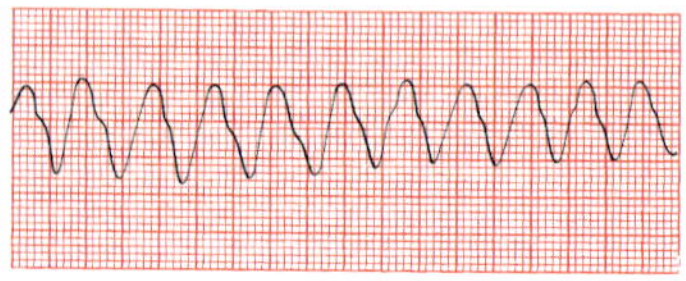

Ventricular tachycardia

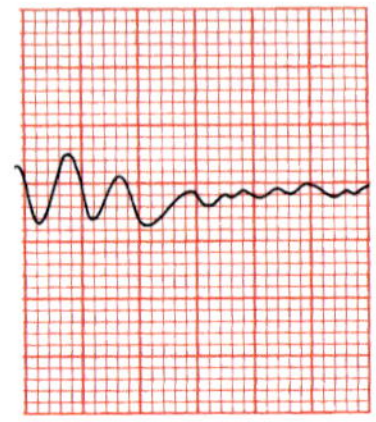

Ventricular fibrillation

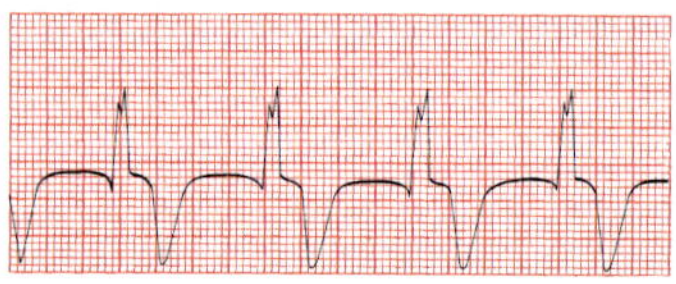

Accelerated idioventricular rhythm

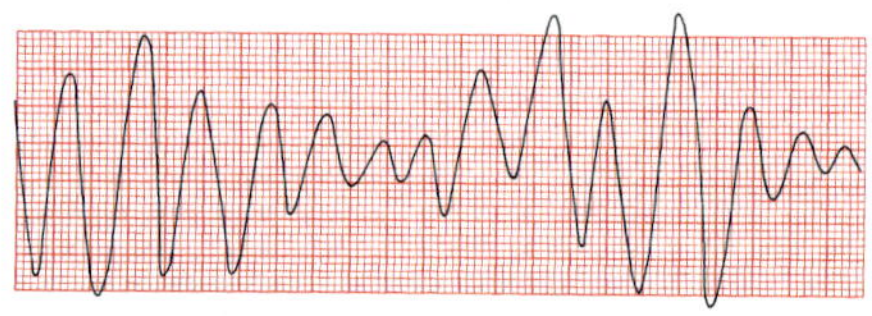

Torsades de pointes

Supraventricular Versus Ventricular Arrhythmias: It's Often But Not Always Easy to Tell Them Apart

The distinction between supraventricular arrhythmias and ventricular arrhythmias is extremely important because the latter generally carry a far more ominous prognosis, and the therapy is very different. In most cases, the distinction is simple: Supraventricular arrhythmias are associated *with a narrow QRS complex and ventricular arrhythmias with a wide QRS complex.*

There are circumstances, however, in which supraventricular beats can be associated with wide QRS complexes. This can occur, for instance, when patients already have an underlying wide QRS complex (eg, if your patient has a right bundle branch or left bundle branch block; we will discuss these types of blocks in the next chapter, but perhaps you can already intuit that any delay in conduction through the ventricles—which can occur when one of the bundle branches isn't firing on all cylinders—will widen the QRS complex. Thus, wide QRS complexes can sometimes be seen in patients with normal sinus rhythm or any supraventricular arrhythmia).

But there is another way in which a supraventricular tachycardia can produce a wide QRS complex in patients whose baseline QRS complex is initially narrow. This is important, so please pay attention. Here's how it happens.

Aberrancy

Sometimes, an atrial premature beat occurs so early in the next cardiac cycle that the Purkinje fibers in the ventricles have not had a chance to repolarize fully in preparation for the next electrical impulse. The right bundle branch, in particular, can be sluggish in this regard, and when the premature atrial impulse reaches the ventricles, the right bundle branch is still refractory. The electrical impulse is therefore prevented from passing down the right bundle branch but is able to pass quite freely down the left bundle branch (Figure *A*). Those areas of the ventricular myocardium ordinarily supplied by the right bundle branch must receive their electrical activation from elsewhere, namely, from those areas already depolarized by the left bundle branch (Figure *B*). The complete process of ventricular depolarization, therefore, takes an unusually long time; the vector of current flow is distorted; and the result is a wide, bizarre QRS complex that looks, for all the world, like a PVC (Figure *C*).

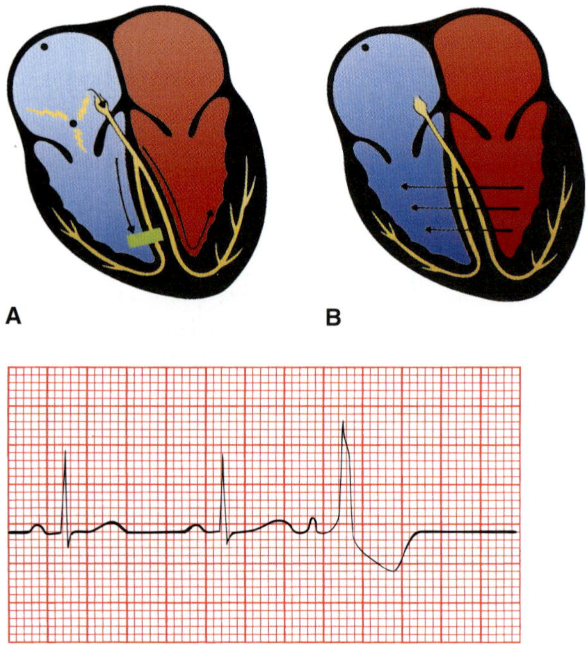

A B C

(*A*) A premature atrial impulse catches the right bundle branch unprepared. Conduction down the right bundle is blocked, but proceeds smoothly down the left bundle. (*B*) Right ventricular depolarization occurs only when the electrical forces can make their way over from the left ventricle—a slow, tedious process. This mode of transmission is very inefficient and results in a wide, bizarre QRS complex. (*C*) The third P wave—a pretty funky looking P wave, but that's beside the point—is a premature atrial contraction. It is conducted aberrantly through the ventricles, generating a wide, bizarre QRS complex.

A wide QRS complex can therefore signify one of several things:

- A beat originating within the ventricles, that is, a PVC
- A supraventricular beat occurring in a patient whose baseline QRS complexes are already wide (eg, in patients with a bundle branch block)
- A supraventricular beat conducted aberrantly

How do you tell these apart? The second possibility is easy—all the QRS complexes will be wide. Also, in the case of a single premature atrial contraction, it's easy because there is a P wave preceding the wide QRS complex. Look especially closely at the T wave of the preceding beat to see if a premature P wave is hidden within it. On the other hand, and rather obviously, there is no P wave preceding a PVC.

However, when there are *several consecutive beats occurring in rapid succession*, or a *lengthy, sustained arrhythmia*, the distinction can be much more difficult. AVNRT and ventricular tachycardia can have about the same rates. Thus, the tracing below is consistent with either ventricular tachycardia or AVNRT conducted aberrantly.

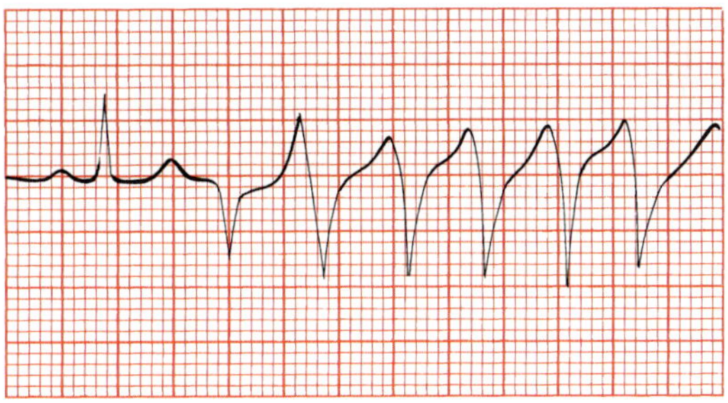

In this tracing, normal sinus rhythm degenerates into a new rhythm, but is it ventricular tachycardia or supraventricular tachycardia conducted aberrantly? Don't feel bad if you can't tell. From this strip alone, as you will see, it is impossible to know for sure.

As you can see from the preceding rhythm strip, it is sometimes very difficult to tell these two entities apart. There are, however, several clinical and electrocardiographic clues that can be helpful.

Clinical Clues

1. Ventricular tachycardia is usually seen in diseased hearts (eg, in a patient with a prior myocardial infarction or congestive heart failure). AVNRT is usually seen in otherwise normal hearts.
2. A Valsalva maneuver may terminate AVNRT, whereas it has no effect on ventricular tachycardia.
3. More than 75% of cases of ventricular tachycardia are accompanied by *AV dissociation*. In AV dissociation, the atria and ventricles beat independently of each other. There is a ventricular pacemaker driving the ventricles and producing ventricular tachycardia on the EKG and an independent sinus (or atrial or nodal) pacemaker driving the atria; the atrial rhythm may sometimes be seen but often is not, hidden on the EKG by the much more prominent ventricular tachycardia. The AV node is kept constantly refractory by the ceaseless bombardment of impulses from above and below, and therefore, no impulse can cross the AV node in either direction. If, as will occur from time to time, the ventricles contract just before the atria, the atria will find themselves contracting against closed mitral and tricuspid valves. This results in a sudden back flooding of blood into the jugular veins, producing the classic *cannon A waves* of AV dissociation. Cannon A waves are not seen in AVNRT.

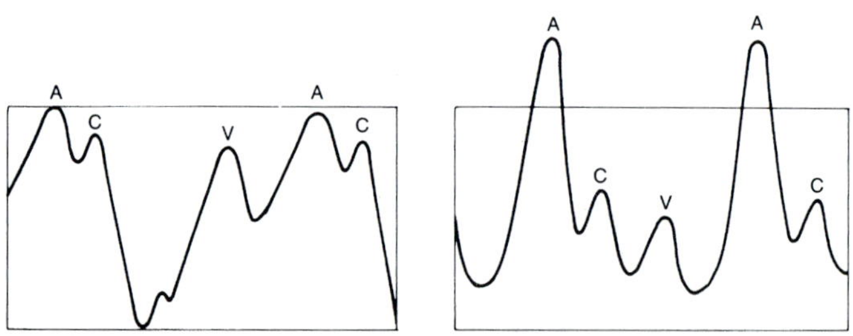

Normal jugular venous tracing

Cannon A waves in a patient with AV dissociation

A wave: right atrial contraction

C wave: closure of the tricuspid valve

V wave: passive filling of the right atrium during diastole

Electrocardiographic Clues

1. AV dissociation accompanying ventricular tachycardia can sometimes be seen on the EKG. The P waves and QRS complexes march along the rhythm strip completely independently of each other. In AVNRT, if P waves are seen, they bear a 1:1 relation to the QRS complexes. And remember, the P waves of AVNRT will be retrograde P waves, with a positive deflection in lead aVR and a negative deflection in lead II.
2. *Fusion beats* may be seen in ventricular tachycardia only. A fusion beat (or capture beat) occurs when an atrial impulse manages to slip through the AV node at the same time that an impulse of ventricular origin is spreading across the ventricular myocardium. The two impulses jointly depolarize the ventricles, producing a QRS complex that is morphologically part supraventricular and part ventricular.
3. In AVNRT with aberrancy, the initial deflection of the QRS complex is usually in the same direction as that of the normal QRS complex. In ventricular tachycardia, the initial deflection is often in the opposite direction.
4. If you have copies of your patient's previous EKGs and can find a PVC on at least one of them, should they appear morphologically similar to the one on your new tracing, chances are you are looking at a PVC.

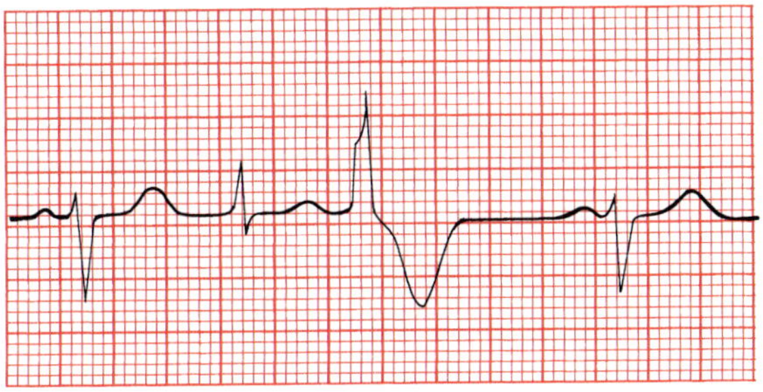

The second beat is a fusion beat, a composite of an atrial (sinus) beat (beats 1 and 4) and a PVC beat (beat 3).

None of these criteria is infallible, and sometimes it remains virtually impossible to identify a tachyarrhythmia as ventricular or supraventricular in origin. In patients with recurrent tachycardias whose origin (and, hence, treatment) remains obscure, *electrophysiologic* testing may be necessary (see page 181). However, if your patient is hemodynamically unstable, you likely don't have time to leisurely pursue additional diagnostic tests; in this situation, assume the worst—treat your patient as if he or she has ventricular tachycardia, which can be lethal. This approach may prove lifesaving and will not be harmful should your patient ultimately prove instead to have a supraventricular tachycardia with aberrant conduction.

The Ashman Phenomenon

We aren't quite ready to leave the subject of aberrancy (sorry, but this is important). The *Ashman phenomenon* is another example of aberrant conduction of a supraventricular beat. It is commonly seen in patients with atrial fibrillation.

The Ashman phenomenon describes a wide, aberrantly conducted supraventricular beat occurring *after a QRS complex that is preceded by a long pause.*

This is why it happens. The bundle branches reset their rate of repolarization according to the length of the preceding beat. If the preceding beat occurred a relatively long time ago, then the bundles repolarize somewhat leisurely. So imagine a normal beat (the second beat on the tracing on the next page) followed by a long pause before the next beat (the third beat on the tracing). The bundle branches anticipate another long pause following this beat and repolarize slowly. If, before repolarization is complete, another supraventricular impulse should pass through the AV node, conduction will be blocked along one of the normal bundle branch pathways, and a wide, bizarre QRS complex will be inscribed (the fourth and obviously abnormal beat). The result may be a single abnormal beat or a sequence of abnormal beats resembling ventricular tachycardia.

Atrial fibrillation, with its variable, irregular conduction producing long and short pauses between QRS complexes, is the perfect setting for this to occur. However, the Ashman phenomenon can occur with any rhythm originating above the AV node, including any supraventricular tachycardia and even normal sinus rhythm.

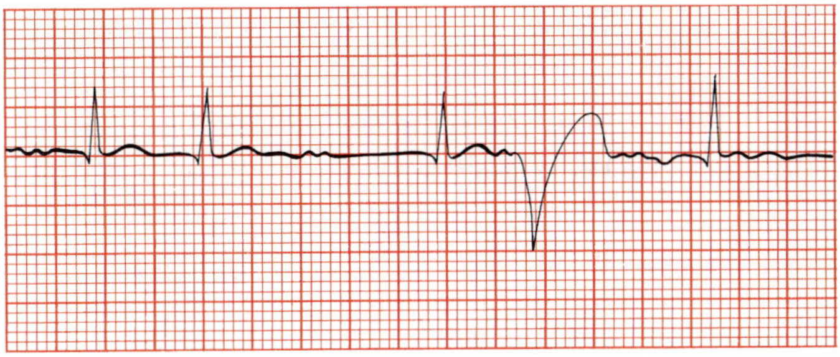

The Ashman phenomenon. The fourth beat looks like a PVC, but it could also be an aberrantly conducted supraventricular beat. Note the underlying atrial fibrillation, the short interval before the second beat, and the long interval before the third beat—all in all, a perfect substrate for the Ashman phenomenon.

Fortunately, most supraventricular arrhythmias are associated with narrow QRS complexes; aberrancy, although not uncommon, is at least the exception, not the rule. The point to take home is this: **A narrow QRS complex virtually always implies a supraventricular origin, whereas a wide QRS complex usually implies a ventricular origin but may reflect aberrant conduction of a supraventricular beat.**

SUMMARY

Ventricular Tachycardia Versus Supraventricular Tachycardia With Aberrancy

	Ventricular Tachycardia	Supraventricular Tachycardias
Clinical Clues		
Clinical history	Diseased heart	Usually healthy heart
Carotid massage	No response	May terminate
Cannon A waves	May be present	Not seen
EKG Clues		
AV dissociation	May be seen	Not seen
Fusion beats	May be seen	Not seen
Initial QRS deflection	May differ from normal QRS complex	Same as normal QRS complex

Electrophysiology Studies (EPS)

Before the introduction of EPS, a patient with an arrhythmia requiring treatment was given a drug empirically, and after several days, when therapeutic levels had been achieved, a 24-hour Holter monitor would be used to see whether the frequency of the arrhythmia had been reduced. This hit-or-miss approach was time consuming and exposed patients to the potential side effects of drugs that might prove of no benefit.

With EPS, the patient is taken to the electrophysiology laboratory where the particular arrhythmia is induced with intracardiac electrodes. Tiny catheters are inserted through peripheral veins or arteries and are then advanced to various locations within the chambers of the heart. A catheter placed at the junction of the right atrium and ventricle at the upper posterior portion of the tricuspid ring will record a His bundle potential, which can help to define the electrical relationship of the atria and ventricles during the propagation of an arrhythmia. For example, if with atrial activation a His potential precedes every QRS complex, then a supraventricular origin is likely. In this way, the source of an arrhythmia can be mapped to determine the most appropriate therapy.

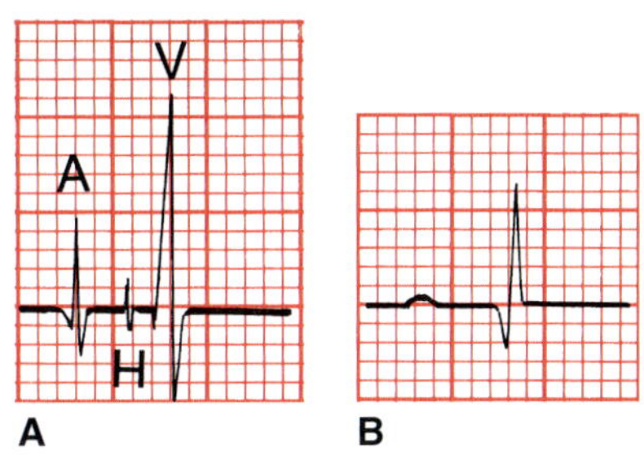

(*A*) A His bundle recording and (*B*) the corresponding EKG. In *A*, the small spike (H) between the spikes of atrial (A) and ventricular (V) activation reflects activation of the bundle of His.

EPS has been used most successfully in managing patients who have recurrent ventricular tachycardia or who have experienced a previous episode of sudden death requiring cardiopulmonary resuscitation. It is also used to identify an arrhythmia in patients with syncope of unknown cause.

EPS mapping techniques have become extremely precise and, combined with the technique of *catheter ablation*, are often used to treat atrial fibrillation, atrial flutter, AVNRT, and (to be discussed in Chapter 5) AV reciprocating tachycardia.

Antiarrhythmic Agents

Since we have devoted this chapter to recognizing and diagnosing arrhythmias, we should at least take this opportunity to familiarize you with the basic categories of antiarrhythmic agents that are still widely used in their treatment. There are various ways to classify them, but the oldest and simplest is probably the best:

- Class I: Sodium channel blockers. This category is actually broken down into three basic subcategories based on their precise mode of action: Ia—these drugs can increase the QT interval and thus, while still highly useful, can paradoxically cause arrhythmias in some patients; among them are quinidine, procainamide and disopyramide; Ib—mild channel blockers that actually can shorten the QT interval, including lidocaine and mexilitine; and Ic—these generally do not prolong the QT interval and include flecainide and propafenone (which also have class 3 activity).
- Class 2: Beta blockers. These act primarily by blocking the activity of the sympathetic nervous system and include drugs such as metoprolol and propranolol (there are many others).
- Class 3: Potassium channel blockers. These can also increase the QT interval. The one to know is amiodarone, but there are others you will encounter. Amiodarone actually has properties of all the classes listed here and is among the most widely used antiarrhythmic agent.
- Class 4: Calcium channel blockers. Only some of these drugs have antiarrhythmic properties. Verapamil and diltiazem are the ones to be aware of.
- There are now additional classes as we've come to identify new targets on the cell membrane and designed drugs to interact with them. These are (fortunately) beyond the scope of this brief introduction.

Implantable Defibrillators

Even when EPS-guided drug therapies or catheter ablation techniques are used, the recurrence rates for ventricular tachycardia are still unacceptably high. For this reason, *implantable cardioverter–defibrillators* have become the standard form of protection for most patients with life-threatening arrhythmias. These small devices are surgically implanted, like a pacemaker, under the skin below the clavicle. There they continuously monitor the heart rhythm and, when they sense a dangerous arrhythmia, deliver either a rapid pacing rhythm or an electric shock to the heart through an electrode that rests in the right ventricle.

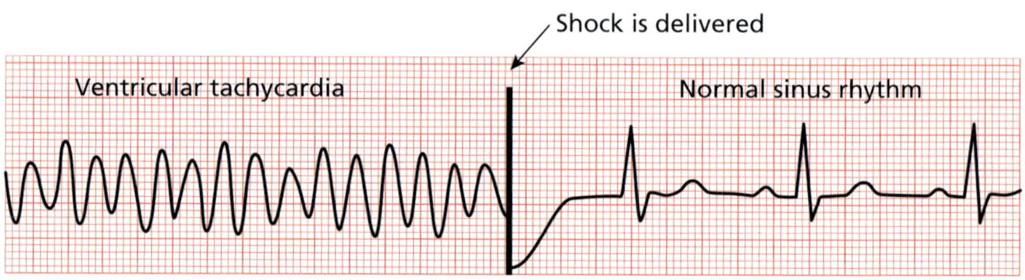

EKG tracing of a patient with ventricular tachycardia who is rescued by a shock delivered by an implantable cardioverter–defibrillator.

External Defibrillators

Automatic external defibrillators are small portable devices that come equipped with patches that attach to the chest wall. Once hooked up, these devices can quickly determine whether the rhythm of an individual who has collapsed is ventricular fibrillation and, if so, can deliver defibrillation shocks that may be lifesaving. Minimal training is required to learn how to operate the defibrillator and place the patches properly. You've certainly encountered these as they are now widely available in police cars, on airplanes, and in public venues.

***

On the following page is an opportunity to review the arrhythmias we have been discussing. For each tracing, use the four-step method discussed previously. Always ask the following questions:

1. Are normal P waves present?
2. Are the QRS complexes narrow or wide?
3. What is the relationship between the P waves and QRS complexes?
4. Is the rhythm regular or irregular?

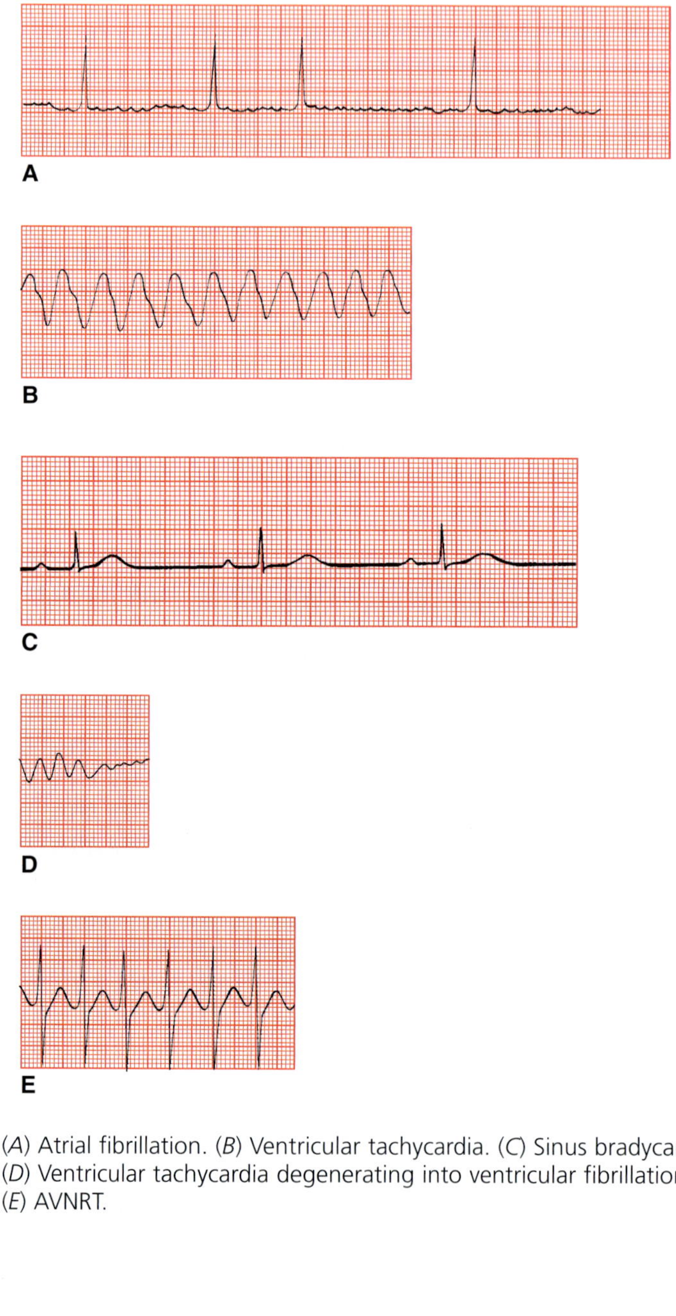

(*A*) Atrial fibrillation. (*B*) Ventricular tachycardia. (*C*) Sinus bradycardia. (*D*) Ventricular tachycardia degenerating into ventricular fibrillation. (*E*) AVNRT.

Evaluating Patients With Syncope

In patients with tachyarrhythmias that result in syncope, further evaluation following the episode is usually warranted because of the high likelihood of recurrence. This evaluation usually includes at the very least appropriate laboratory studies (eg, to rule out electrolyte imbalances and hyperthyroidism), a baseline EKG, a stress echocardiogram (to look for valvular disease and coronary artery disease), and an ambulatory monitor to capture any further rhythm disturbances. Prolonged seizure activity associated with the syncopal event or any persistent neurologic deficits will necessitate a neurologic evaluation. In many states and countries, if no treatable cause for the syncopal event is found, the patient will not be permitted to drive for at least several months.

CASE 3

George M., irascible and older than time, comes to see you late one Friday afternoon (he always comes late on Friday afternoons, probably because he knows you like to get an early start on the weekend). This time, he tells you that he fainted the day before and now is feeling a bit light headed. He also has a strange fluttering sensation in his chest. George is always complaining of something, and you have yet to find anything the matter with him in the many years you have known him, but just to be careful, you obtain an EKG.

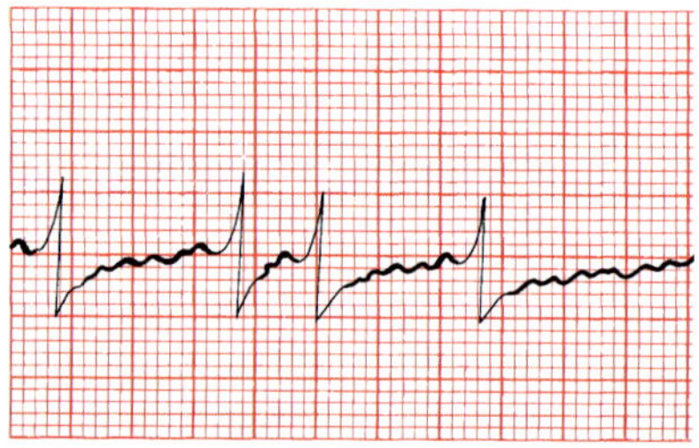

You quickly recognize the arrhythmia and are reaching for your stethoscope when George's eyes roll back in his head and he drops unconscious to the floor. Fortunately, the EKG is still running, and you see

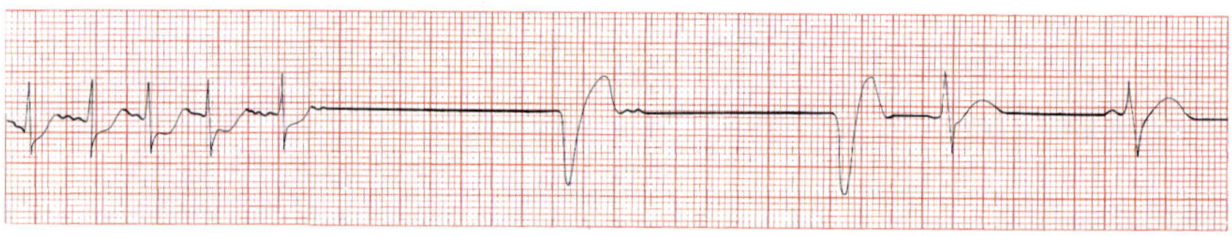

You drop down to his side, ready, if need be, to begin cardiopulmonary resuscitation, when his eyes pop open and he mutters something under his breath. The EKG now shows

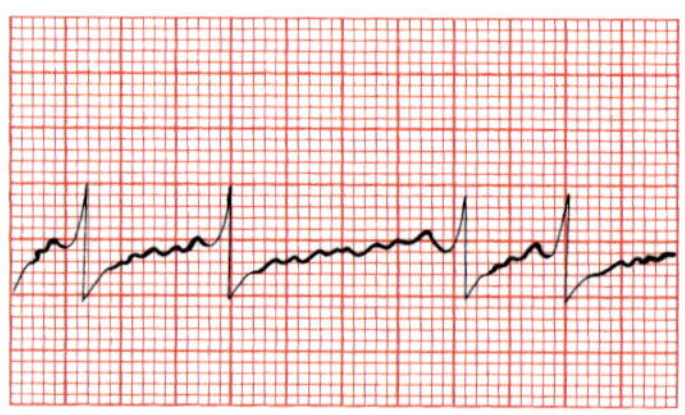

You may not know precisely what's going on, but at least you can identify the three tracings. Right?

The first and third tracings are the same, showing classic atrial fibrillation. The baseline is undulating, without clear-cut P waves, and the QRS complexes appear irregularly. The second tracing is more interesting. It shows the atrial fibrillation terminating abruptly and then a long pause. (It was during such a pause that George dropped to the floor, a result of brain hypoxia caused by the lack of significant cardiac output.) The beats that you see next are ventricular escape beats. The QRS complexes are wide and bizarre, there are no P waves, and the rate is about 33 beats per minute, exactly what you would expect of a ventricular escape rhythm. The final thing you see on the strip is the sinus node kicking in. The last strip shows him once again in atrial fibrillation.

George has *sick sinus syndrome*, also called the *tachy–brady syndrome*. It is typified by alternating episodes of a supraventricular tachycardia, such as atrial fibrillation, and bradycardia. Often, when the supraventricular arrhythmia terminates, there is a long pause (>4 seconds) before the sinus node fires again (hence, the term sick sinus). Fortunately for George, a few ventricular escape beats came to a timely rescue.

Sick sinus syndrome usually reflects significant underlying disease of the conduction system of the sort that we will be studying in the next chapter. It is one of the leading reasons for pacemaker insertion.

George M. revives in your office and insists on going home. Fortunately, wiser heads prevail and he is taken by ambulance to the hospital. A short stay in the cardiac care unit confirms that he has not had a heart attack, but his heart monitor shows numerous episodes of prolonged bradycardia alternating with various supraventricular arrhythmias. It is decided that George should have a pacemaker placed, and he reluctantly agrees. The pacemaker provides a safety net, giving George's heart an electrical "kick" every time his own electrical mechanism fails him. George is discharged, and no further episodes of symptomatic bradycardia occur.

CASE 4

Frederick van Z. is a renowned (and highly strung) orchestral conductor whose delusions of grandeur are tempered by a small regular dose of citalopram, an antidepressant medication. Late one night, after a triumphant all-Beethoven performance at the large concert hall in your town, he is rushed to the hospital with a high fever, confusion, and blood in his urine (hematuria). In the emergency room, he is found to be hypotensive from urosepsis. He is treated with the intravenous antibiotic, levofloxacin. Here is lead II from his cardiac monitor in the emergency room. Can you identify his rhythm?

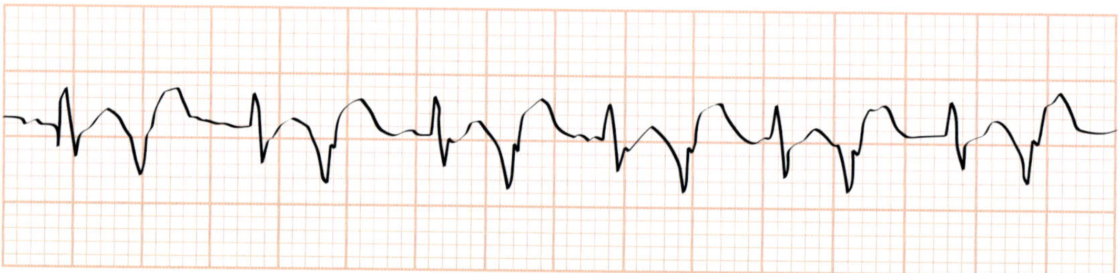

You should recognize two different types of beats of very different morphology, alternating with one another. The maestro is in bigeminy, with supraventricular beats (junctional beats, with a narrow QRS complex, and no visible P wave) occurring in a 1:1 ratio with ventricular beats (PVCs, with a wide QRS complex).

He is transferred to the intensive care unit where you confidently take over his case. As soon as you hook him up to the heart monitor, you see this. What has happened?

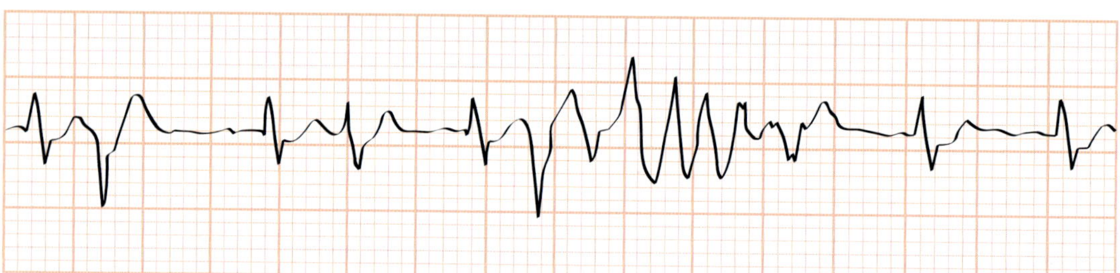

Let's read this left to right. The first beat is a junctional beat, the second a PVC, and the third and fourth beats two more junctional beats. He clearly is no longer in strict bigeminy. On the fifth beat, right after the QRS complex, a PVC has landed on the vulnerable QT interval and triggered a short run of a ventricular tachycardia that is fortunately self-terminating.

Moments later, his blood pressure collapses, his body seizes up in bed, and you see the following arrhythmia. In a flash, you recognize it and prepare to swing into action. What does the tracing show?

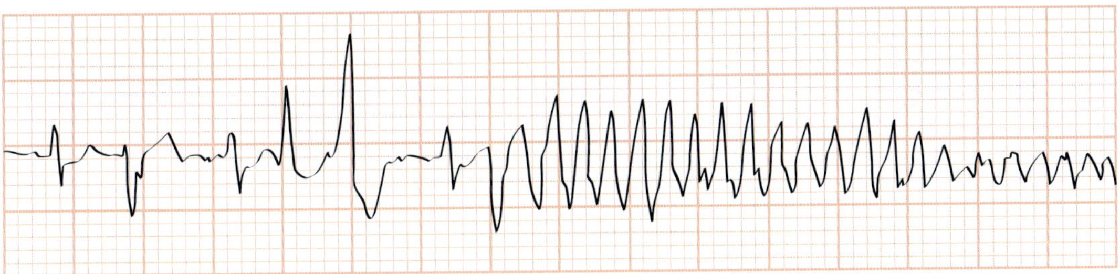

As in the previous tracing, a PVC has fallen on a QT interval, but now, the resulting ventricular tachycardia persists. The changes in amplitude of the QRS complexes (reflecting a change in axis as the QRS complexes spiral around the baseline) identify the arrhythmia as torsade de pointes, a medical emergency.

The great conductor is successfully treated and his vital signs return to normal. Several hours later, his rhythm strip now shows this. What do you see (hint: look closely at the lengths of the various intervals)?

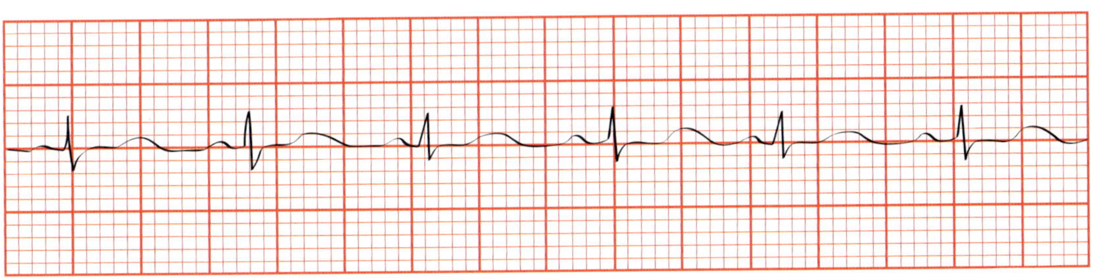

He is in normal sinus rhythm—note the presence of P waves—but take a close look at his QT interval. Normally, it should constitute about 40% of the cardiac cycle, but here, it measures well over 50% of one cardiac cycle. This prolonged QT interval was the perfect substrate for torsade de pointes. The patient was on two drugs that can prolong the QT interval—citalopram, which he was taking on a chronic basis, and levofloxacin, the antibiotic he was given in the emergency room that acutely lengthened his QT interval even more and set up the great master for the nearly fatal events that followed. You immediately discontinue both medications, and his QT interval normalizes. There will be no more episodes of torsade de pointes on your watch!

4 Conduction Blocks

In this chapter, you will learn:

1 | what a conduction block is

2 | that there are several types of conduction blocks that can occur between the sinus node and the atrioventricular (AV) node, some that are of little concern and others that can be life threatening

3 | how to recognize each of these *AV Blocks* on the EKG

4 | that conduction blocks can occur in the ventricles as well, and these *bundle-branch blocks* are also easily identified on the EKG

5 | that sometimes, conduction along only one fascicle of the left bundle branch can be blocked

6 | how to recognize *combined* AV blocks and bundle-branch blocks on the EKG

7 | what pacemakers are used for, and how to recognize their bursts of electrical activity on an EKG

8 | about the cases of Sally M., Jamar N., and Jeong O., which will illustrate the importance of knowing when conduction disturbances are truly disturbing

What Is a Conduction Block?

Any obstruction or delay of the flow of electricity along the normal pathways of electrical conduction is called a *conduction block*.

> Technically, not all of what we call conduction blocks are true blocks; whereas some actually do bring the flow of current to a complete halt, in many cases, they only slow it down. Nevertheless, the term stands, and we will use it throughout this chapter.

A conduction block can occur anywhere in the conduction system of the heart. There are three types of conduction blocks, defined by their anatomic location.

1. *Sinus node block*—This is the sinus exit block that we discussed in the last chapter. In this situation, the sinus node fires normally, but the wave of depolarization is immediately blocked and is not transmitted into the atrial tissue. On the EKG, it looks just like a pause in the normal cardiac cycle. There is no need to discuss it further here.
2. *AV block*—This term refers to any conduction block between the sinus node and the terminal Purkinje fibers. Note that this includes the AV node and His bundle.
3. *Bundle-branch block*—As the name indicates, bundle-branch block refers to a conduction block in one or both of the ventricular bundle branches. Sometimes, only a part of the relatively more complicated left bundle branch is blocked; this circumstance is called a *fascicular block* or a *hemiblock*.

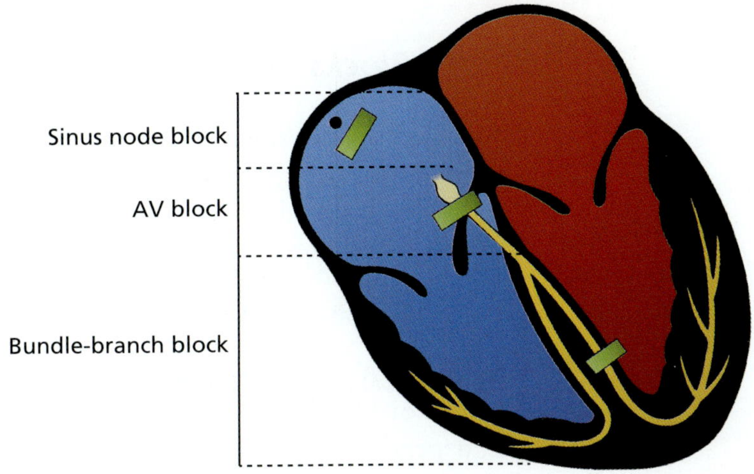

To a rough approximation, this picture shows typical sites of the three major conduction blocks.

AV Blocks

AV blocks come in three varieties, termed (with a sad lack of imagination) *first degree*, *second degree*, and *third degree*. They are diagnosed by carefully examining the relationship of the P waves to the QRS complexes.

First-Degree AV Block

First-degree AV block is characterized by a delay in conduction at the AV node or His bundle (recall that the His bundle—or bundle of His, depending on your grammatical preference—is the part of the conducting system located just below the AV node. A routine 12-lead EKG cannot distinguish between a block in the AV node and one in the His bundle). The wave of depolarization spreads normally from the sinus node through the atria, but upon reaching the AV node, it is held up for longer than usual. As a result, the PR interval—the time from the start of atrial depolarization to the start of ventricular depolarization, a time period that encompasses the delay at the AV node—is prolonged.

The diagnosis of first-degree AV block requires only that the PR interval be longer than 0.2 seconds.

In first-degree AV block, despite the delay at the AV node or His bundle, every atrial impulse does eventually make it through the AV node to activate the ventricles. Therefore, to be precise, first-degree AV block is not really a "block" at all, but rather a "delay" in conduction. Every QRS complex is preceded by a single P wave.

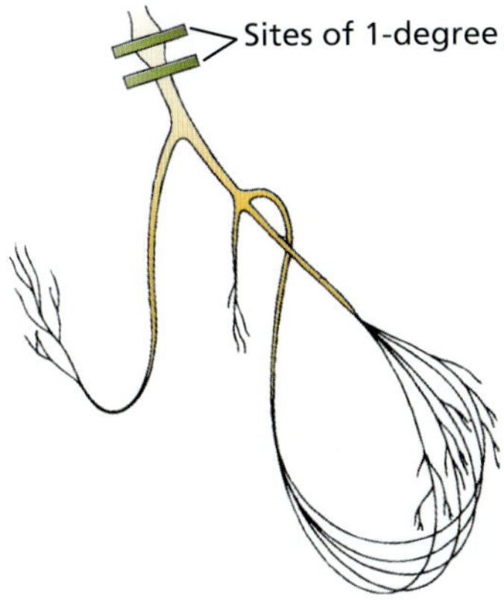

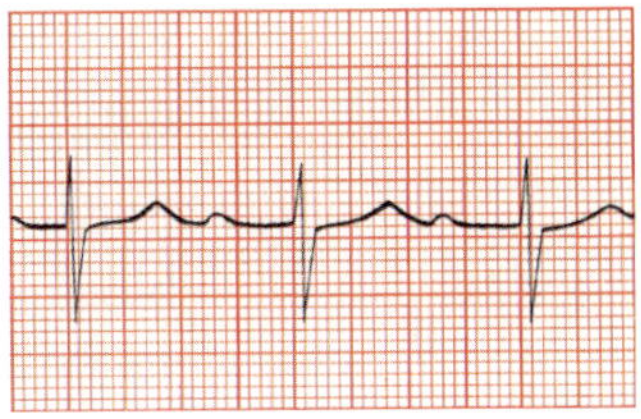

First-degree AV block. Note the prolonged PR interval.

First-degree AV block is a common finding in normal hearts, particularly during sleep, but it can also be an early sign of degenerative disease of the conduction system or a transient manifestation of myocarditis or drug toxicity. By itself, it does not require treatment (but, for one important exception, see our discussion of Lyme disease on page 206).

Second-Degree AV Block

In *second-degree AV block*, not every atrial impulse is able to pass through the AV node into the ventricles. Because some P waves fail to conduct through to the ventricles, the ratio of P waves to QRS complexes is greater than 1:1 (see the tracing on the next page). The distance from one P wave to the next does not change, because the sinus node is not affected.

Just to make things a little more interesting, there are two types of second-degree AV block: *Mobitz type I second-degree AV block*, more commonly called *Wenckebach block*, and *Mobitz type II second-degree AV block*.

If these names sound arbitrary and needlessly obscure, they are actually rooted in electrocardiographic history. In 1942, Woldemar Mobitz, a Russian–German physician, first classified the different types of second-degree AV block. Karel Frederik Wenckebach, "Venky" to his friends (really), was a Dutch anatomist who, in 1899, first recognized the AV block that now bears his name.

Wenckebach Block (Mobitz Type I Second-Degree AV Block)

Wenckebach block is almost always due to a block *within* the AV node. The electrical effects of Wenckebach block are unique. The block, or delay, is variable, increasing with each ensuing impulse. **Each successive atrial impulse encounters a longer and longer delay in the AV node until one impulse (usually every third or fourth) fails to make it through.** What you see on the EKG is a progressive lengthening of the PR interval with each beat and then suddenly a P wave that is not followed by a QRS complex (a "dropped beat"). After this dropped beat, during which no QRS complex appears, the sequence—the gradual lengthening of the PR interval until one QRS complex is dropped—repeats itself, over and over, and often with impressive regularity.

Sometimes it may be difficult to tell that the PR interval is prolonging from one PR to the next. It is then best to look at the PR intervals just before and just after the dropped beat. These should be the longest and shortest PR intervals and therefore the easiest to contrast.

The following tracing shows a 4:3 Wenckebach block, in which the PR interval grows longer with each beat until the fourth atrial impulse fails to stimulate the ventricles, producing a ratio of four P waves to every three QRS complexes. Because the block occurs within the AV node and above the ventricular conducting system, the QRS complexes are usually narrow. One important exception—the QRS complexes will be wide if there is a coexisting bundle-branch block, but we will get to this later in the chapter.

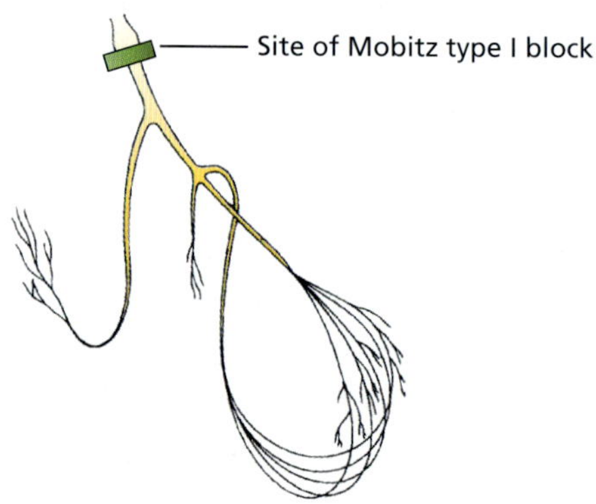

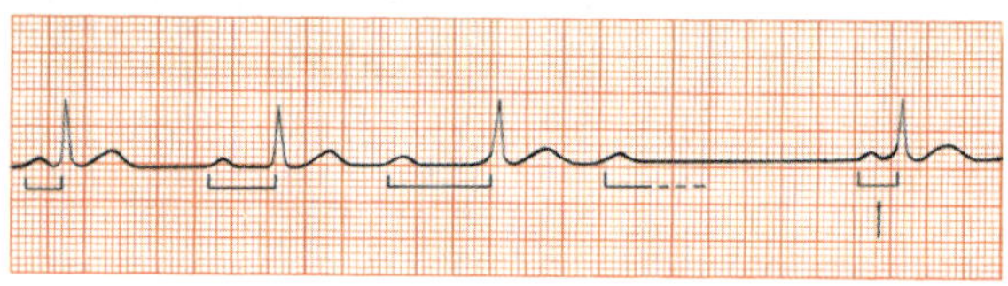

Mobitz type I second-degree AV block (Wenckebach block). The PR intervals become progressively longer until one QRS complex is dropped.

Here's another example of Wenckebach block. Again, you can clearly see the PR intervals increasing until one is no longer conducted and fails to generate a QRS complex. Are you confused by what appears to be an absent P wave following the fourth and seventh QRS complexes? Don't be–the P wave is hidden in the T waves, which, if you look closely, as a result, appear somewhat taller and more pointy than the other T waves, as if there were something inside trying to poke its way out. If you don't believe me, map out the P-to-P intervals, and you will see that a P wave should appear right in the middle of those T waves.

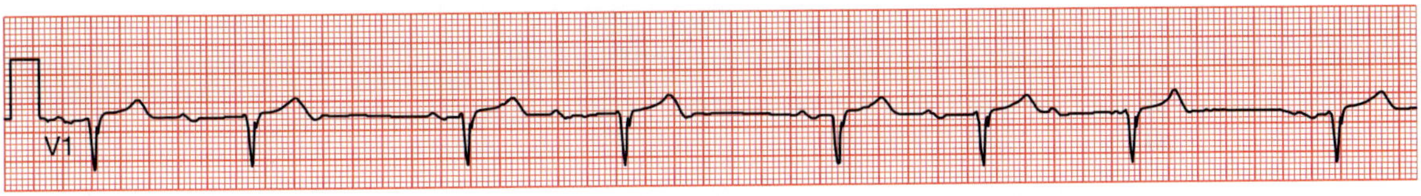

Another example of Wenckebach block. The PR intervals get longer and longer until one P wave, in this case hidden within the T wave, fails to conduct to the ventricles.

The diagnosis of Wenckebach block requires the progressive lengthening of each successive PR interval until one P wave fails to conduct through the AV node and is therefore not followed by a QRS complex.

Mobitz Type II Second-Degree AV Block

Mobitz type II block is usually due to a block *below* the AV node in the His bundle. It resembles Wenckebach block in that some, but not all, of the atrial impulses are transmitted to the ventricles. However, progressive lengthening of the PR interval does *not* occur. Instead, conduction is an all-or-nothing phenomenon. The EKG shows two or more normal beats with normal PR intervals and then a P wave that is not followed by a QRS complex (a dropped beat). The cycle is then repeated. The ratio of conducted beats to nonconducted beats is rarely constant, with the ratio of P waves to QRS complexes varying, from 2:1 to 3:2 and so on. Because the block is infranodal, that is, below the AV node, the QRS complexes are often wide.

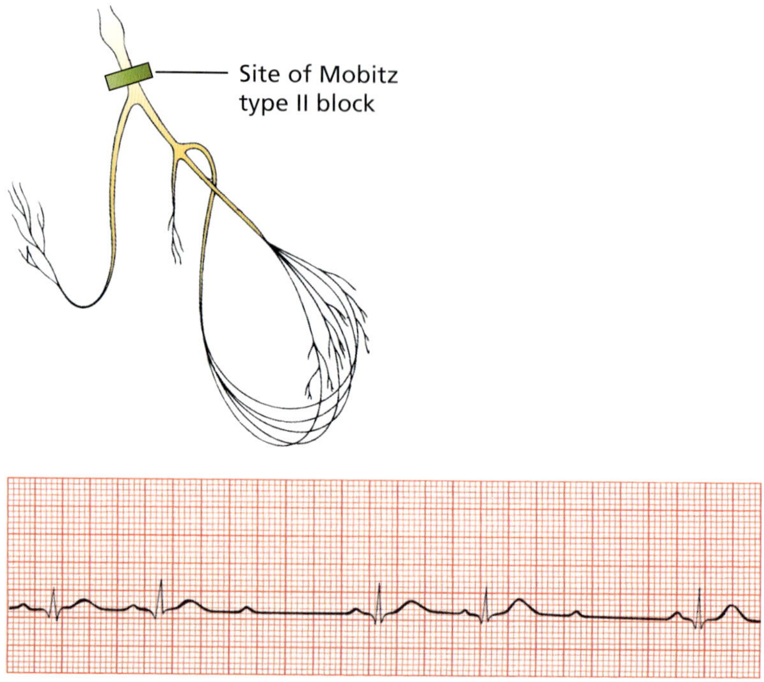

Mobitz type II second-degree AV block. On this EKG, each third P wave is not followed by a QRS complex (dropped beat).

The diagnosis of Mobitz type II block requires the presence of a dropped beat without progressive lengthening of the PR interval.

Is It a Wenckebach Block or a Mobitz Type II Block?

Compare the electrocardiographic manifestations of Wenckebach block and Mobitz type II block on the following EKGs:

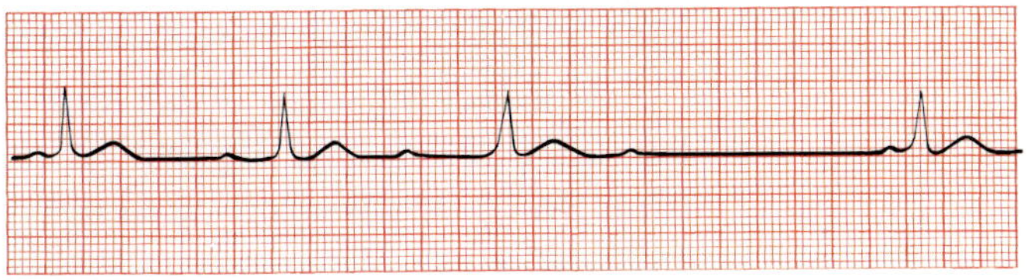

A

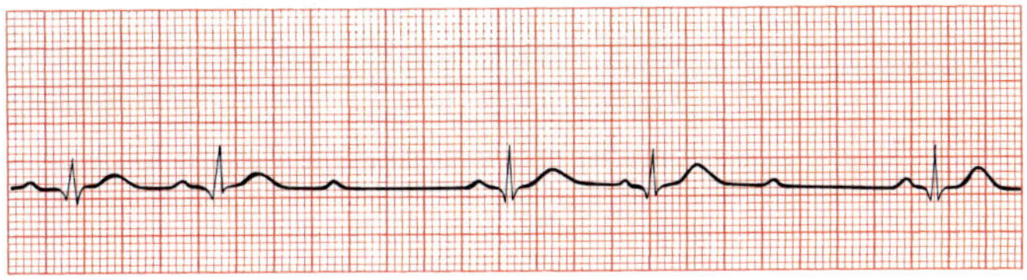

B

(*A*) Wenckebach block, with progressive lengthening of the PR interval.
(*B*) Mobitz type II block, in which the PR interval is constant.

Now that you are an expert, look at the following EKG. Is this an example of Wenckebach block or Mobitz type II block?

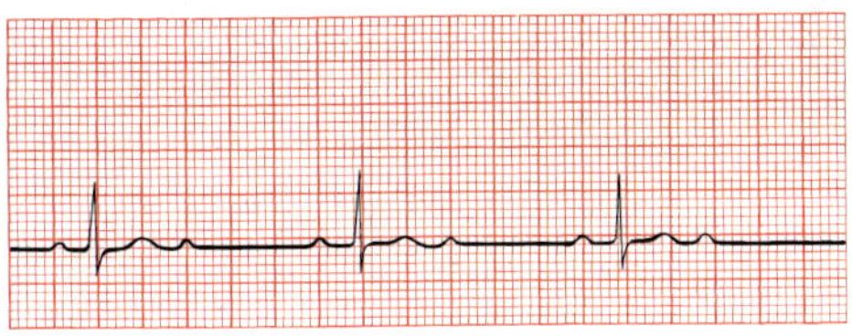

Well, it certainly is an example of second-degree heart block. The ratio of P waves to QRS complexes is 2:1, but you were pretty clever if you realized that it is impossible to tell whether it is due to Wenckebach block or Mobitz type II block. The distinction between these two types of second-degree heart block depends on whether or not there is progressive PR lengthening, but with a 2:1 ratio in which every other QRS complex is dropped, it is impossible to make this determination. This should simply—and most accurately—be called 2:1 AV block.

Here is a bit of technical esoterica that, unless you plan to become a cardiologist, you can probably safely ignore. In cases of 2:1 second-degree AV block, as shown on the previous page, there actually are two ways—one clinical and one invasive—to localize the site of the block and determine how serious the problem may be.

The bedside approach: Vagal tone affects the AV node more than the His bundle, so anything that increases vagal tone—for example, a Valsalva maneuver—can increase AV nodal block. However, it will either not affect or may even possibly improve an infranodal block; it does so by slowing the heart rate, thereby allowing the infranodal tissue time to recover between beats and conduct more efficiently. Thus, depending on the location of the block, the degree of block will respond differently to vagal stimulation, thus allowing you to distinguish Wenckebach from Mobitz type II heart block.

The invasive approach: An electrophysiologic study is the definitive way to make the distinction. A small electrode introduced into the region of the His bundle can identify whether the site of the block is above, within, or below the His bundle.

The distinction between Wenckebach block and Mobitz type II second-degree AV block is an important one to make. Wenckebach block is typically transient and benign, and rarely progresses to third-degree heart block (see next page), which can be dangerous and even life threatening.

Mobitz type II block is far more serious, although less common than Wenckebach block, often signifying underlying heart disease and capable of progressing suddenly to third-degree heart block.

Whereas pacemaker placement is only uncommonly needed for Wenckebach block unless patients are symptomatic (eg, experiencing syncope), Mobitz type II heart block mandates insertion of a pacemaker.

Third-Degree AV Block

Third-degree heart block is the ultimate in heart blocks. No atrial impulses at all make it through to activate the ventricles. For this reason, it is often called *complete heart block*. The site of the block can be either at the AV node or lower. The ventricles respond to this dire situation by generating an escape rhythm, usually a barely adequate 30 to 45 beats per minute. The atria and ventricles continue to contract, but they now do so at their own intrinsic rates—about 60 to 100 beats per minute for the atria and 30 to 45 beats per minute for the ventricles. The atria and ventricles have virtually nothing to do with each other, separated by the absolute barrier of the complete conduction block. We have already described this type of situation in our discussion of ventricular tachycardia: It is called *AV dissociation* and refers to any circumstance in which the atria and ventricles are being driven by independent pacemakers. Both the atrial and ventricular rhythms are regular, so that the R-R intervals and P-P intervals do not vary (although there may be some slight variation in the P-P intervals due to the presence of normal sinus arrhythmia, the variation of the sinus rate with respiration, see page 124).

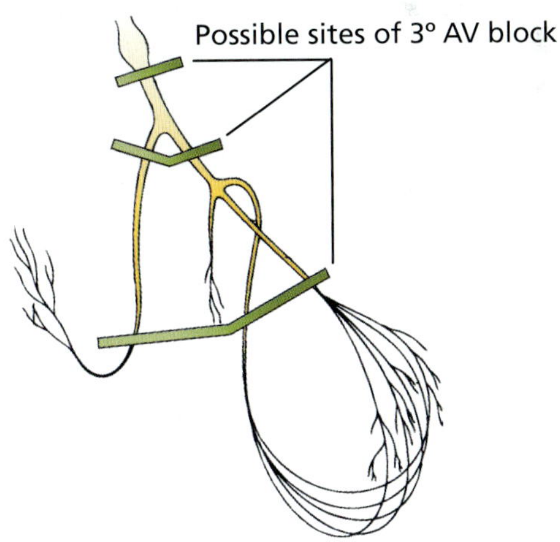

The EKG in third-degree heart block shows P waves marching across the rhythm strip at their usual rate (60 to 100 waves per minute) but bearing no relationship to the QRS complexes that appear at a much slower escape rate. The QRS complexes usually appear wide and bizarre, looking just like premature ventricular contractions (PVCs), because they arise from a ventricular source.

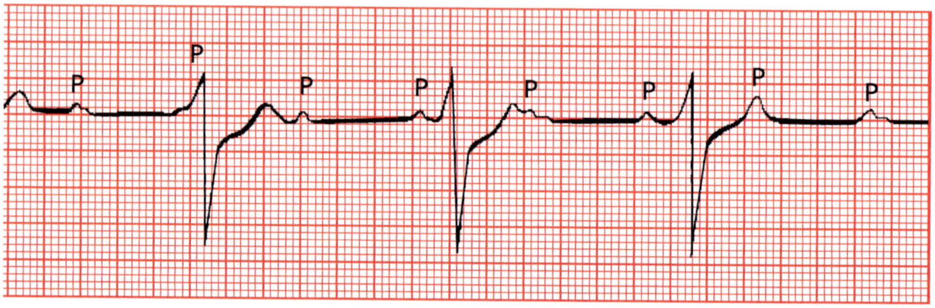

Third-degree AV block. The P waves appear at regular intervals, as do the QRS complexes, but they have nothing to do with one another. The QRS complexes are wide, implying a ventricular origin.

With the onset of third-degree heart block, there may be a delay (or, in the most unfortunate circumstances, even complete absence) in the appearance of a ventricular escape rhythm. The EKG will then show sinus beats (P waves) activating the atria with no ventricular activity at all for several seconds before either normal AV conduction resumes or a ventricular escape rhythm finally appears. When there are 4 or more seconds without ventricular activity, the patient may experience a near or complete faint. These faints have been termed Stokes–Adams attacks and almost always require a pacemaker (see page 227).

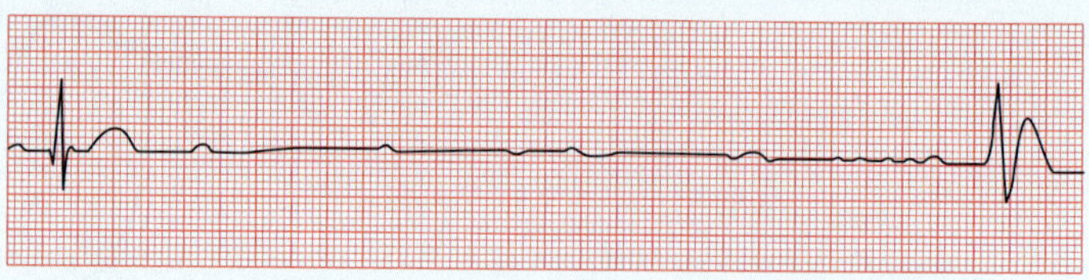

This patient was in normal sinus rhythm (see the first complex) when he suddenly went into complete heart block. There is a long pause during which you can see nothing but P waves; no escape beats can be seen for several seconds. Finally, the first ventricular escape beat saves the day, but during the long pause, the patient experienced a Stokes–Adams attack.

Although a ventricular escape rhythm may look like a slow run of PVCs (accelerated idioventricular rhythm, see page 170), there is one important difference: PVCs are *premature*, occurring before the next expected beat, and even the slowest ventricular tachycardia will be faster than the patient's normal rhythm. On the other hand, a ventricular escape beat occurs after a long pause and is therefore never premature, and a sustained ventricular escape rhythm is always *slower* than the normal beats. PVCs, being premature intrusions, can be suppressed with little clinical consequence. A ventricular escape rhythm, however, may be lifesaving, and suppression could be fatal.

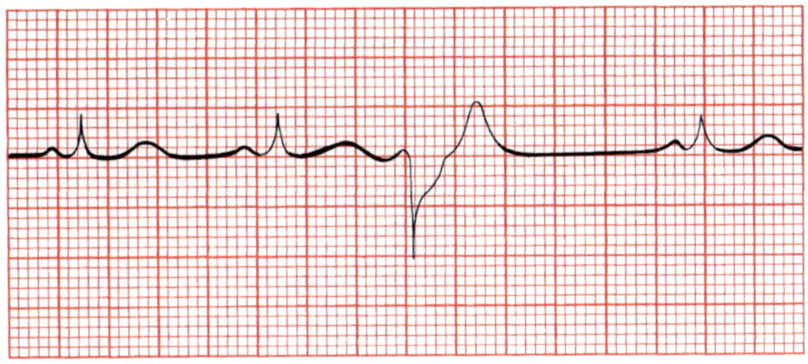

A

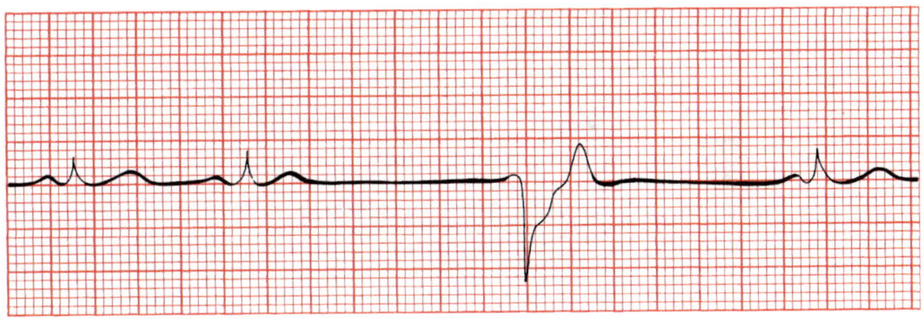

B

(*A*) The third beat is a PVC, occurring before the next anticipated normal beat. (*B*) The third ventricular complex occurs late, after a prolonged pause. This is a ventricular escape beat.

Atrioventricular dissociation can also occur when there is a block high in the AV node, but in this case, there is an accelerated *junctional* rhythm to drive the ventricles that is faster than the sinus rhythm. The QRS complexes may appear narrow in this instance. This situation rarely requires a pacemaker. It occurs most often in patients experiencing an acute myocardial infarction with high vagal tone and in those who have received an overdose of an antiarrhythmic medication.

The diagnosis of third-degree heart block requires the presence of AV dissociation, in which the ventricular rate is slower than the sinus or atrial rate.

Degenerative disease of the conduction system, seen most often in elderly patients, is the leading cause of third-degree heart block. Complete heart block can also complicate an acute myocardial infarction. Pacemakers are virtually always required when third-degree heart block develops. It is a true medical emergency.

Most complete heart blocks are permanent. One of the more common causes of *reversible* complete heart block is Lyme disease, caused by infection with the spirochete, *Borrelia burgdorferi*. The heart block is caused by inflammation of the myocardium and conducting system, and any level of AV block can occur. Patients with type 1 AV block, ordinarily benign, in which the PR interval is >300 ms, can progress rapidly to complete heart block and may require hospitalization. In patients with Lyme disease who develop complete heart block, the block typically occurs within the AV node and is associated with a narrow QRS complex *junctional* escape rhythm. A stat Lyme titer can avoid the need for a permanent pacemaker, although temporary pacing may be needed. Treatment includes antibiotics and corticosteroids.

Some forms of complete heart block develop prenatally (congenital heart block), most commonly in maternal systemic lupus erythematosus. Congenital heart blocks are often associated with an adequate and stable ventricular escape rhythm. Permanent pacemakers are only implanted in these children if there is clear-cut developmental impairment that can be attributed to an inadequate cardiac output.

SUMMARY

AV Blocks

AV block is diagnosed by examining the relationship of the P waves to the QRS complexes.

1. *First degree:* The PR interval is >0.2 seconds; *all* beats are conducted through to the ventricles.

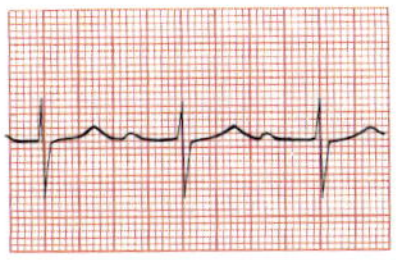

2. *Second degree:* Only *some* beats are conducted through to the ventricles.

   A. *Mobitz type I* (Wenckebach): Progressive prolongation of the PR interval until a QRS is dropped.

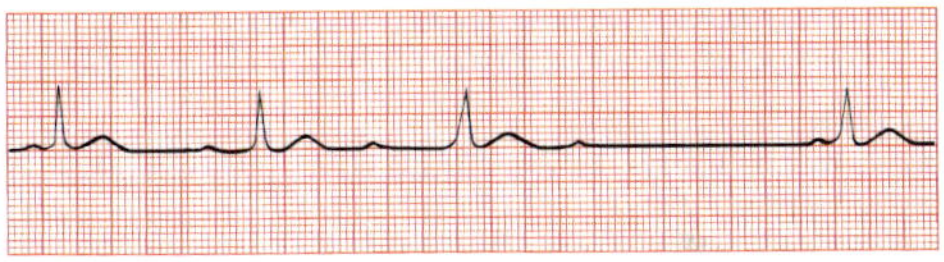

   B. *Mobitz type II:* All-or-nothing conduction, in which QRS complexes are periodically dropped without prolongation of the PR interval.

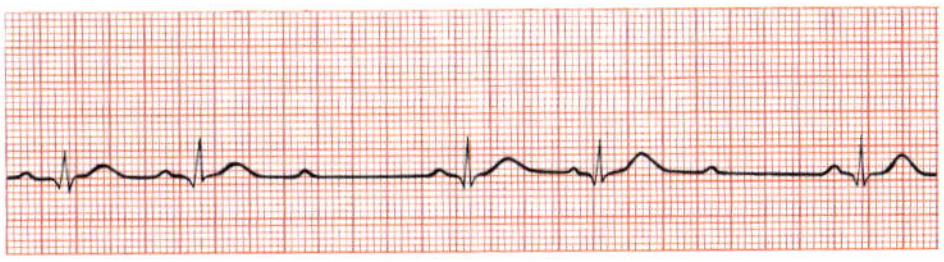

3. *Third degree:* No beats are conducted through to the ventricles. There is complete heart block with AV dissociation. No impulses reach the ventricles from above, and the ventricles are driven by a ventricular escape rhythm.

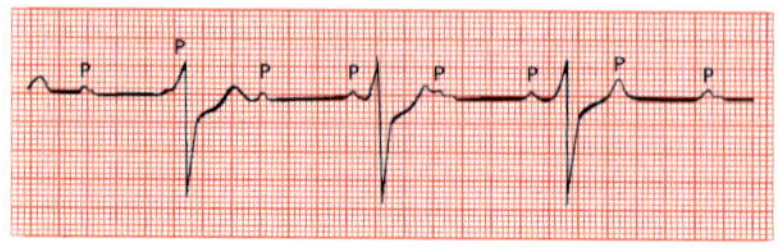

Note: Different degrees of AV block can coexist in the same patient. Thus, for example, a patient can have both first-degree and Mobitz type II heart blocks at different times. Blocks also can be transient—a patient with Lyme carditis can bounce back and forth between different degrees of AV block within seconds!

Bundle-Branch Block

The term *bundle-branch block* refers to a conduction block (or slowing) of current flow in either the left or right bundle branches. The figure below reviews the anatomy of the ventricular bundle branches.

A Quick Review of Ventricular Depolarization

The normal sequence of ventricular activation should be familiar to you by now. The wave of depolarization sweeps out of the AV node and bundle of His into the bundle-branch system. The right and left bundle branches deliver the current to the right and left ventricles, respectively. This is the most efficient means of dispersing the electrical current, and the resultant QRS complex, representing ventricular depolarization from start to finish, is narrow—less than 0.10 seconds in duration. Also, because the muscle mass of the left ventricle is so much larger than that of the right ventricle, left ventricular electrical forces dominate those of the right ventricle, and the resultant electrical axis is leftward, lying between 0° and +90°.

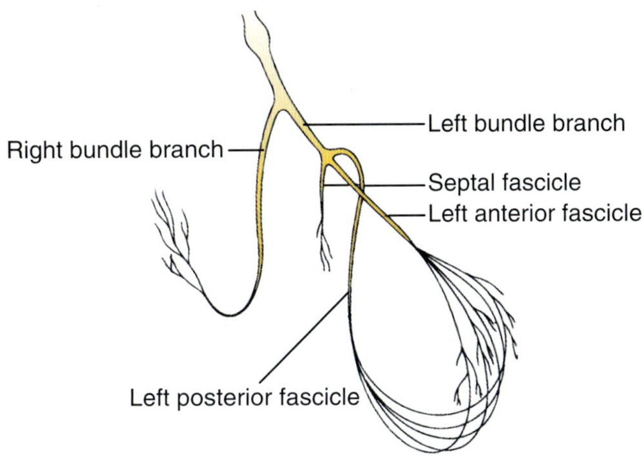

The anatomy of the ventricular bundle branches.

Thus, with normal ventricular depolarization, the QRS complex is narrow, and the electrical axis lies between 0° and 90°. *All of this changes with bundle-branch block.*

Bundle-branch block is diagnosed by looking at the width, axis, and configuration of the QRS complexes.

Right Bundle-Branch Block

In *right bundle-branch block*, conduction through the right bundle is delayed. As a result, right ventricular depolarization is slowed; it does not begin until the left ventricle is almost fully depolarized. This causes two things to happen on the EKG:

1. The delay in right ventricular depolarization prolongs the total time for ventricular depolarization. As a result, the QRS complex widens beyond 0.12 seconds.

2. The wide QRS complex assumes a unique, virtually diagnostic shape in those leads overlying the right ventricle, V1 and V2. The *normal* QRS complex in these leads consists of a small positive R wave, due to normal left-to-right depolarization of the interventricular septum, and a deep negative S wave, reflecting the electrical dominance of the left ventricle. With *right bundle-branch block*, you may still see the initial R and S waves as the left ventricle depolarizes. However, as the right ventricle then begins its delayed depolarization, unopposed by the now fully depolarized and electrically silent left ventricle, the electrical axis of current flow swings sharply back toward the right. This inscribes a *second* R wave, called R′ (pronounced "R prime"), in leads V1 and V2. The whole complex is called RSR′ ("R-S-R prime"), and its appearance has been likened to rabbit or bunny ears. Meanwhile, in the left lateral leads overlying the left ventricle (I, aVL, V5, and V6), late right ventricular depolarization causes reciprocal late deep S waves to be inscribed.

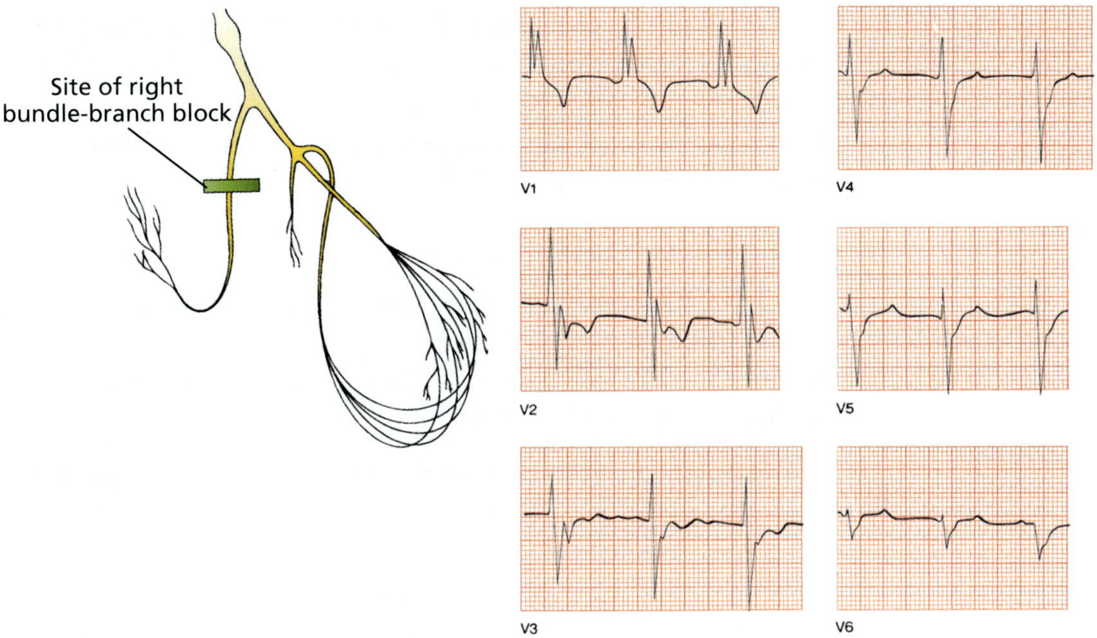

Right bundle-branch block. The QRS complex in lead V1 shows the classic wide RSR′ configuration. Note, too, the S waves in V5 and V6.

In fairness, and in the spirit of full disclosure, you should know that you will not always see a beautiful pair of rabbit ears with right bundle-branch block. Sometimes, as in the tracing below, you will only see tall R waves in leads V1 and V2, but the QRS complexes will certainly be wide.

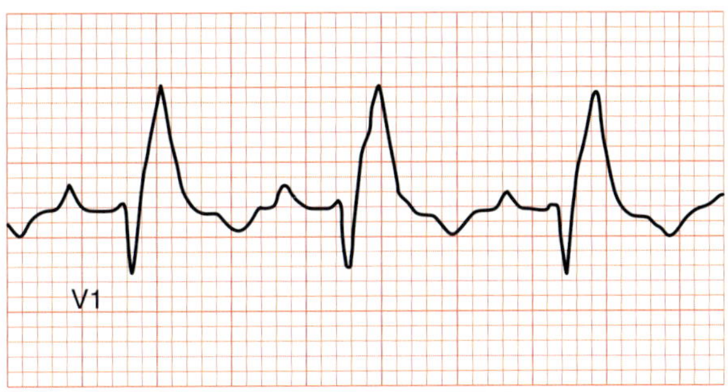

Lead V1 showing right bundle-branch block without rabbit ears but with a tall R wave and wide QRS complex.

Left Bundle-Branch Block

In *left bundle-branch block*, it is *left* ventricular depolarization that is delayed. Again, there are two things to look for on the EKG:

1. The delay in left ventricular depolarization causes the QRS complex to widen beyond 0.12 seconds in duration.
2. The QRS complex in the leads overlying the left ventricle (I, aVL, V5, and V6) will show a characteristic change in shape. The QRS complexes in these leads already have tall R waves. Delayed left ventricular depolarization causes a marked prolongation in the rise of those tall R waves, which will either be broad on top or notched. True rabbit ears are less common than in right bundle-branch block. Those leads overlying the right ventricle, V1 and V2, will show reciprocal, broad, deep S waves. The left ventricle is so dominant in left bundle-branch block that left axis deviation may also be present, but this is variable.

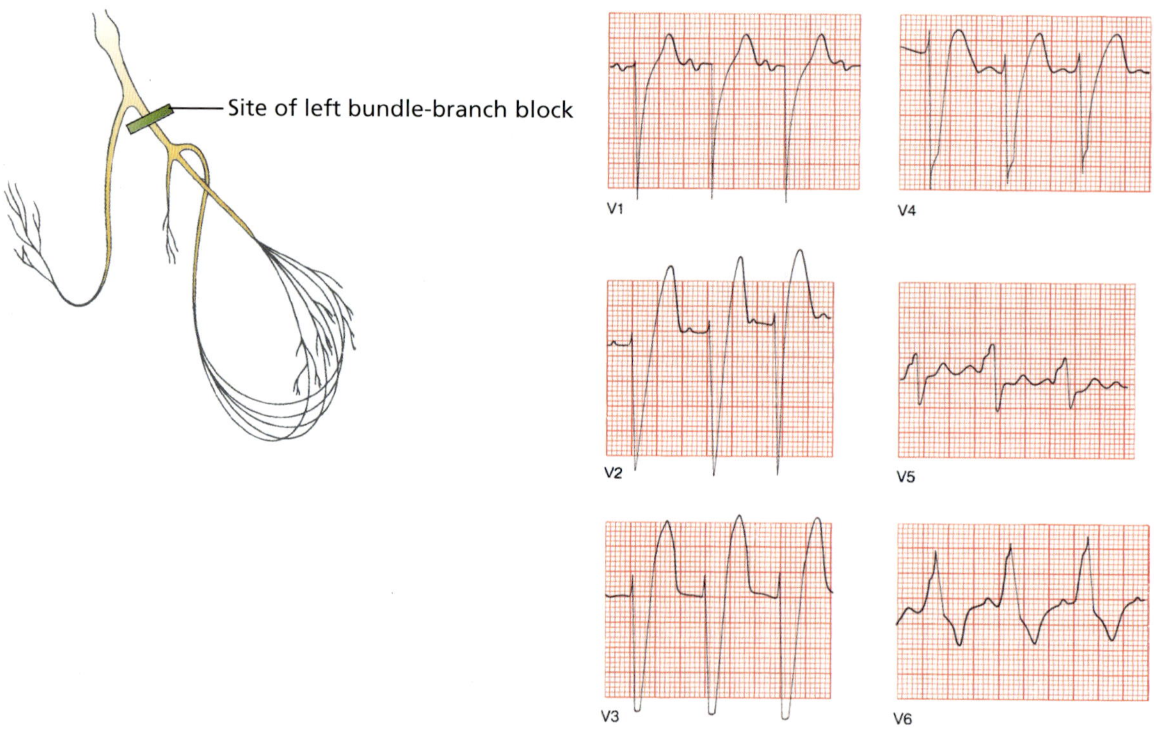

Left bundle-branch block.

Bundle-Branch Block and Repolarization

In the previous EKGs, did you notice the depressed ST segments and flipped T waves in leads V1 through V3 with right bundle-branch block and in leads V5 and V6 with left bundle-branch block? These ST-segment and T-wave changes occur because the *repolarization* sequence is also affected by the conduction block.

In right bundle-branch block, the right precordial leads will show ST-segment depression and T-wave inversion, just like the repolarization abnormalities we saw with ventricular hypertrophy (see page 100).

Similarly, in left bundle-branch block, ST-segment depression and T-wave inversion can be seen in the left lateral leads.

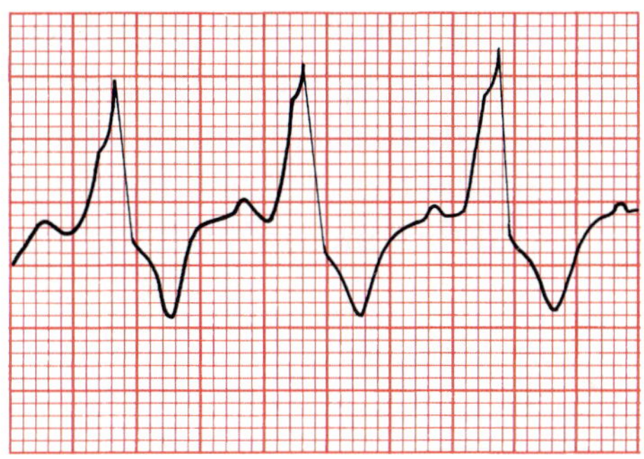

ST-segment depression and T-wave inversion in lead V6 in a patient with left bundle-branch block.

Who Gets Bundle-Branch Blocks?

Although right bundle-branch block can be caused by diseases of the conducting system, it is also a fairly common phenomenon in otherwise normal hearts.

Left bundle-branch block, on the other hand, rarely occurs in normal hearts and almost always reflects underlying cardiac disease, such as degenerative disease of the conduction system or ischemic coronary artery disease.

Critical Rate

Both right and left bundle-branch blocks can be intermittent or fixed. In some individuals, bundle-branch block only appears when a particular heart rate, called the *critical rate*, is achieved. In other words, the ventricles conduct the electrical impulse normally at slow heart rates, but above a certain rate, bundle-branch block develops.

The development of a rate-related bundle-branch block is directly related to the time it takes a particular bundle branch to repolarize and thus prepare itself for the next electrical impulse to arrive. If the heart rate is so rapid that a particular bundle branch cannot repolarize in time, there will be a temporary block to conduction, resulting in the classic EKG appearance of a rate-related bundle-branch block.

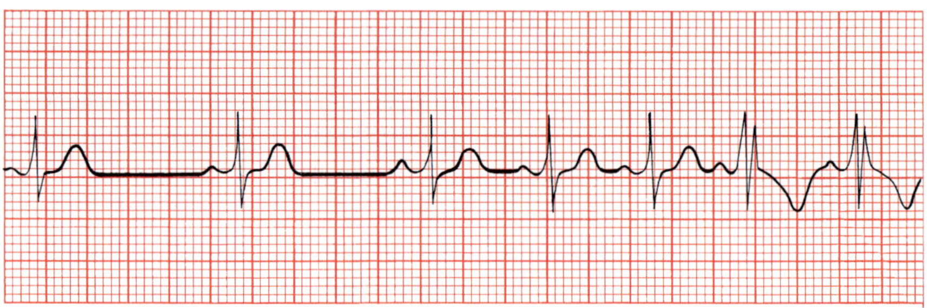

An example of critical rate (lead V2). As the heart accelerates, the pattern of right bundle-branch block appears.

The occurrence of rate-related bundle-branch block depends on the same physiology that accounts for aberrant conduction of supraventricular arrhythmias (see page 173), in which the aberrantly conducted supraventricular beat results from some portion of the bundle branch system failing to repolarize in a timely fashion.

SUMMARY

Bundle-Branch Block

Bundle-branch block is diagnosed by looking at the width and configuration of the QRS complexes.

Criteria for right bundle-branch block

1. QRS complex widened to >0.12 seconds
2. RSR′ (rabbit ears) or a tall R wave in V1 and V2 with ST-segment depression and T-wave inversion
3. Reciprocal changes in V5, V6, I, and aVL

Criteria for left bundle-branch block

1. QRS complex widened to >0.12 seconds
2. Broad or notched R wave with prolonged upstroke in leads V5, V6, I, and aVL, with ST-segment depression and T-wave inversion
3. Reciprocal changes in V1 and V2
4. Left axis deviation may be present

Note: Because bundle-branch block affects the size and appearance of R waves, the criteria for diagnosing ventricular hypertrophy discussed in Chapter 2 cannot be used when bundle-branch block is present. Specifically, right bundle-branch block precludes the diagnosis of right ventricular hypertrophy, and left bundle-branch block precludes the diagnosis of left ventricular hypertrophy. In addition, the diagnosis of a myocardial infarction can be extremely difficult in the presence of left bundle-branch block; we will see why in Chapter 6.

Hemiblocks

Here again is a picture of the ventricular conduction system. The left bundle branch is composed of three separate fascicles—the septal fascicle, the left anterior fascicle, and the left posterior fascicle. The term *hemiblock* refers to a conduction block of just one of these fascicles. The right bundle branch does not divide into separate fascicles; thus, the concept of hemiblock only applies to the left ventricular conducting system.

Septal blocks need not concern us here. Hemiblocks of the anterior and posterior fascicles, however, are both common and important.

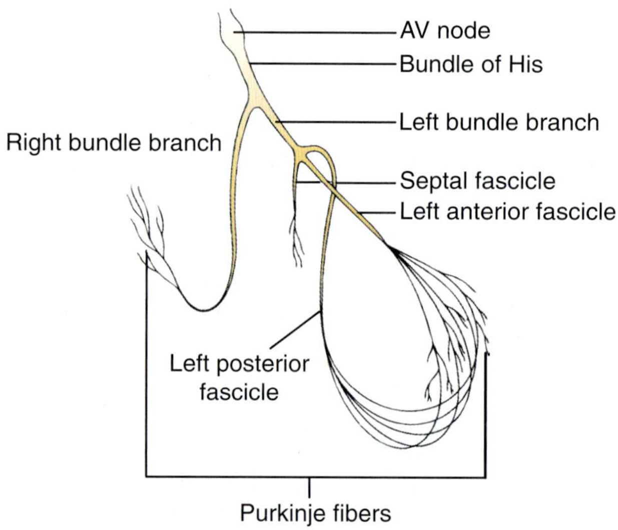

The ventricular conduction system. The right bundle branch remains intact, whereas the left bundle branch divides into three separate fascicles.

Hemiblocks Cause Axis Deviation

The major effect that hemiblocks have on the EKG is *axis deviation.* Here is why.

As illustrated on the previous page, the left anterior fascicle lies superiorly and laterally to the left posterior fascicle. With *left anterior hemiblock*, conduction down the left anterior fascicle is blocked. All the current, therefore, rushes down the left posterior fascicle to the inferior surface of the heart. Left ventricular myocardial depolarization then occurs, progressing in an inferior-to-superior and right-to-left direction.

The axis of ventricular depolarization is therefore redirected upward and slightly leftward, inscribing tall positive R waves in the left lateral leads and deep S waves inferiorly. This results in *left axis deviation* in which the electrical axis of ventricular depolarization is redirected between −30° and −90°.

Do you remember how to identify left axis deviation? The simplest method is to look at the QRS complex in leads I and aVF. The QRS complex will be positive in lead I and negative in lead aVF. However, this analysis will define a range from 0° to −90°, and the diagnosis of left anterior hemiblock requires left axis deviation of greater than −30°. Therefore, look at lead II, which is angled at +60°; if its QRS complex is negative, then the axis must lie more negative than −30°.

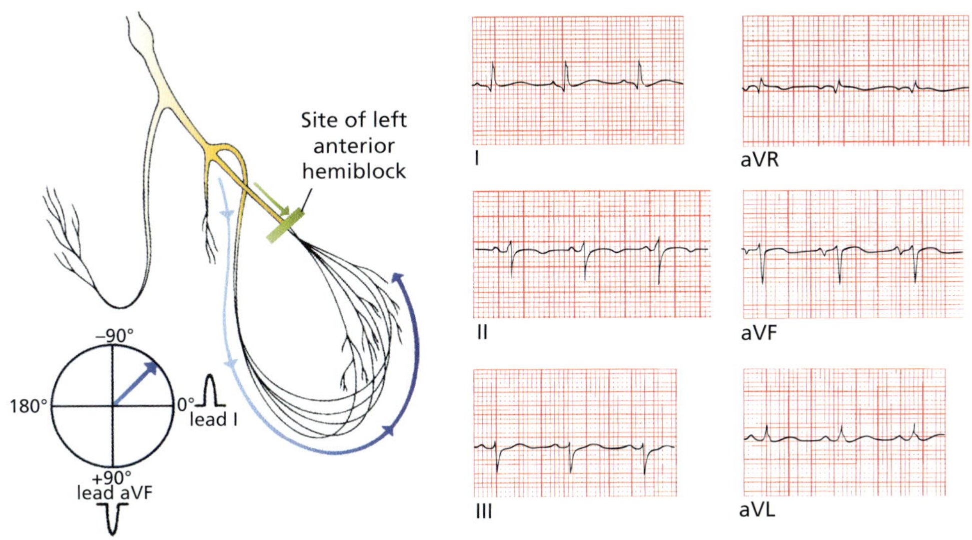

Left anterior hemiblock. Current flow down the left anterior fascicle is blocked; hence, all the current must pass down the posterior fascicle. The resultant axis is redirected upward and leftward (left axis deviation).

There are many causes of left axis deviation. Can you think of one we have previously discussed? How about left ventricular hypertrophy? And there are others that we have yet to explore. **You can only diagnose left anterior hemiblock when no other cause of left axis deviation is present.**

In *left posterior hemiblock*, the reverse occurs. All of the current rushes down the left anterior fascicle, and ventricular myocardial depolarization then ensues in a superior-to-inferior and left-to-right direction. The axis of depolarization is therefore directed downward and rightward, writing tall R waves inferiorly and deep S waves in the left lateral leads. The result is *right axis deviation* (ie, the electrical axis of ventricular depolarization is between +90° and 180°). The QRS complex will be negative in lead I and positive in lead aVF.

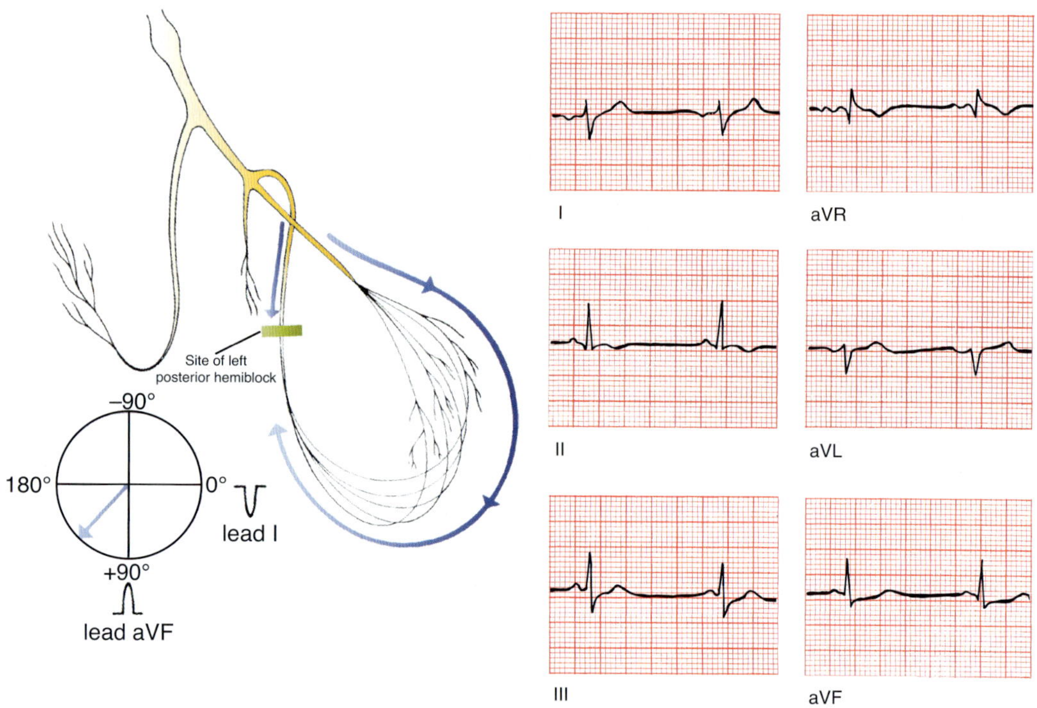

Left posterior hemiblock. Current flow down the left posterior fascicle is blocked; hence, all the current must pass down the right anterior fascicle. The resultant axis is redirected downward and rightward (right axis deviation).

Just as in the case of left axis deviation with left anterior hemiblock, there are other causes of right axis deviation than just left posterior hemiblock. One common cause is chronic lung disease, which we will encounter in Chapter 7. **You can only diagnose left posterior hemiblock if no other cause of right axis deviation is present.**

Hemiblocks Do Not Prolong the QRS Complex

Whereas the QRS complex is widened in *complete* left and right bundle-branch block, the QRS duration in both left anterior and left posterior hemiblocks is normal. (Actually, there is a very minor prolongation, but not enough to widen the QRS complex appreciably.) There are also no ST-segment and T-wave repolarization changes.

Left anterior hemiblock is far more common than left posterior hemiblock, possibly because the anterior fascicle is longer and thinner and has a more tenuous blood supply than the posterior fascicle. Left anterior hemiblock can be seen in both normal and diseased hearts, whereas left posterior hemiblock is virtually the exclusive province of sick hearts.

Is hemiblock present in the following EKG?

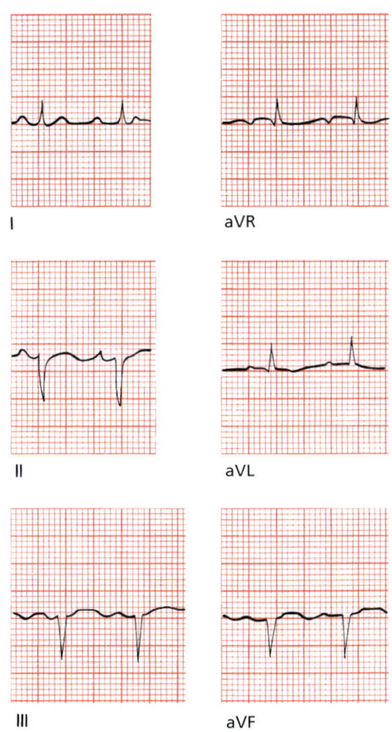

Left axis deviation >–30° seen in a patient with left anterior hemiblock.

Remember, before settling on the diagnosis of hemiblock, it is always necessary to make sure that other causes of axis deviation, such as ventricular hypertrophy, are not present. For most individuals, however, if the tracing is normal except for the presence of axis deviation, you can feel reasonably confident that hemiblock is responsible.

Criteria for Hemiblock

Hemiblock is diagnosed by looking for left or right axis deviation.

Left Anterior Hemiblock

1. Normal QRS duration and no ST-segment or T-wave changes.
2. Left axis deviation between −30° and −90° (tall R wave in lead I and a small R wave and deep S wave in lead II).
3. No other cause of left axis deviation is present.

Left Posterior Hemiblock

1. Normal QRS duration and no ST-segment or T-wave changes.
2. Right axis deviation (small R wave and deep S wave in lead I and tall R wave in lead aVF).
3. No other cause of right axis deviation is present.

Combining Right Bundle-Branch Block and Hemiblocks

Right bundle-branch block and hemiblocks can occur together. The term *bifascicular block* refers to the combination of right bundle-branch block with either left anterior or left posterior hemiblock. The EKG findings include a combination of features of both hemiblock and right bundle-branch block. Patients with this combination are at increased risk of progressing to complete heart block.

Criteria for Bifascicular Block

The features of right bundle-branch block combined with left anterior hemiblock are as follows:

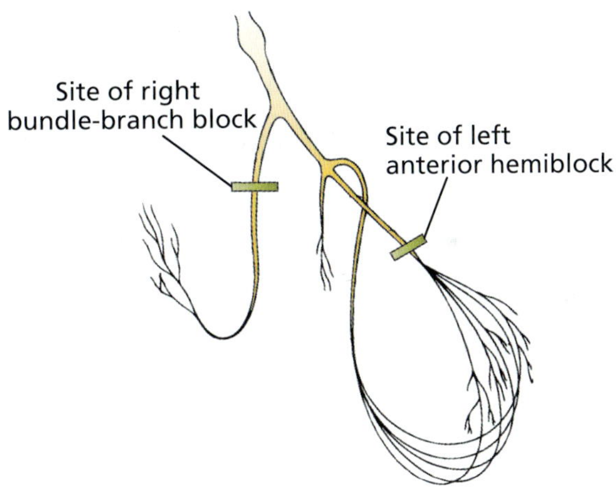

Right Bundle-Branch Block

- QRS wider than 0.12 seconds
- RSR′ in V1 and V2

Left Anterior Hemiblock

- Left axis deviation between −30° and −90°

The features of right bundle-branch block combined with left posterior hemiblock are as follows:

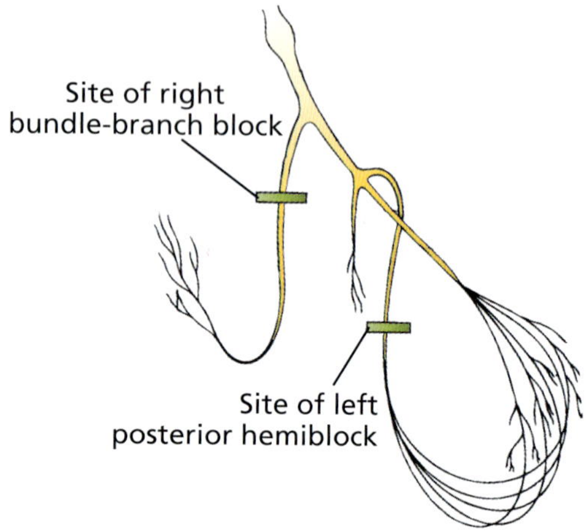

Right Bundle-Branch Block

- QRS wider than 0.12 seconds
- RSR′ in V1 and V2

Left Posterior Hemiblock

- Right axis deviation

Can you identify a bifascicular block on this EKG?

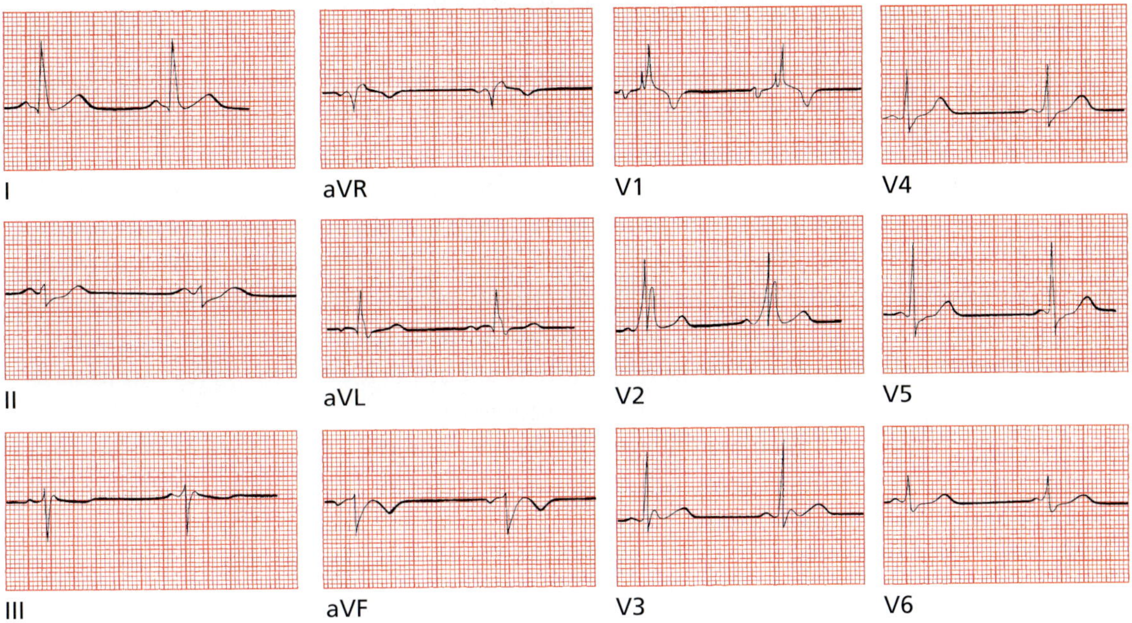

This is an example of right bundle-branch block combined with left anterior hemiblock. Note the widened QRS complex and rabbit ears in leads V1 and V2, characteristic of right bundle-branch block, and the left axis deviation in the limb leads (the QRS complex is predominantly positive in lead I and negative in leads aVF and II) that suggests left anterior hemiblock.

Blocks That Underachieve

Not every conduction block meets all the criteria for a bundle-branch block or bifascicular block. These are extremely common and generally fall into two types:

A *nonspecific intraventricular conduction delay* (abbreviated IVCD) is said to occur when there is QRS widening >0.10 seconds without the other criteria for either bundle-branch block or bifascicular block.

An *incomplete bundle-branch block* is said to occur when the EKG tracing shows a left or right bundle branch appearance (eg, rabbit ears in V1 in right bundle-branch block), but the QRS duration is between 0.10 and 0.12 seconds.

These conduction blocks are caused by the same disease processes that cause the other conduction blocks.

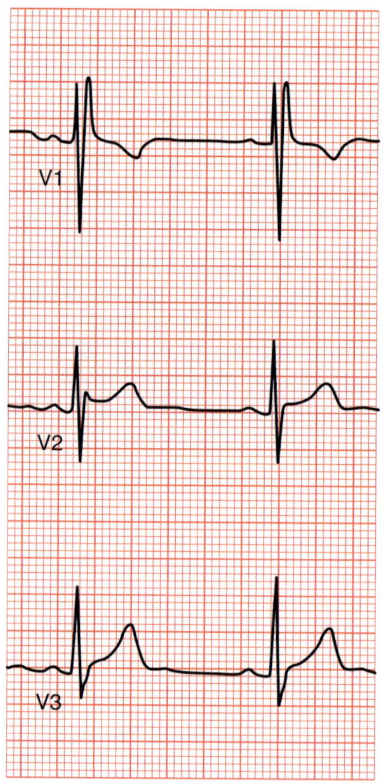

Incomplete right bundle-branch block; the QRS complex is not widened beyond 0.12 seconds, but note the classic rabbit ears configuration in leads V1 and V2.

The Ultimate in Playing With Blocks: Combining AV Blocks, Right Bundle-Branch Block, and Hemiblocks

Right bundle-branch block, hemiblocks, and bifascicular blocks can also occur in combination with AV blocks. (Are you sure you're ready for this?) Take a look at the following EKG and see if you can identify the different conduction blocks that are present. An orderly approach is essential.

1. Is there an AV block? Look at the relationship between the P waves and QRS complexes.
2. Is there a bundle-branch block? Look in the precordial leads for wide QRS complexes with their distinctive configurations; are there any ST-segment and T-wave changes?
3. Is there a hemiblock? Look for axis deviation.

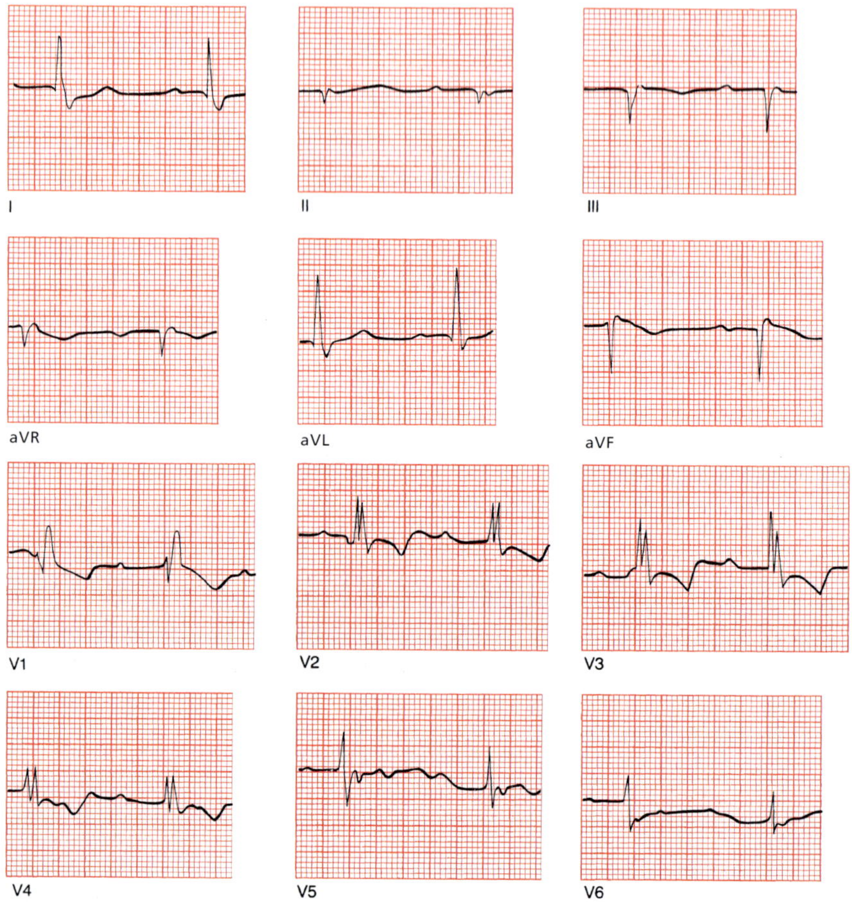

This EKG shows:

1. First-degree AV block (the PR interval exceeds 0.20 seconds)
2. Right bundle-branch block (there are wide QRS complexes with rabbit ears in leads V1 through V4)
3. Left anterior hemiblock (left axis deviation is present)

Pacemakers

Many pacemakers, both temporary and permanent, are inserted every year, and in the right circumstances, they can relieve symptoms of inadequate cardiac output and prevent sudden death from a complete conduction block. Clinical evidence strongly supports their use in patients with:

- third-degree (complete) AV block
- a lesser degree of AV block or bradycardia (eg, sick sinus syndrome) if the patient is symptomatic (especially in atrial fibrillation)
- the sudden development of various combinations of AV block and bundle-branch block in patients who are in the throes of an acute myocardial infarction (this situation usually only requires a temporary pacemaker that can be removed after the acute incident has resolved)
- recurrent ventricular tachycardias that can be overdriven and thereby terminated by pacemaker activity
- a patient who has strong indication for therapy with an AV nodal blocker, for example, a high burden of PVCs, but who is unable to use these drugs without developing a clinically intolerable bradycardia (shortness of breath, dizziness, etc.)

Pacemakers are nothing more than a power source controlled by a microchip and connected to electrodes. The power source is usually placed subcutaneously, and the electrodes are threaded into the right atrium and right ventricle through veins that drain to the heart. Pacemakers provide an alternate source of electrical stimulation for a heart whose own intrinsic source of electricity (the sinus node) or whose ability to conduct electrical current is impaired.

Whereas early pacemakers were capable of firing only at a single predetermined rate (*fixed rate pacemakers*) no matter what the heart itself was doing, today's pacemakers are responsive to the moment-to-moment needs of the heart. They are programmable in terms of sensitivity, rate of firing, refractory period, and so on. The present generation of pacemakers can also increase the heart rate in response to movement for those patients who cannot increase their own heart rate appropriately during activity, either because of disease of the sinus node or the effects of medications; this pacemaker function is referred to as *rate response*.

The most widely used pacemaker is a *demand pacemaker*. A demand pacemaker fires only when the patient's own intrinsic heart rate falls below a threshold level. For example, a demand pacemaker set at 60 beats per minute will remain silent as long as the patient's heart rate remains above 60 beats per minute. As soon as there is a pause between beats that translates into a rate below 60, the pacemaker will fire.

Pacemaker electrodes can be placed in the atrium or ventricle alone (single-chamber pacemakers) or, more commonly, in both chambers (dual-chamber pacemakers). Dual-chamber pacemakers are also called A-V sequential pacemakers.

Among the recent developments in pacemaker technology is the leadless pacemaker, a self-contained pacemaker placed through the femoral vein and screwed into the right ventricle. This type of pacemaker eliminates the need for any leads and for any incisions. At present, these devices pace only in the ventricles, but newer technologies are under development to allow for atrial pacing and even for coordination between leadless devices in the atria and ventricles.

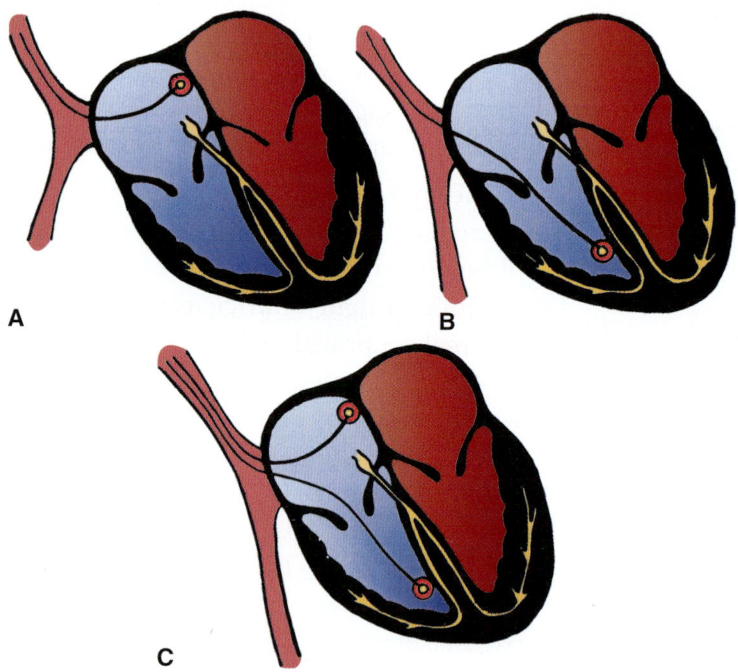

(*A*) Site of atrial pacemaker implantation. (*B*) Ventricular pacemaker. (*C*) Sequential pacemaker with atrial and ventricular leads.

When a pacemaker fires, a small spike can be seen on the EKG (be careful not to confuse these with the transition lines used to separate the tracings of the different leads that are present on most EKGs). With a ventricular pacemaker, the ensuing QRS complex will be wide and bizarre, just like a PVC. Because the electrodes are located in the right ventricle, the right ventricle will contract first, and then the left ventricle. This generates a pattern identical to left bundle-branch block, with delayed left ventricular activation. A retrograde P wave may or may not be seen.

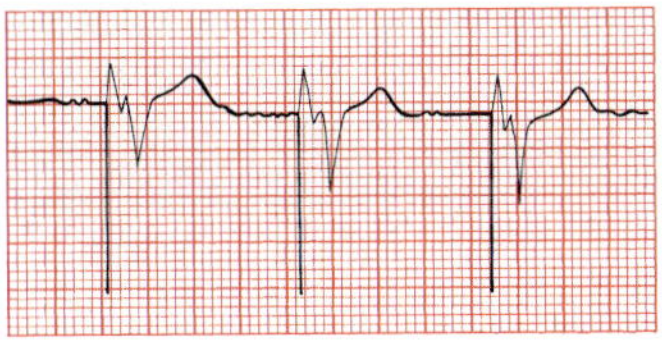

EKG from a patient with a ventricular pacemaker. The sharp downward line is the pacemaker spike.

An atrial pacemaker will generate a spike followed by a P wave, a normal PR interval, and a normal QRS complex.

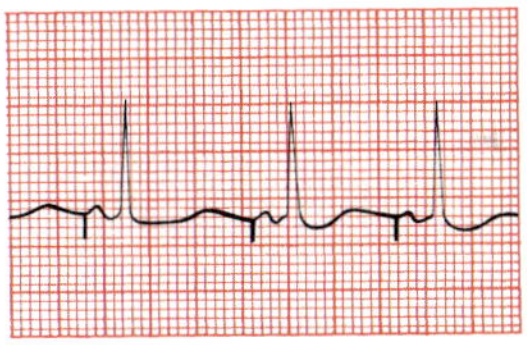

EKG from a patient with an atrial pacemaker.

With a sequential pacemaker, two spikes will be seen, one preceding a P wave and one preceding a wide, bizarre QRS complex.

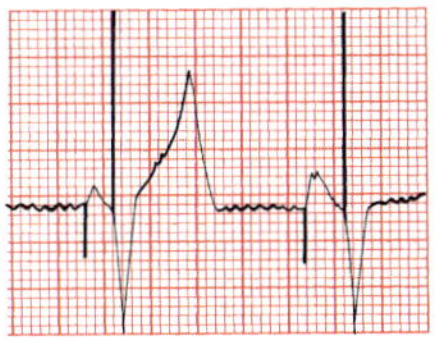

EKG from a patient with an AV sequential pacemaker.

In some patients, pacemaker spikes can be difficult to see on a standard EKG because their amplitude may be very small. If you are examining an EKG from a patient unknown to you that demonstrates wide QRS complexes and left axis deviation, you must always suspect the presence of a pacemaker even if the tiny pacemaker spikes cannot be seen. Obviously, examination of the patient, a review of the chest x-ray, or—if the patient is lucid—a simple question or two will reveal the presence or absence of an electrical pacemaker.

CASE 5

Sally M. works at your hospital as a volunteer. One day, she is instructed to take some intravenous solutions from the pharmacy in the hospital basement to the intensive care unit (ICU) on the third floor. At the same time, you just happen to be standing at the third-floor elevator, waiting impatiently for a ride down to the cafeteria. When the elevator door opens, you find Sally collapsed on the floor. A quick assessment of her vital signs reveals that she is breathing adequately, has a strong pulse, and is slightly tachycardic. You grab a gurney that is conveniently parked nearby and rush her to the ICU.

On the way to the unit, you try talking to her. She is confused and disoriented, and you notice that she has been incontinent. In the ICU, this rhythm strip is obtained.

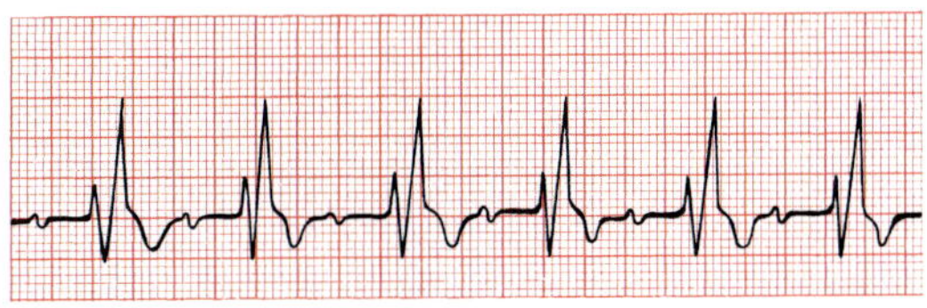

V1

Does this rhythm strip tell you what happened to Sally on the elevator?

In a word, no. The rhythm strip reveals a modest sinus tachycardia, first-degree AV block, and the rabbit ears of right bundle-branch block. Nothing here can account for her collapse. Had you found significant bradycardia, a ventricular arrhythmia, or an advanced degree of heart block, you would certainly have cause to suspect Stokes–Adams syncope, a sudden faint from inadequate cardiac output. The prolonged period of disorientation following her collapse is also not typical of Stokes–Adams syncope but is much more indicative of the postictal state seen after a seizure.

About 15 minutes after her collapse, Sally's mental state has returned to normal, and she is anxious to return to work. You are able to persuade her that a short stay in the ICU for observation would be a good idea. Continual cardiac monitoring reveals no significant arrhythmias or conduction blocks, but a magnetic resonance imaging (MRI) scan of her head reveals a meningioma. It is likely, therefore, that Sally suffered a seizure caused by an expanding (but fortunately not malignant) brain lesion. The meningioma is excised without complication, and several months later, you see Sally happily plying her trade once again, a joyful reminder to all that performing a service for others is the surest way to achieve true satisfaction in life.

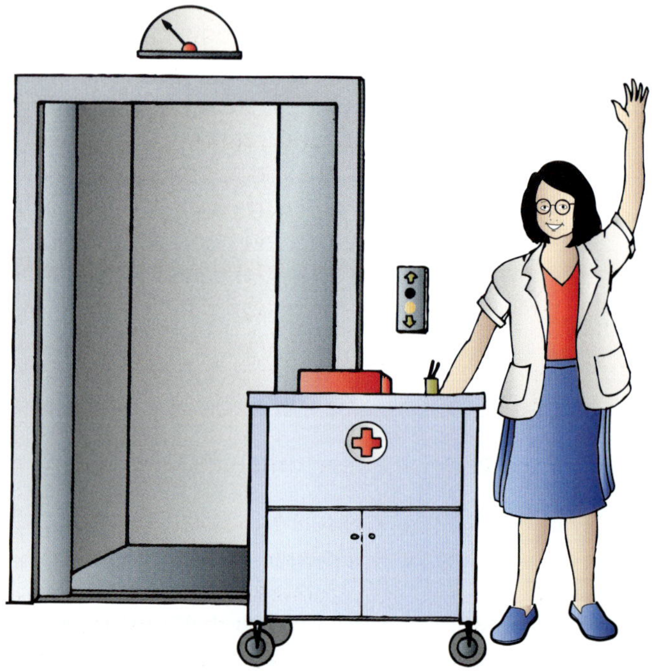

CASE 6

Jamar N., dressed in a magnificent three-piece bespoke suit and wearing hand-sewn shoes whose cost could fund an overseas medical clinic for a month, is the chief executive officer of a large investment firm, a position he describes as "more stressful than anything you, my friend, could ever imagine." He is new to your practice and tells you that he has recently been suffering from some exertional shortness of breath but doesn't have time for "all the nonsense of a history and physical." He insists that you simply run an EKG and tell him if he is having a heart attack. Taking a deep breath, you hook him up to your EKG machine. The 12-lead EKG does not show any acute ischemia, but lead V1 does show this:

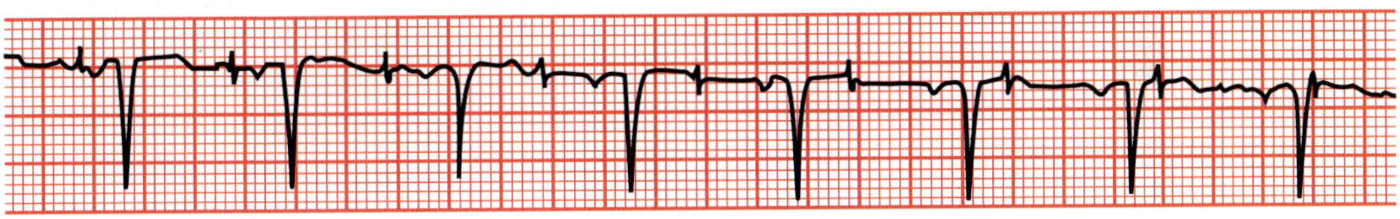

What do you see, what do you infer, and what do you do?

The most striking finding is the procession of pacemaker spikes marching across the EKG bearing no relation whatsoever to the P waves and QRS complexes. The pacemaker is failing to capture the heart. You can infer a heart history that required the pacemaker in the first place. Because the rate and rhythm appear to be otherwise well maintained, it is not at all clear that this consummate executive's shortness of breath is related to the failure of the pacemaker to adequately capture and drive the heart. What you do, of course, is now insist on a careful history and physical examination to guide your next move (you are not surprised when you discover that he has a history of high degrees of AV block that necessitated placement of the pacemaker, and a prior myocardial infarction, items he neglected to mention in your initial conversation).

CASE 7

Jeong O. is a 60-year-old biochemist who presents to your office with fever, chills, and dysuria. Her history is notable for a prior aortic valve replacement several years ago for a congenital bicuspid valve. You suspect urosepsis—soon confirmed—but you also hear a loud systolic murmur and a prominent diastolic murmur on cardiac auscultation, consistent with aortic valve stenosis and insufficiency. Her EKG is shown below—what do you see?

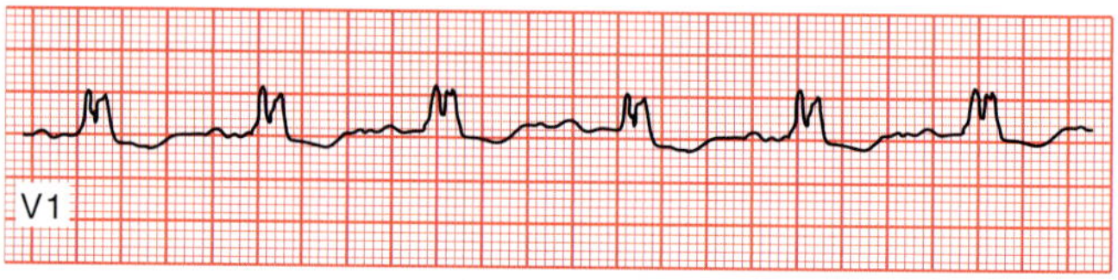

Her EKG shows a normal PR interval (look closely; the P waves are tiny, but they are there) and the classic rabbit ears of right bundle-branch block. Fortunately, you have an old EKG taken a year ago, and it appears identical.

Based on her history and physical, you suspect bacterial endocarditis (fever, chills, and new heart murmurs in someone with a valve replacement), you draw blood cultures and send her to the hospital. An echocardiogram reveals an aortic valve vegetation, and the blood cultures grow out *Enterococcus Faecium*, a common culprit in this setting. Antibiotics are begun, and an EKG taken 24 hours later looks like this—now what do you see?

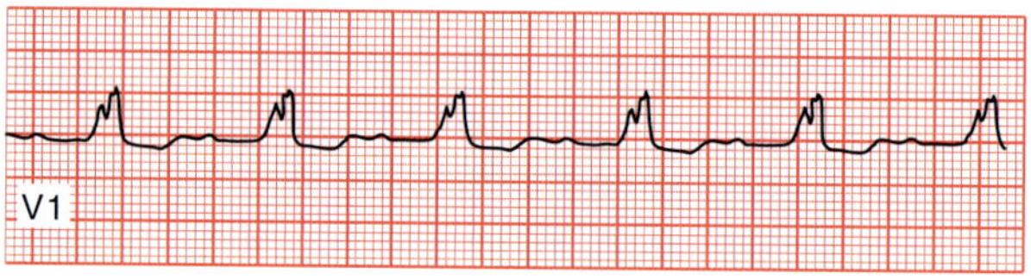

Her PR interval has increased—she now has first-degree AV block. Although in most settings this is a benign finding, in a patient with bacterial endocarditis it is not and may indicate extension of the infection into the conducting system.* Anatomy fans, please note: The aortic valve lies adjacent to the bundle of His. The infection has extended and is now disrupting electrical conduction. This is a poor prognostic sign and mandates aggressive intervention; in Jeong's case, the need for urgent surgical aortic valve replacement.

---

*Just a quick note: widening of the QRS complex can also be a sign of conduction system disease in endocarditis.

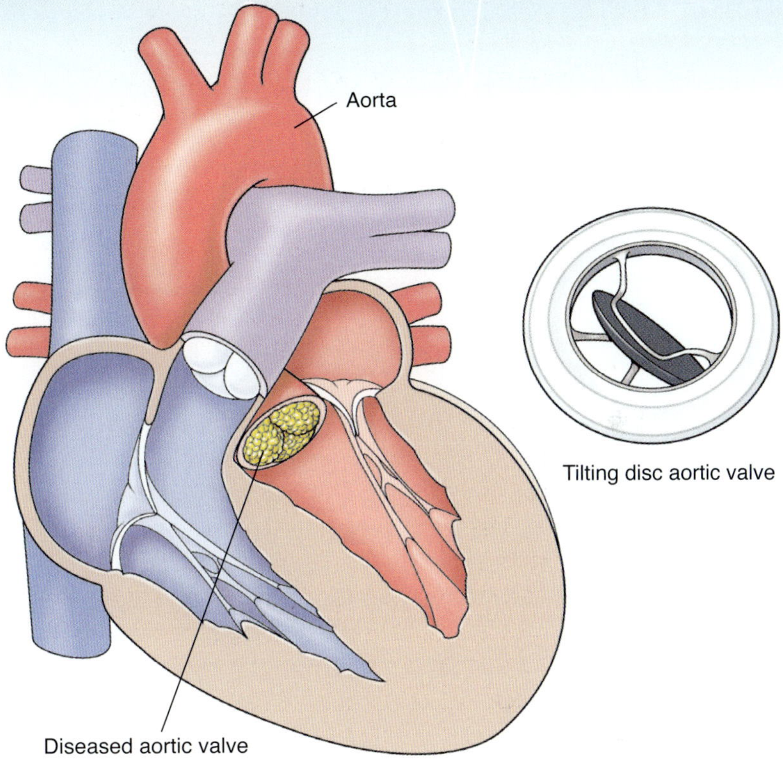

Because of your careful attention to Jeong's EKG and recognition of the relatively subtle progression to first-degree AV block, you have helped to save her life!

5 Preexcitation Syndromes

In this chapter, you will learn:

1. what an accessory pathway is
2. what happens when electrical current is conducted to the ventricles more rapidly than usual
3. that Wolff–Parkinson–White is not the name of a law firm
4. why accessory pathways predispose to arrhythmias
5. about the case of Alejandro T., a *preexcitable* personality

What Is Preexcitation?

In the last chapter, we discussed what happens when conduction from the atria to the ventricles is delayed or blocked. This chapter presents the other side of the coin: what happens when the electrical current is conducted to the ventricles *more quickly than usual.*

How can such a thing happen?

With normal conduction, the major delay between the atria and the ventricles is in the atrioventricular (AV) node, where the wave of depolarization is held up for long enough for the atria to contract and empty their content of circulating blood into the ventricles. In the *preexcitation syndromes*, there are *accessory pathways* by which the current can bypass the AV node and thus arrive at the ventricles without the delay and ahead of time.

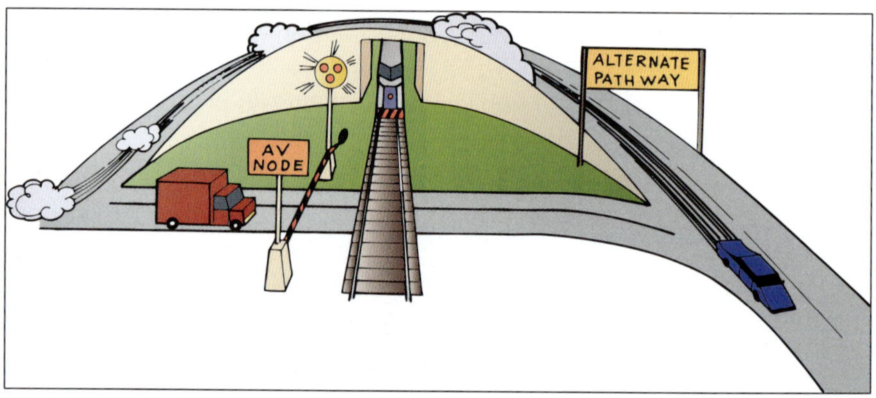

A number of different accessory pathways have been discovered. Probably fewer than 1% of individuals possess one of these pathways. There is a decided male preponderance. Accessory pathways may occur in normal healthy hearts as an isolated finding, or they may occur in conjunction with mitral valve prolapse, hypertrophic cardiomyopathies, and various congenital disorders.

The most important preexcitation syndrome is *Wolff–Parkinson–White (WPW)*. It is named after three gentlemen—Louis Wolff, Sir John Parkinson, and Paul Dudley White—who reported some unusual EKG findings in fourteen otherwise healthy individuals who were experiencing episodes of palpitations and prone to rapid supraventricular tachycardias.

Wolff–Parkinson–White

In WPW, the bypass pathway is a discrete, aberrant conducting pathway that connects the atria and ventricles. It can be left sided (connecting the left atrium and left ventricle), right sided (connecting the right atrium and right ventricle), or even along the septum.

Premature ventricular depolarization through the accessory pathway causes two things to happen on the EKG:

1. The PR interval, representing the time from the start of atrial depolarization to the start of ventricular depolarization, is shortened. The specific criterion for the diagnosis of *a short PR interval is <0.12 seconds (120 ms).*

2. The QRS complex is widened to more than 0.1 second by the presence of what is called a delta wave. Unlike bundle-branch block, in which the QRS complex is widened because of *delayed* ventricular activation, in WPW, it is widened because of *premature* activation. The QRS complex in WPW actually represents a combination (fusion) beat: some of the ventricular myocardium is activated through the normal conduction pathways, and some *is depolarized early* through the accessory pathway. The region of myocardium that is depolarized early gives the QRS complex a characteristic slurred initial upstroke called a *delta wave*. A true delta wave may be seen in only a few leads, so scan the entire EKG.

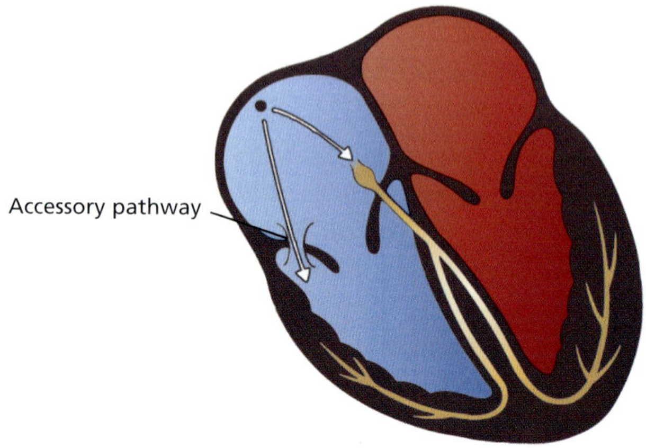

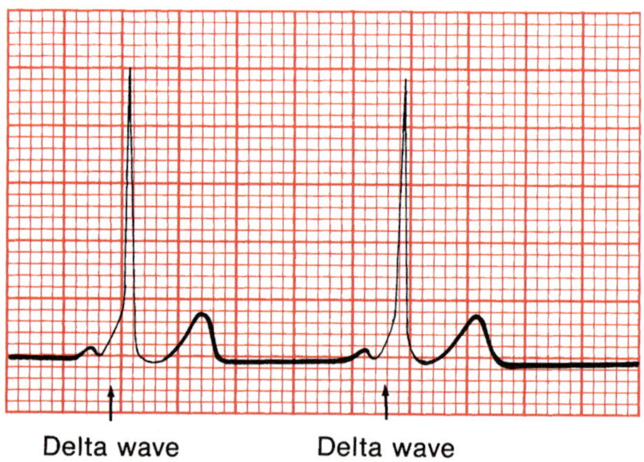

Wolff–Parkinson–White (WPW). Current is held up by the normal delay at the AV node but races unimpeded down the accessory pathway. The EKG shows the short PR interval and delta wave.

A Short PR Interval Without a Delta Wave

Even more common than WPW is the presence of a short PR interval without an accompanying delta wave. No single anatomic pathway has been consistently identified to explain this finding, and it is probably the result of a variety of structural abnormalities. Some patients may have a small bypass pathway within or very close to the AV node. Others may simply have an AV node that conducts more rapidly than normal. Still others may have a low ectopic atrial focus that lies close to the AV node, and thus, has a shorter distance to traverse than normal sinus beats.

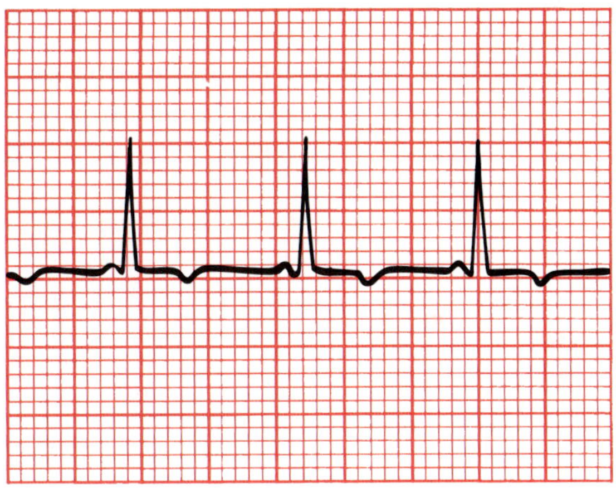

The PR interval is short, but there is no delta wave.

Why Do We Care About Preexcitation?

In many individuals with WPW, preexcitation poses few, if any, clinical problems. However, preexcitation does predisposes to various tachyarrhythmias. Only some individuals with WPW experience at least one supraventricular arrhythmia. These patients may then develop symptoms such as palpitations, shortness of breath, and so on. The presence of both the classic EKG abnormalities and symptoms is referred to as *WPW syndrome.**

The two tachyarrhythmias most often seen in WPW are a *supraventricular tachycardia* and *atrial fibrillation.*

Supraventricular Tachycardia in WPW

In normal hearts, supraventricular tachycardias usually arise through a reentrant mechanism (AV nodal reentrant tachycardia [AVNRT], see page 142). A similar mechanism occurs in WPW.

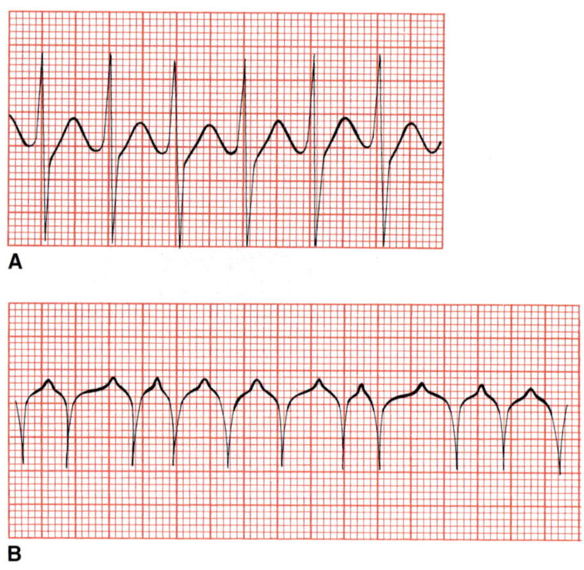

(*A*) Supraventricular tachycardia; note the regular rhythm. (*B*) Atrial fibrillation, with the classic irregularly irregular rhythm.

*The presence of an EKG showing a short PR interval plus a delta wave in a patient without symptoms is referred to as an "EKG with WPW pattern".

In fact, the presence of an accessory bundle—an alternate pathway of conduction—is the *perfect* substrate for reentry. Here is how it works.

One cautionary note: WPW can be intermittent, and the EKG findings can come and go, so your level of suspicion should remain high even in the absence of the classic features we just described.

We have described how, in WPW, a normal beat generates a QRS complex that is a combination of two waves, one conducted through the accessory pathway and one through the AV node and along the normal pathway of conduction. Although the accessory pathway usually conducts current faster than the AV node, it also tends to have a longer refractory period once it has been depolarized. What happens, then, if a normal sinus impulse is followed abruptly by a premature atrial beat? This premature beat will be conducted normally through the AV node, but the accessory pathway may still be refractory, blocking conduction through the alternate route. The wave of depolarization will move through the AV node and into the bundle branches and ventricular myocardium. By the time it encounters the accessory pathway on the ventricular side, the accessory pathway may no longer be refractory, and the current can pass back into the atria. It is then free to pass right back down through the AV node, and a self-sustaining, revolving reentrant mechanism is established. The result is a supraventricular tachycardia. The QRS complex during the arrhythmia is narrow because ventricular depolarization occurs via the normal bundle branches.

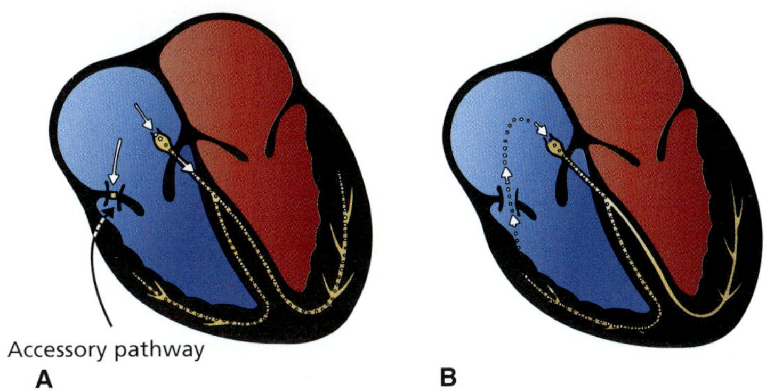

The formation of a reentry circuit in WPW. (*A*) A premature atrial beat sends current down the normal conduction pathways but not through the refractory accessory pathway. (*B*) Current then circles back through the accessory pathway, which is no longer refractory to conduction, forming a complete reentrant circuit.

Less commonly, the reentrant mechanism circles the other way, that is, down the accessory pathway and back up through the AV node. The result, again, is a supraventricular tachycardia, but now, the QRS complex is wide and bizarre because ventricular depolarization does not occur along the normal bundle branches. This arrhythmia may be indistinguishable from ventricular tachycardia on the EKG.

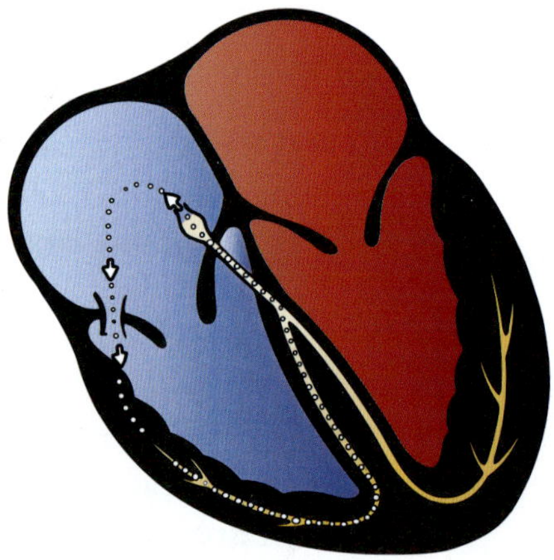

A second type of reentry circuit in WPW. Current moves antegrade down the accessory pathway and then retrograde through the AV node, establishing an independent revolving circuit.

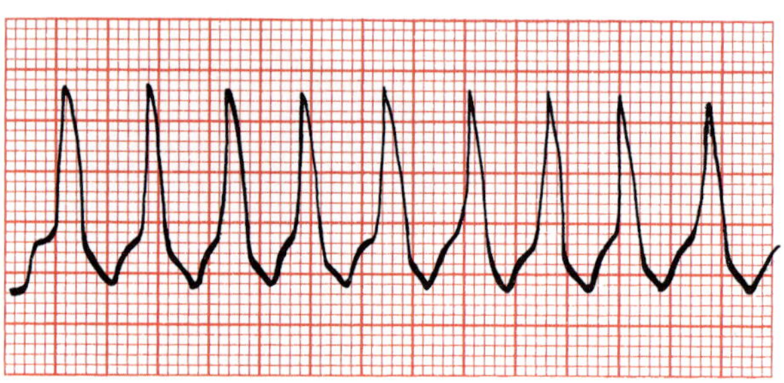

Wide-complex supraventricular tachycardia in WPW.

Let's again recall that the "usual" form of supraventricular tachycardia in normal hearts is most often caused by a reentry loop within the AV node and is called AVNRT. Here, in patients with the WPW pattern on their EKG, because the reentrant loop reciprocates between the atria and ventricles, the arrhythmia is more accurately termed **AV reciprocating tachycardia (AVRT)**. Remember back in Chapter 3 (page 142) that we first mentioned the AVRT is one of the causes of a sustained supraventricular tachycardia, one that we would discuss later? No? Well, I can hardly blame you. But that is what we are talking about now!

When the tachycardia activates the ventricles in an antegrade manner through the AV node, generating a narrow QRS complex, the arrhythmia is further subcategorized as an **orthodromic tachycardia** (the prefix *ortho* conveys the meaning of correct, or orthodox). Reciprocating tachycardias that activate the ventricles through the accessory pathway, generating a wide QRS complex, are subcategorized as **antidromic tachycardia**.

In 10% to 15% of patients with WPW, there is more than one accessory pathway, permitting the formation of multiple reentry loops as the current passes up and down through the different accessory pathways and the AV node.

So what do you do if a hemodynamically unstable patient—whose history you do not know and for whom there is no baseline EKG—shows up in your emergency room with a wide QRS complex tachycardia, and the various techniques we discussed on page 144 don't help you distinguish ventricular tachycardia from a wide complex supraventricular tachycardia? Maybe your patient has WPW, maybe not. You can't rely on looking for delta waves—you will almost never see them in patients with WPW while they are experiencing a supraventricular arrhythmia until you restore them to normal sinus rhythm. The answer is this: Assume the patient has ventricular tachycardia and treat it accordingly. Ventricular tachycardia is much more common than AVRT and can be lethal.

Atrial Fibrillation in WPW

Atrial fibrillation, the other arrhythmia commonly seen in WPW, can be particularly devastating. The accessory pathway can act as a free conduit for the rapid, chaotic atrial activity. Without the AV node to act as a barrier between the atria and ventricles, ventricular rates can rise as high as 300 beats per minute! The precise rate will depend on the refractory period of the accessory pathway.

The QRS complexes often show varying morphology, as some are triggered via normal conduction through the AV node and others via conduction through the accessory pathway. Still others may represent fusion beats fed by both the AV node and accessory pathway at the same time.

This very rapid atrial fibrillation has been known to induce ventricular fibrillation, because of the lack of normal filtering by the AV node and the rapid ventricular response. Fortunately, atrial fibrillation is rare in WPW, but it must be considered a diagnostic possibility in patients who have been resuscitated from an episode of sudden death or syncope and are found to have preexcitation on their cardiograms.

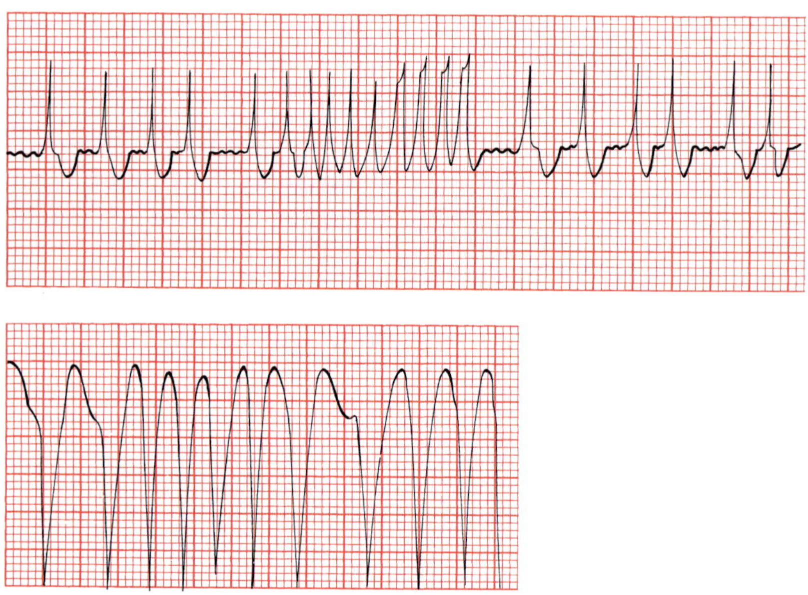

Two examples of atrial fibrillation in WPW. The ventricular rate is extremely fast.

Mapping the aberrant pathways in patients with WPW can be accomplished with an electrophysiology study (EPS) and has become routine in patients who are symptomatic, for example, those with a history of syncope or who have documented arrhythmias. During the mapping procedure, the aberrant pathway can be ablated, thereby resolving the problem.

Patients with WPW have an increased risk of sudden cardiac death, but this is only very rarely its first manifestation, allowing time for successful clinical intervention before an episode of sudden death can occur. The overall prognosis today for patients with WPW is excellent.

Patients with a short PR interval without a delta wave may also have an increased risk of tachyarrhythmias. The risk, however, appears to be exceedingly small, and there is no evidence that these patients are at increased risk of sudden cardiac death. Patients with a short PR interval without delta waves and who have had at least one tachyarrhythmia are said to have Lown–Ganong–Levine (LGL) syndrome.

If you get one take home lesson from this chapter, it is this: Always look for a short PR interval and a delta wave on the EKG of any patient who presents with a history suggestive of a tachyarrhythmia, for example, palpitations or syncope. And look at all 12 leads; you may only see clear-cut delta waves in some of them.

SUMMARY

Preexcitation

The diagnosis of preexcitation is made by looking for a short PR interval.

Criteria for WPW Pattern

1. PR interval <0.12 seconds
2. Wide QRS complexes
3. Delta wave seen in some leads

Arrhythmias may include the following:

1. AVRT—narrow QRS complexes (orthodromic tachycardia) are more common than wide ones (antidromic tachycardia).
2. Atrial fibrillation can be very rapid and rarely can lead to ventricular fibrillation.

Differential Diagnosis of Wide Complex Tachycardias

1. Ventricular tachycardia
2. A supraventricular tachycardia with aberrant conduction (eg, supraventricular tachycardia with underlying bundle-branch block); often rate related, appearing only with fast heart rates
3. AVRT (antidromic tachycardia) in a patient with preexcitation (eg, WPW)
4. Paced rhythms

When you see what appears to be a wide complex tachycardia and you did not run the EKG yourself—for example, if you are looking at the tracing on a hospital monitor—make sure you are not seeing an artifact caused by the patient's activity; it could be caused by something as simple as patients brushing their teeth!

Because the presence of an accessory pathway in WPW alters the vectors of current flow to at least some degree, you cannot assess axis or amplitude with any precision, and hence, any attempt to determine the presence of ventricular hypertrophy or bundle-branch block is bound to be unreliable.

CASE 8

Alejandro T., a young biochemical engineer, is brought to the emergency room by his partner. During dinner, he became light headed and nauseous.

In the emergency room, Alejandro denies any chest pain or shortness of breath.

The medical student who is the first to examine him has seen just enough patients to feel overconfident in his diagnostic abilities. Tired and overworked, he listens to Alejandro's story and is ready to send him home with a diagnosis of food poisoning when an astute nurse takes the trouble to put a hand on his pulse and discovers it is extremely rapid. An EKG reveals the following:

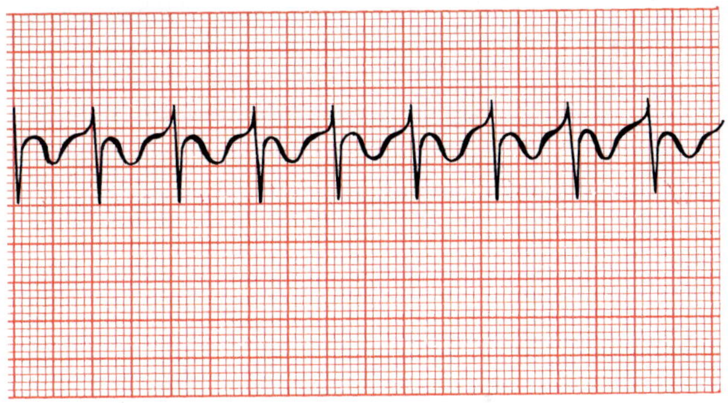

Distraught by his carelessness, the medical student becomes somewhat pallid himself. The emergency room doctor takes over, notes the patient's rapid, regular pulse, glances at the rhythm strip, and immediately orders electrical cardioversion. The tachycardia breaks at once, and the new rhythm strip looks like this:

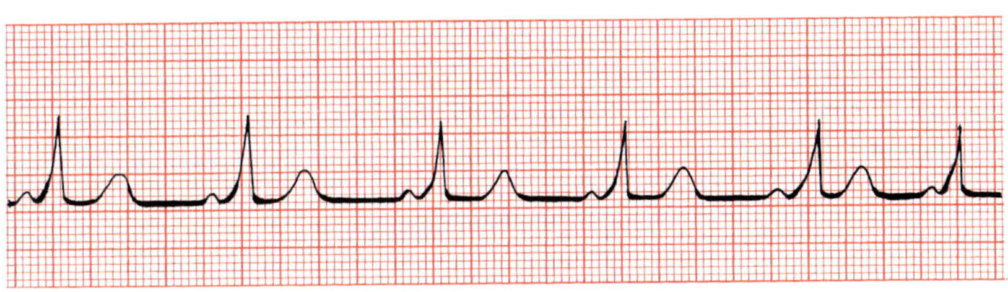

Can you match the emergency room doctor's heady acumen with erudition of your own and figure out exactly what has happened?

Of course you can! Alejandro has WPW. This is readily apparent from the second EKG, which reveals the characteristic short PR interval, delta wave, and prolonged QRS complex. The initial strip shows the typical narrow QRS complex AV reciprocating tachycardia that can occur in these individuals. The rapid tachycardia was responsible for Alejandro's symptoms, not his undercooked Cornish game hen.

This was Alejandro's first attack, and because most patients with WPW have only infrequent episodes of tachycardia, chronic antiarrhythmic therapy is not indicated at this time.

As for what became of the medical student, he learned from his experience and went on to become a model of thoroughness and efficiency, eventually graduating at the top of his class. He also has never forgotten the first rule of medicine: **always take the vital signs**. There is a good reason why they are called "vital."

6 Myocardial Ischemia and Infarction

In this chapter, you will learn:

1 | the three major things that can happen to the EKG during a myocardial infarction (T-wave peaking and inversion, ST-segment elevation or depression, and the appearance of new Q waves)

2 | how to distinguish normal Q waves from the Q waves of infarction

3 | how the EKG can localize an infarct to a particular region of the heart

4 | how to recognize the EKG changes that will allow you to distinguish among the most common acute coronary syndromes, including angina without infarction, ST-segment elevation myocardial infarction (STEMIs) and non–ST-segment elevation myocardial infarction (non-STEMI or NSTEMI)

5 | the value of stress testing in diagnosing coronary artery disease

6 | about the cases of Joan L., who is experiencing an acute myocardial infarction and has a number of complications requiring your acute attention, and Saul S., who feels fine, but what is that we see on his EKG?

Stable Angina and Acute Coronary Syndromes

Let's start by defining a few key terms:

Angina is the classic symptom of cardiac ischemia. Patients most often describe it as diffuse chest pain or pressure that may radiate to the neck, arms, or back and may be accompanied by shortness of breath, nausea, vomiting, dizziness, or diaphoresis (sweating). Some patients with cardiac ischemia may have no chest-related symptoms at all, particularly females, individuals with diabetes, and the elderly.

The underlying pathophysiology in most patients with angina is progressive narrowing of the coronary arteries by atherosclerosis, which impedes blood flow to the heart muscle (other less common causes of angina include, among others, aortic stenosis and hypertrophic cardiomyopathy). With physical exertion, the limited blood supply is inadequate to meet the increased demands of the heart. Although there is variability among patients, blockage of about 70% of the cross-sectional area of the lumen is sufficient to cause exertional angina. Patients whose chest discomfort is brought about only by a given level of exertion (eg, walking up a flight of stairs) and relieved with rest have what is called *stable angina*. These patients are not at immediate risk of a myocardial infarction.

The term *acute coronary syndrome* is used to describe urgent situations when the blood supply to the heart is acutely compromised. Acute coronary syndromes are most often caused by acute rupture or erosion of an atherosclerotic plaque, which in turn prompts the formation of a thrombus in the coronary artery, further limiting or completely blocking blood flow. The result can be either what is called *unstable angina* or a *myocardial infarction* (aka, heart attack).

It is important to know that the *size* of the plaque is less important in the genesis of acute coronary syndrome than the *vulnerability* of the plaque to rupture or erosion. The size of the fibrous cap (thin is dangerous), the extent of the lipid core (large is dangerous), and the presence of inflammatory cells within the plaque can predispose to an unstable plaque with subsequent rupture. Even small plaques can become unstable, rupture, and cause a myocardial infarction (see

Figure on page 254). Why is this important to know? Because neither stress tests—which we will be discussing on page 295—nor standard cardiac catheterizations can tell you if a plaque is stable or unstable, thus limiting their utility in predicting a patient's risk for infarction.

Patients with *unstable angina* experience the same type of symptoms as those with stable angina, but it can occur with much less—or even no—exertion, and is typically more severe and lasts longer. Many of these patients may have a history of stable angina, and a change in their typical pattern of symptoms or the new onset of symptoms at rest is what marks it as unstable.

Myocardial infarctions occur in two basic varieties. If blood flow through a coronary artery is totally occluded, the result can be what we call an *ST-segment elevation myocardial infarction* or *STEMI*. As you might suspect from the name, its most characteristic feature is elevation of the ST segments on the EKG. We'll be talking about the ST segment in diagnosing myocardial infarctions in the pages to come. A STEMI is a true emergency because the heart muscle is starved of blood supply.

If, however, blood flow is reduced but not totally blocked, the result can be either unstable angina or a *non–ST-segment myocardial infarction (non-STEMI or NSTEMI)*. In non-STEMIs and unstable angina, the ST segments do not elevate, may remain normal, but more often are depressed (in the morphologic, not emotional, sense).

So what's the story with these ST segments? They clearly are a key diagnostic feature in diagnosing ischemic heart disease, and we will be spending a lot of time with them in this chapter. Now is therefore a good time to ask why they sometimes elevate and sometimes depress in response to impaired blood flow. The answer is complex and not fully understood, but we know that depriving myocardium of blood flow and oxygen alters the electrical properties of the myocardial cells, leading to voltage gradients between normal myocardium and ischemic myocardium. These gradients create injury currents within the heart tissue, and it is these that appear to move the ST segments one way or another.

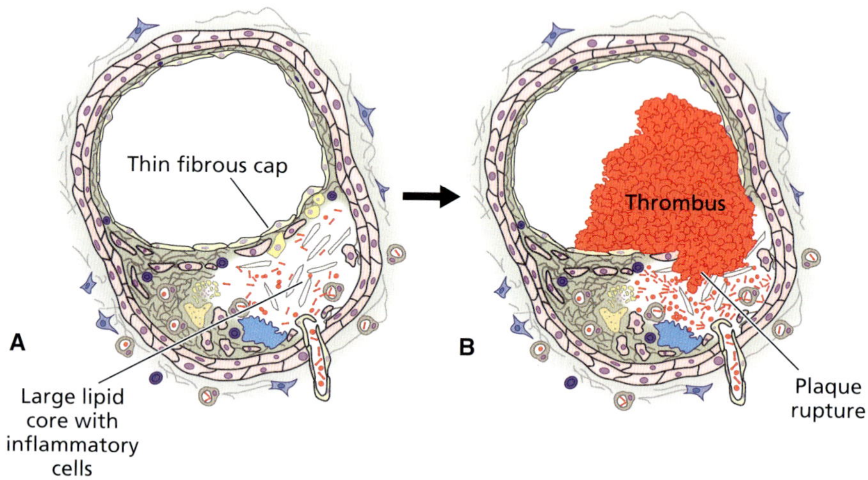

Figure (*A*) shows the lumen of a coronary artery with a vulnerable plaque that has a thin fibrous cap and a thick inflammatory lipid core; Figure (*B*) shows formation of a thrombus at the site of plaque rupture, which can lead to a myocardial infarction.

Not all myocardial infarctions occur because of obstruction of one of the coronary arteries. Some happen when the oxygen demand of the myocardium exceeds the body's ability to deliver the necessary blood supply. These patients may or may not have obstructive coronary artery disease. Causes include extreme tachycardias and severe hypotension due to blood loss (shock). The EKG cannot distinguish between the different causes of heart attack, although the changes on the EKG—as well as the patient's symptoms—tend to be less dramatic when the primary cause is not coronary artery occlusion.

How to Diagnose a Myocardial Infarction

There are three components to the diagnosis of a myocardial infarction: (1) history and physical examination, (2) cardiac enzyme determinations, and (3) the EKG.

History and Physical Examination

When a patient presents with the typical features of infarction—the sudden onset of prolonged, crushing substernal chest pain radiating to the jaw, shoulders, or left arm, associated with nausea, diaphoresis, and shortness of breath—there can be little doubt about the diagnosis. However, many patients may not have all of these symptoms, or their symptoms may be atypical, described instead as burning, a knot in the throat, or a sensation of fullness in the neck. As we stated earlier, some patients may only complain of nausea, shortness of breath, or other symptoms remote from the chest, such as abdominal pain. And it is estimated that up to one-third of all myocardial infarctions are "silent"; that is, they are not associated with any overt clinical manifestations whatsoever. When angina is present, its severity is not an accurate predictor of either the likelihood of a myocardial infarction or the size of the infarct.

Cardiac Enzymes

Dying myocardial cells leak their internal contents into the bloodstream. Historically, elevated blood levels of *creatine kinase* (CK), particularly the MB isoenzyme, were among the first to be used as a diagnostic tool for infarction. Today, elevated levels of the cardiac *troponin* enzymes occupy the prominent role in the laboratory diagnosis of myocardial infarction. Troponin enzyme determinations are the go-to blood test to help rule in or rule out a myocardial infarction. Troponin levels rise earlier than the CK-MB isoenzyme (high-sensitivity troponin assays, now widely available, can start to peak within 1 hour after the onset of an infarction) and may stay elevated for several days. CK levels do not usually rise until 6 hours after an infarction and return to normal within 48 hours.

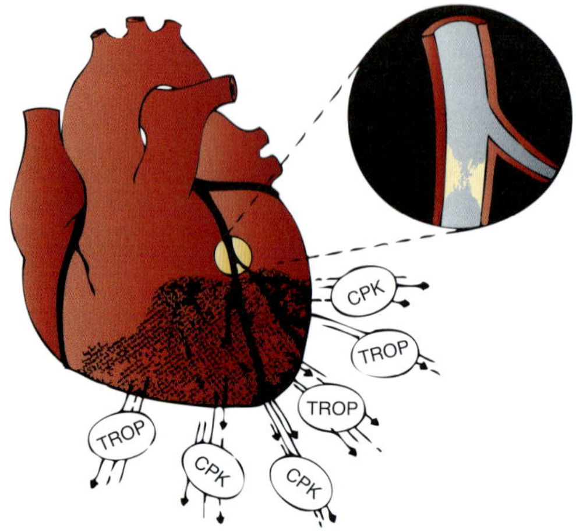

Intracellular enzymes are released by the dying myocardial cells after complete coronary occlusion, resulting in acute infarction.

Although testing for cardiac troponins has increased our ability to diagnose a myocardial infarction, they have by no means supplanted the EKG as an equally valuable tool. In emergency settings, if the EKG shows changes of a STEMI in a patient with a consistent history, no one waits around for the enzyme levels to come back—that patient is off to the catheterization lab!

In addition, cardiac troponins can be elevated in conditions other than an infarction, for example, with pulmonary embolism, sepsis, respiratory failure, and renal impairment. They can also arise from other disorders associated with myocardial injury, such as congestive heart failure, myocarditis, or pericarditis. Thus, although normal troponin levels make it very unlikely that the patient is having a myocardial infarction, false positives are not uncommon. Depending on where you define your cutoff, some patients with an elevated troponin level will prove to have something other than a myocardial infarction.

The EKG

In most infarctions, the EKG will reveal the correct diagnosis. Characteristic electrocardiographic changes accompany a myocardial infarction, and the earliest changes occur almost at once with the onset of myocardial compromise. An EKG should be performed immediately on anyone in whom an infarction is even remotely suspected. However, the initial EKG may not always be diagnostic, and the evolution of electrocardiographic changes varies from person to person; therefore, it is important to obtain serial cardiograms.

> If you suspect a patient may be in the early stages of a myocardial infarction but the EKG is not conclusively diagnostic, repeat the EKG. Most guidelines suggest getting the second EKG 15 to 30 minutes after the first, and even getting a third or fourth, if necessary. As many as 20% of STEMIs are diagnosed only on a repeat EKG.

ST-Segment Elevation Myocardial Infarctions

During an acute STEMI, the EKG evolves through three stages:

1. T-wave peaking followed by T-wave inversion (*A* and *B*, below)
2. ST-segment elevation (*C*)
3. The appearance of new Q waves (*D*)

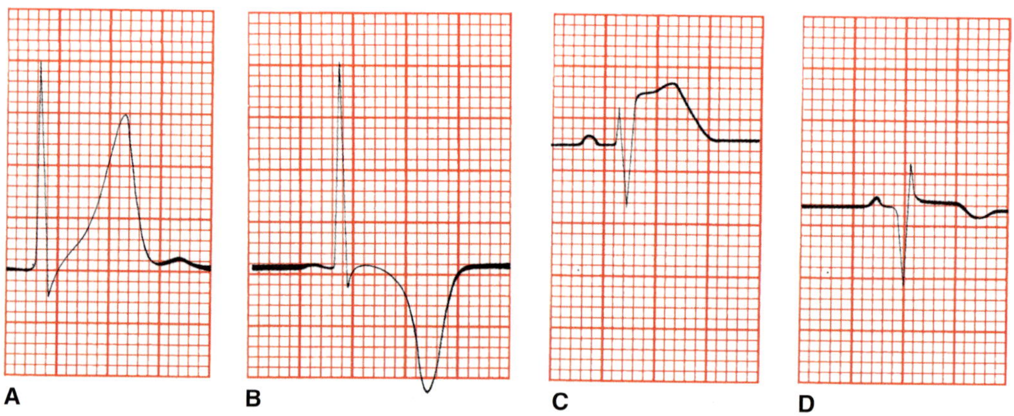

(*A*) T-wave peaking, (*B*) T-wave inversion, (*C*) ST-segment elevation, and (*D*) formation of a new Q wave.

One caveat before we proceed: Although the EKG typically evolves through these three stages during an acute STEMI, it does not always do so, and any one of these changes may be present without any of the others. Thus, for example, it is not at all unusual to see ST-segment elevation without T-wave inversion. Nevertheless, if you learn to recognize each of these three changes and keep your suspicion of myocardial infarction high, you will almost never go wrong.

The T Wave

With the onset of infarction, the T waves become tall, nearly equaling or even exceeding the height of the QRS complexes in the same lead. This phenomenon is called *peaking*. These peaked T waves are often referred to as *hyperacute T waves*. How tall does a T wave have to become to be considered hyperacute? There is no specific definition, but any T wave that approaches or exceeds the height of the QRS complex in the same lead is suspect. In addition, the upslope of the T wave, which is normally gradual and smooth, may straighten out. The clinical context, for example, if the patient is experiencing chest pain, will also help.

Shortly afterward, usually a few hours later, the T waves invert; that is, positive peaked T waves will become negative.

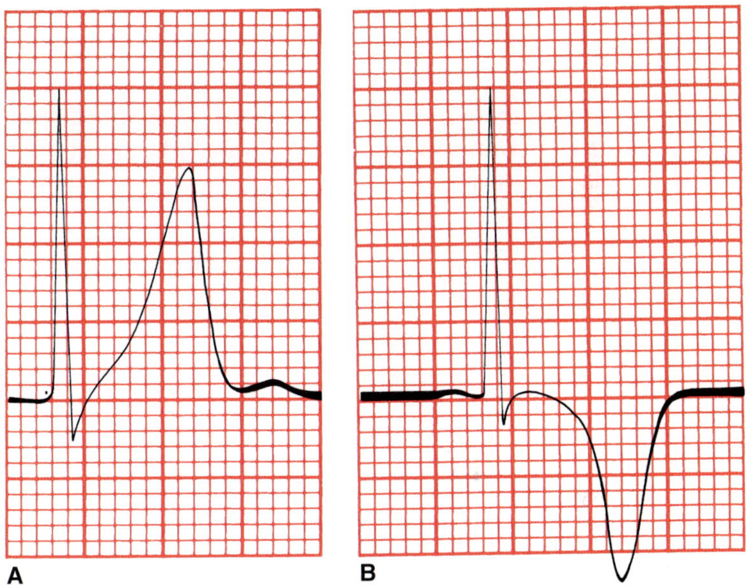

(*A*) T-wave peaking in a patient undergoing acute infarction. (*B*) The same lead in a patient 2 hours later shows T-wave inversion.

These T-wave changes reflect myocardial *ischemia*, the lack of adequate blood flow to the myocardium. Reduced blood flow affects the cardiac membrane ion channels, compromising the repolarization process (particularly the flow of potassium ions) and leading to the T wave changes that we observe.

Ischemia is potentially reversible: If blood flow is restored or the oxygen demands of the heart are eased, the T waves will revert to normal. On the other hand, if actual myocardial cell death (true infarction) has occurred, T-wave inversion may persist for months to years.

T-wave inversion by itself is not diagnostic of myocardial infarction. It is a very nonspecific finding. Many things can cause a T wave to flip; for example, we have already seen that both bundle-branch block and ventricular hypertrophy with repolarization abnormalities are associated with T-wave inversion. T-wave inversions are the most common EKG finding with pulmonary emboli (more on this on page 331). Hyperventilation, which is a common and understandable response to being hooked up to an EKG machine and having folks in white coats telling you they are worried about your heart, can itself be sufficient to flip T waves! T-wave inversion can also be seen after a run of ventricular tachycardia or ventricular pacing (this particular type of T-wave inversion is called "T-wave memory"). But perhaps the most common cause is improper placement of leads V1 and V2; T-wave inversions in those leads can occur when they are placed too high on the chest.

One helpful diagnostic feature is that the T waves of myocardial ischemia are inverted *symmetrically*, whereas in most other circumstances, they are asymmetric.

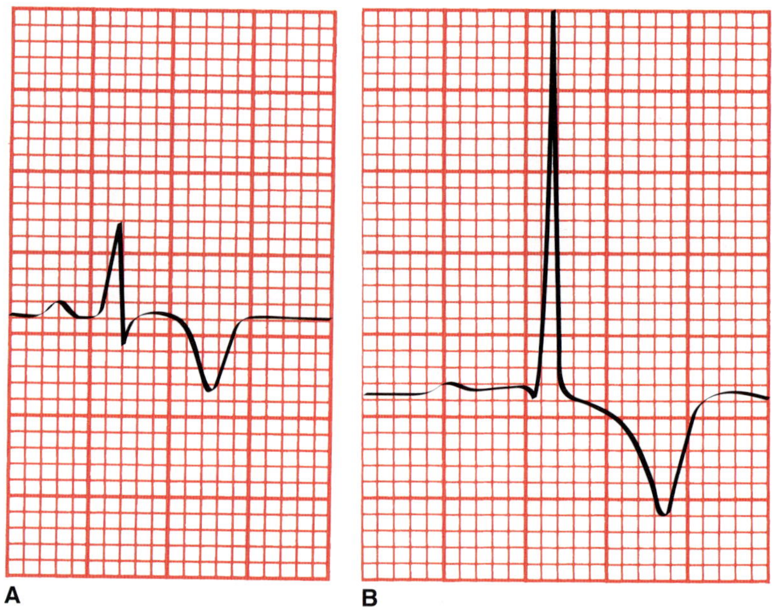

(*A*) The symmetric T-wave inversion in a patient with ischemia. (*B*) An example of asymmetric T-wave inversion in a patient with left ventricular hypertrophy and repolarization abnormalities.

In patients whose T waves are already inverted, ischemia may cause them to revert to normal, a phenomenon called *pseudonormalization*. Recognition of pseudonormalization requires comparing the current EKG with a previous tracing.

It is normal to see inverted T waves in leads V1, V2, and V3 in perfectly healthy children and young adults. In some instances, these T waves may remain inverted into adulthood, a finding referred to as *persistent juvenile T-wave pattern.* It is seen most often in young women in whom it can persist into their mid-40s. These T waves are asymmetric and usually shallow, not more than 3 mm in depth; they may be fully inverted or biphasic. Persistent juvenile T-wave pattern is completely benign, and its importance lies in its mimicry of ischemia, so don't be fooled. If you have a young adult patient, especially a female, with chest pain and inferior T-wave inversions, repeat EKGs (they will not evolve with persistent juvenile T-wave pattern but will with ischemia), and cardiac troponins will quickly get you the right answer.

It is important to note that inverted T waves are a completely normal finding in all people in those leads that overlie the right side of the heart, notably III, aVR, and V1.

And just a heads up: we are not quite done with T waves and infarction. Later in this chapter (see page 277) when we discuss anterior myocardial infarctions, we will revisit the T wave and discuss a couple of important situations in which the T wave is a major player: de Winter T waves and Wellens waves. But for now, we are sticking to the basics, so on to the ST segment.

The ST Segment

ST-segment elevation is the second change that occurs acutely in the evolution of a STEMI.

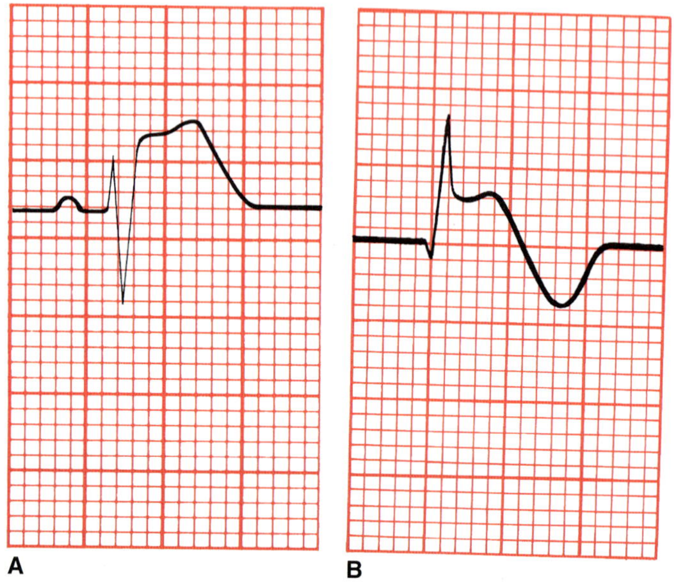

Two examples of ST-segment elevation during an acute STEMI: (*A*) without T-wave inversion and (*B*) with T-wave inversion.

ST-segment elevation often signifies myocardial *injury*. Injury probably reflects a degree of cellular damage beyond that of mere ischemia, but it, too, is potentially reversible, and in some cases, the ST segments may rapidly return to normal even without treatment. *In most instances, however, ST-segment elevation is a reliable sign that true infarction has occurred and that the complete electrocardiographic picture of infarction will evolve unless there is immediate and aggressive therapeutic intervention.*

A logical question to ask is: ST-segment elevation in relation to what? In other words, what is the reference baseline? There are two obvious candidates—the TP segment and the PR segment. Neither is perfect. The PR segment is problematic because it can be depressed in patients with pericarditis, a condition that can clinically mimic ischemia (and which we will discuss in the next chapter). A depressed PR segment will make the ST segment look artificially elevated. On the other hand, the TP segment may not be clearly seen in sinus tachycardia if, as often happens in this setting, the P wave overlaps with (is superimposed on) the T wave. So which one should you use? Most experts would say you should choose the TP segment whenever it is visible.

Even in the setting of a true infarction, the ST segments usually return to baseline within a few hours. Persistent ST-segment elevation often indicates the formation of a *ventricular aneurysm*, a weakening and bulging out of the ventricular wall.

Like T-wave inversion, ST-segment elevation can be seen in a number of other conditions in addition to an evolving myocardial infarction—we will list them at the end of this chapter (page 291). For now, just know that there are a lot of them. The ones you will encounter most often are:

- Left ventricular hypertrophy
- Left bundle-branch block
- Early repolarization/J-point elevation

Let's talk about the last, because it is a very common finding in normal hearts. The *J point*, or *junction point*, is the place where the ST segment takes off from the QRS complex. More specifically, it is the point at which the EKG tracing goes from vertical to horizontal after the QRS complex.

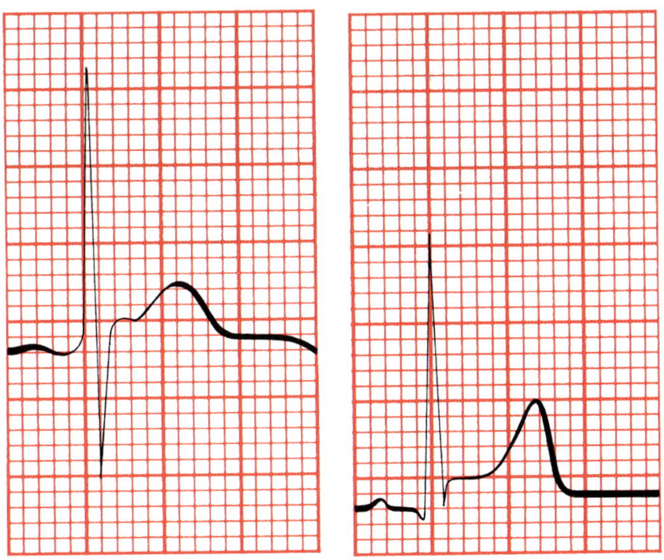

Two examples of J-point elevation, the second showing the notch of early repolarization.

J-point elevation is often seen in young healthy individuals, particularly—but not only—in leads V1, V2, and V3. Sometimes, along with an elevated J point, you will see a small notch or slur in the downslope of the R wave, and this combination of findings is referred to as *early repolarization*. For most patients, J-point elevation by itself appears to have no pathologic significance and carries no risk to the patient. But there are data suggesting that a small subset of patients with early repolarization may have a slightly increased risk of ventricular arrhythmias and sudden cardiac death.

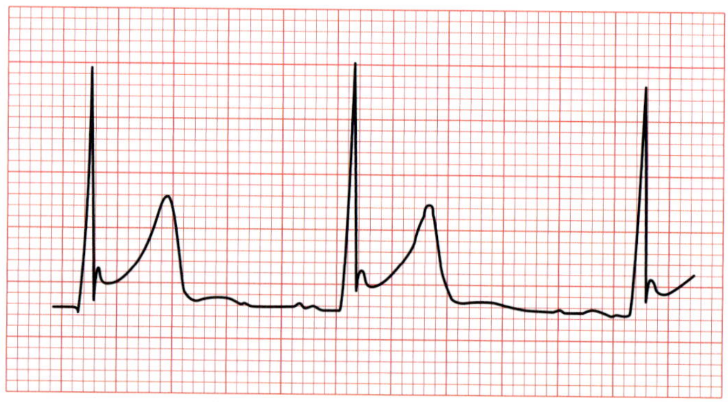

Early repolarization. Note the J-point elevation and the notching at the terminal portion of the R wave.

How can the ST-segment elevation of myocardial injury be distinguished from that of J-point elevation? With myocardial injury, the elevated ST segment has a distinctive configuration. It is bowed upward—picture a frown (or, on a more somber note, a tombstone)—and tends to merge imperceptibly with the T wave. In J-point elevation, the ST segment bows downward—picture a smile—and the T wave maintains its independent waveform.

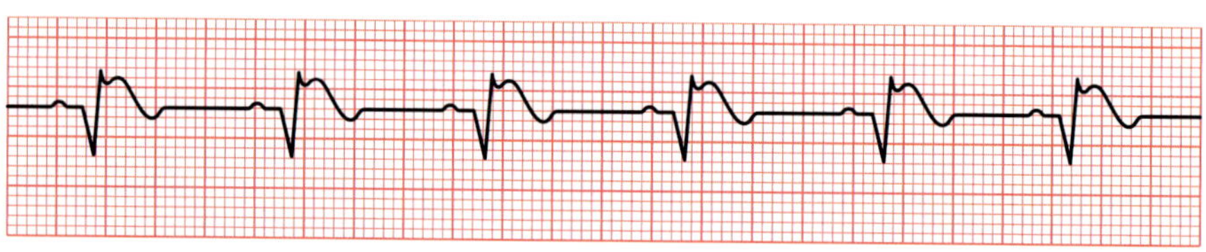

ST-segment elevation during a STEMI. Note how the ST segment and T wave merge into each other without a clear demarcation between them; it is impossible to tell where the ST segment ends and the T wave begins.

Does the amplitude of the ST-segment elevation help? Yes, but only to a limited point. The greater the elevation, the greater the likelihood of ischemia. But some patients, particularly males, without evidence of ischemia, may have ST elevation as high as 3 mm, particularly in the precordial leads (false positives). And, more importantly, some patients with active ischemia will have ST-segment elevation that barely achieves 1 mm in height. The key—and we never tire of making this point—is clinical context. If you are worried about an evolving STEMI, don't waste time dithering over electrocardiographic subtleties—get your patient the urgent care they need.

There are a couple of simple steps that can also help you decide what to do when you are unsure if the ST-segment elevation on a patient's EKG is concerning:

1. If you have access to a previous EKG, just compare the old one to the new one—if the ST elevation is new, you are most likely dealing with an acute coronary syndrome.
2. We have already made this point, but it bears repeating: If the patient is stable and in a monitored environment where emergency care is available, obtain serial EKGs. Any increase in the ST-segment elevation over the ensuing 15 to 60 minutes is indicative of cardiac ischemia. J-point elevation/early repolarization changes will not evolve.

All of the above points are important and useful, but never forget to err always on the side of assuming your patient has a STEMI, and quickly consult your cardiology team to decide immediate next steps whenever there is concern. Remember: Time is myocardium!

Q Waves

The appearance of new Q waves indicates that irreversible myocardial cell death has occurred. The presence of Q waves is diagnostic of myocardial infarction.

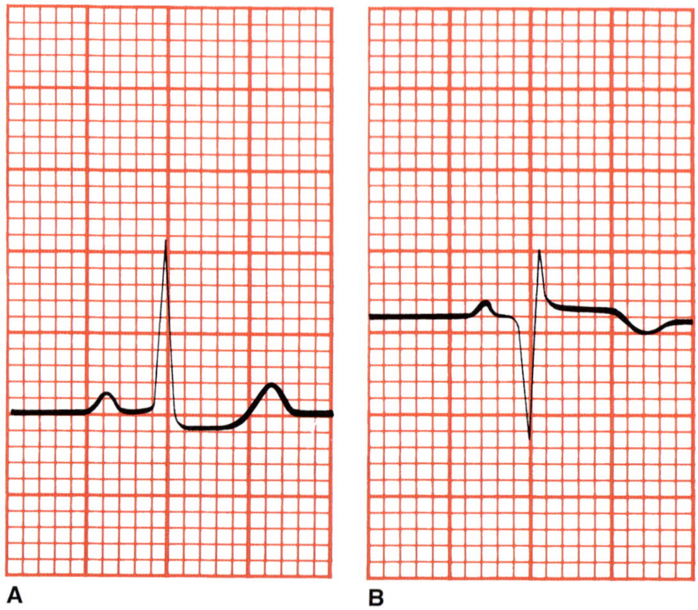

(*A*) Lead III in a healthy patient. (*B*) The same lead in the same patient 2 weeks after undergoing an inferior STEMI. Note the deep Q wave.

Q waves usually appear within several hours of the onset of a STEMI, but in some patients, they may take several days to evolve. The ST segment usually has returned to baseline by the time Q waves have appeared. Q waves usually persist for the lifetime of the patient.

Why Q Waves Form

The genesis of Q waves as a sign of infarction is easy to understand. When a region of myocardium dies, it becomes electrically silent—it is no longer able to conduct an electrical current. As a result, all of the electrical forces of the heart will be directed *away* from the area of infarction. An electrode overlying the infarct will therefore record a deep negative deflection, a Q wave.

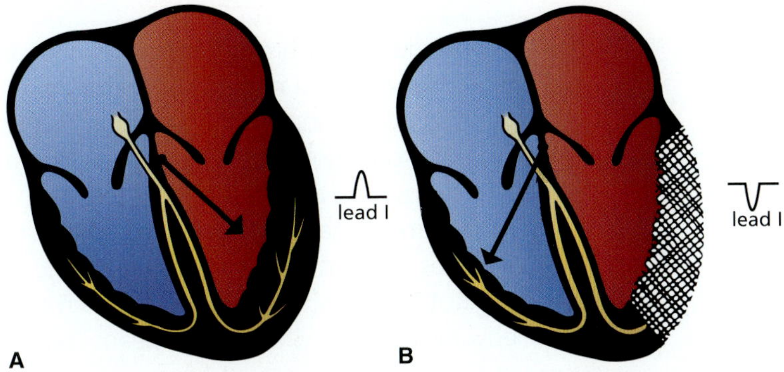

(*A*) Normal left ventricular depolarization with the *arrow* showing the electrical axis. Note the tall R wave in lead I. (*B*) The lateral wall of the left ventricle has infarcted and, as a result, is now electrically silent. The electrical axis, therefore shifts rightward, away from lead I, which now shows a negative deflection (Q wave).

Reciprocal Changes

Other leads, located some distance from the site of infarction, will see an apparent *increase* in the electrical forces moving toward them. They will record tall positive R waves. This makes sense—an injury current moving away from one area of the heart (inscribing deep Q waves) will, of logical necessity, be moving toward another (inscribing tall R waves).

These opposing changes seen by distant leads are called *reciprocal changes*. **The concept of reciprocity applies not only to Q waves but also to ST-segment and T-wave changes**. Thus, a lead distant from a STEMI may record ST-segment *depression*.

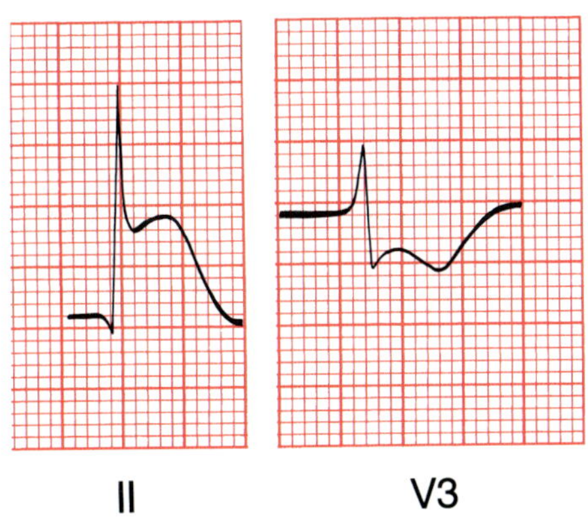

Reciprocal ST-segment and T-wave changes in an inferior infarction. The acute ST elevation and T-wave peaking in lead II are echoed by the ST depression and T-wave inversion in lead V3.

When you see reciprocal changes, the diagnosis of a STEMI is much more likely. J-point elevation/early repolarization is not accompanied by reciprocal changes. However, you do not need to see reciprocal changes to diagnose a STEMI. Whereas virtually all (not all, but most) infarctions involving the inferior surface of the heart are accompanied by reciprocal changes in leads overlying distant areas of the heart, as many as 30% of infarctions involving the anterior surface of the heart will not have any reciprocal changes. This occurs for what should be obvious reasons—there are no leads that directly view the posterior of the heart. The best we have on the standard 12-lead EKG is lead V1, which may record reciprocal changes during an anterior STEMI.

Normal Versus Pathologic Q Waves

Some Q waves are perfectly normal. As we discussed way back in Chapter 1, small Q waves can often be seen in the left lateral leads (I, aVL, V5, and V6). These Q waves are caused by the early left-to-right depolarization of the interventricular septum. Q waves, very prominent Q waves, are normal in lead aVR, which overlies the right side of the heart. Lead aVR should not be considered when using Q waves to assess possible infarction. Large Q waves, also commonly seen in lead III and, when present in that lead but in no other inferior lead, are a normal variant. If you remember this last point, it will save you a lot of unnecessary *agita* in the future.

Pathologic Q waves signifying infarction are *wider* and *deeper* than the small Q waves seen with depolarization of the interventricular septum. They are often referred to as *significant Q waves*. The criteria for significance are the following:

1. The Q wave must be >0.04 seconds in duration.
2. The depth of the Q wave must be at least 25% the height of the R wave in the same QRS complex.

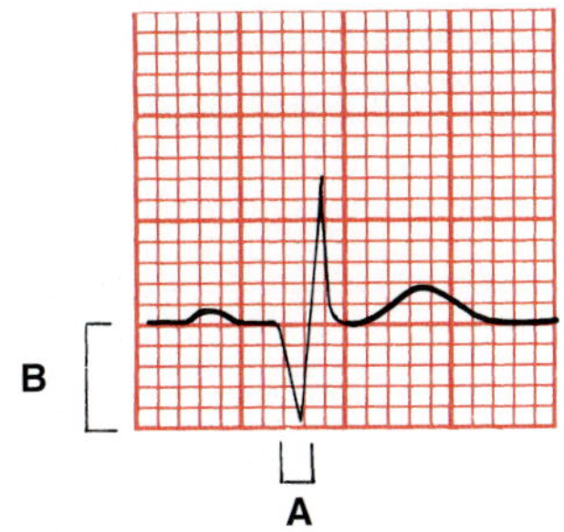

An example of a significant Q wave. Its width (*A*) exceeds 0.04 seconds, and its depth (*B*) exceeds one-third that of the R wave.

Pathologic Q waves are almost never isolated to a single lead but are present in two or more contiguous leads, that is, leads that look at the same geographic region of the heart, such as the inferior leads considered as a group, the anterior leads, or the left lateral leads. As stated above, isolated deep Q waves in lead III are a common normal variant that almost never signifies a myocardial infarction.

When you see significant Q waves meeting the above criteria on the EKG of a patient in whom you have *no reason to suspect a myocardial infarction*, take a closer look. You will be surprised how often you will detect tiny R waves preceding the negative waves, so what at first glance appear to be Q waves are in fact S waves and therefore of no concern.

Are the following Q waves significant?

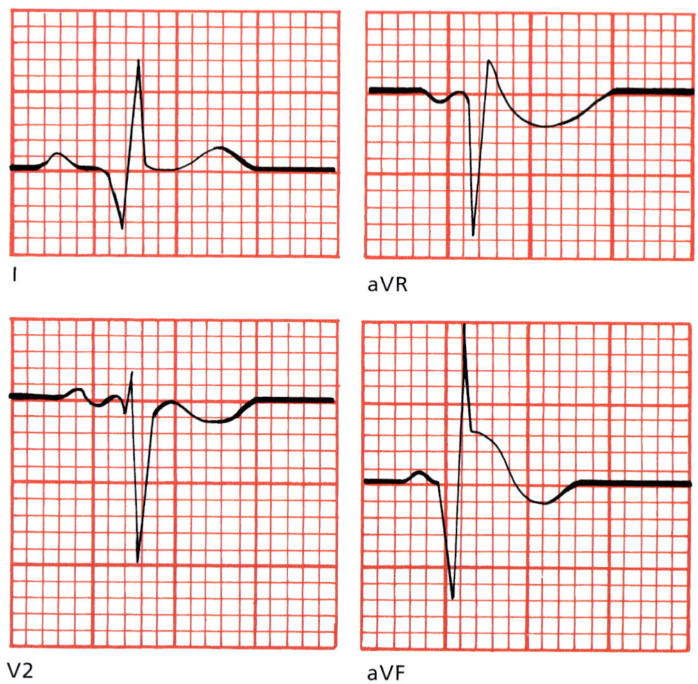

Answers: The Q waves in leads I and aVF are significant. The Q wave in lead V2 is too shallow and narrow to qualify (don't confuse the tiny Q wave with the large S wave). The Q wave in lead aVR is immense, but Q waves in aVR are never significant!

SUMMARY

The EKG Changes of an Evolving STEMI

1. Acutely, the T wave peaks and then inverts. T-wave changes reflect myocardial ischemia. If true infarction occurs, the T wave may remain inverted for months to years.
2. Acutely, the ST segment elevates and merges with the T wave. ST-segment elevation reflects myocardial injury. If infarction occurs, the ST segment usually returns to baseline within a few hours.
3. New Q waves appear within hours to days. They signify myocardial infarction. In most cases, they persist for the lifetime of the patient.

When it comes to saving lives and preventing immediate and future cardiac complications, diagnosing a STEMI early in its evolution is one of the most important things you can do. Therapy is widely available that—when delivered within the first few hours of the onset of the event—can prevent completion of the infarct and improve survival. *Thrombolytic agents* can lyse a clot within the coronary arteries and restore blood flow before myocardial death has occurred. In hospitals with catheterization and angioplasty capabilities, emergency *angioplasty* within the first several hours—ideally within the first 90 minutes—of the onset of infarction offers superior survival to thrombolysis alone, both acutely and in long-term follow-up.

Once angioplasty has been successfully carried out, the placement of stents coated with antiproliferative drugs to prevent reocclusion (which usually occurs as a result of cell proliferation) at the site of the original lesion prevents restenosis. The administration of dual oral antiplatelet therapy and intravenous anticoagulants (eg, bivalirudin) has further improved patient outcomes.

Whichever intervention is chosen, the key to successful therapy is timing: you must intervene quickly. The lives of patients are being saved every day by alert and informed health care providers. The recognition of the acute changes of a threatened or evolving myocardial infarction on the EKG is a critical diagnostic skill.

Localizing the Infarct

The region of myocardium that undergoes infarction depends on which coronary artery becomes occluded and the extent of collateral blood flow. There are two major systems of blood supply to the myocardium, one supplying the right side of the heart and one supplying the left side.

The *right coronary artery* runs between the right atrium and right ventricle and then swings around to the posterior surface of the heart. In most individuals, it gives off a descending branch that supplies the atrioventricular (AV) node.

The *left main artery* divides into a *left anterior descending (LAD) artery* and a *left circumflex artery*. The LAD runs between the two ventricles and supplies the anterior wall of the heart and most of the interventricular septum. The circumflex artery runs between the left atrium and left ventricle and supplies the lateral wall of the left ventricle. In about 10% of the population, it gives off the branch that supplies the AV node.

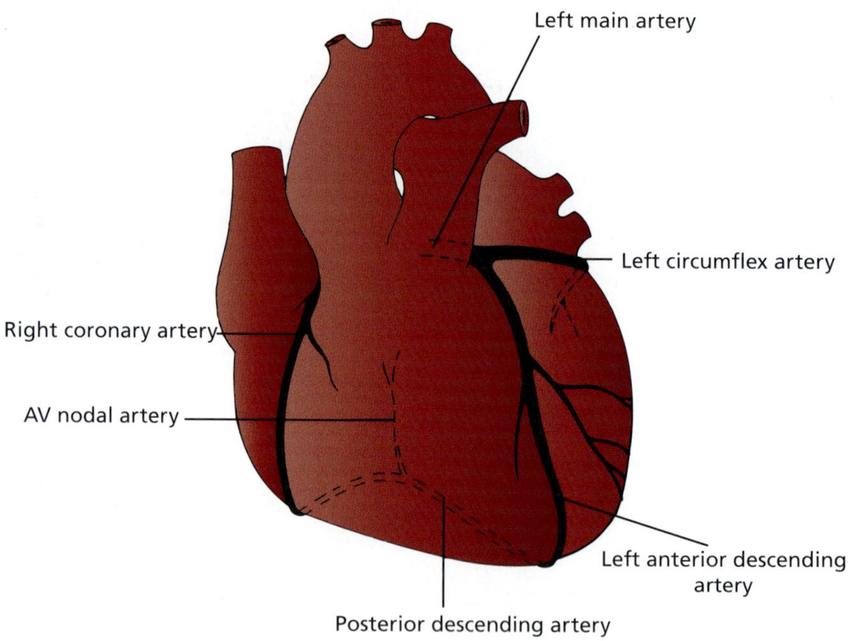

The main coronary arteries.

Does it matter which coronary artery is occluded and what part of the heart is affected? Absolutely! Localization of an infarct is important because the prognostic and therapeutic implications are in part determined by which area of the heart is in jeopardy.

Infarctions can be grouped into several general anatomic categories. These categories include *inferior*, *lateral*, *anterior*, and *posterior* infarctions. Combinations can also be seen, such as *anterolateral* and *inferoposterior* infarctions. Almost all myocardial infarctions involve the left ventricle. This should not be surprising because the left ventricle is the largest and most muscular chamber and is called on to do the most work. It is therefore most vulnerable to a compromised blood supply. Pure *right ventricular infarctions* can occur but are exceedingly rare; they almost always accompany inferior infarctions.

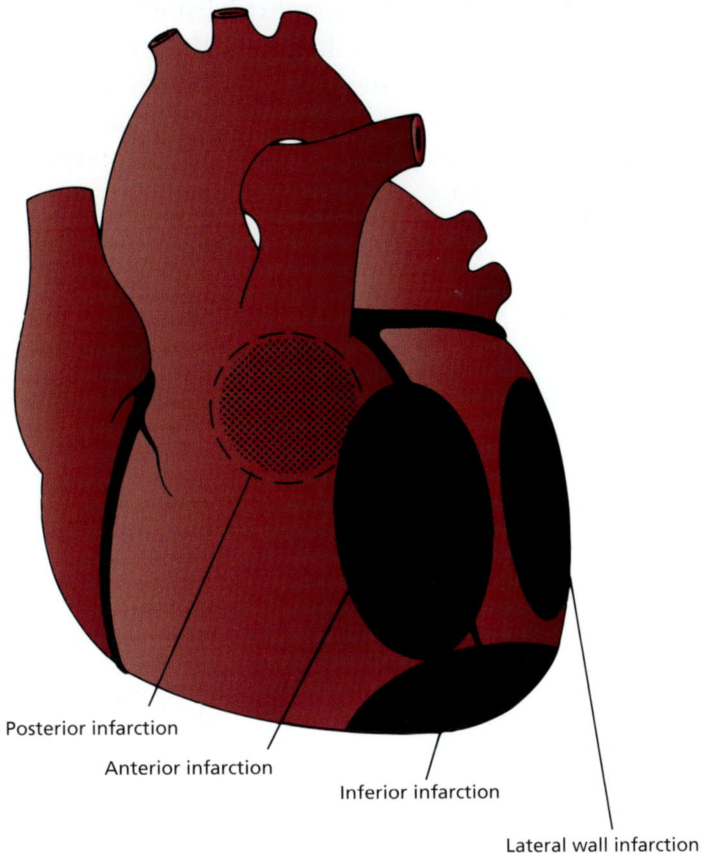

The four basic anatomic sites of myocardial infarction.

The characteristic electrocardiographic changes of infarction occur only in those leads overlying or near the site of infarction:

1. *Inferior infarction* involves the diaphragmatic surface of the heart. It is often caused by occlusion of the *right coronary artery* or its descending branch. The characteristic electrocardiographic changes of infarction can be seen in the inferior leads II, III, and aVF. When accompanied by *right ventricular infarction*, changes may be seen as well in leads V1 and/or V2.

2. *Lateral infarction* involves the left lateral wall of the heart. It is most often due to occlusion of the *left circumflex artery*. Changes will occur in the left lateral leads I, aVL, V5, and V6.

3. *Anterior infarction* involves the anterior surface of the left ventricle and is usually caused by occlusion of the *LAD artery*. Any of the precordial leads (V1 through V6) may show changes. Occlusion of the *left main artery* will characteristically cause an extensive *anterolateral infarction* with changes in the precordial leads plus leads I and aVL.

4. *Posterior infarction* involves the posterior surface of the heart and is usually caused by occlusion of the *right coronary artery*. Posterior infarctions rarely occur in isolation, but usually accompany an inferior infarction or, less commonly, a lateral infarction. There are no leads directly overlying the posterior wall. The diagnosis must therefore be made by looking for reciprocal changes in the anterior leads, for example, a tall R wave in leads V1, V2, or V3 (there is another way that may surprise you, which we will discuss shortly).

A note of caution: Coronary anatomy can vary markedly among individuals, and the precise vessel involved may not always be what one would predict from the EKG.

Inferior Infarcts

Inferior infarction typically results from occlusion of the right coronary artery or its descending branch. Changes occur in leads II, III, and aVF. Reciprocal changes may be seen in the anterior and left lateral leads.

Surprisingly perhaps, T-wave inversion in lead aVL, a lateral lead, is a particularly common change during an inferior infarction. This is a reciprocal change, and **T-wave inversion in aVL may be the first sign of an inferior infarction, appearing before the inferior ST-segment elevation and T-wave inversion we associate with an acute inferior infarction**. Serial EKGs will soon—usually within minutes—show the expected inferior changes.

Although in most infarctions significant Q waves persist for the lifetime of the patient, this is not necessarily true with inferior infarcts. Within half a year, as many as 50% of these patients will lose their criteria for significant Q waves. The presence of small Q waves inferiorly may therefore suggest an old inferior infarction. Remember, however, that a Q wave in a single inferior lead, particularly lead III, may be seen in normal hearts. The clinical history of the patient must be your guide.

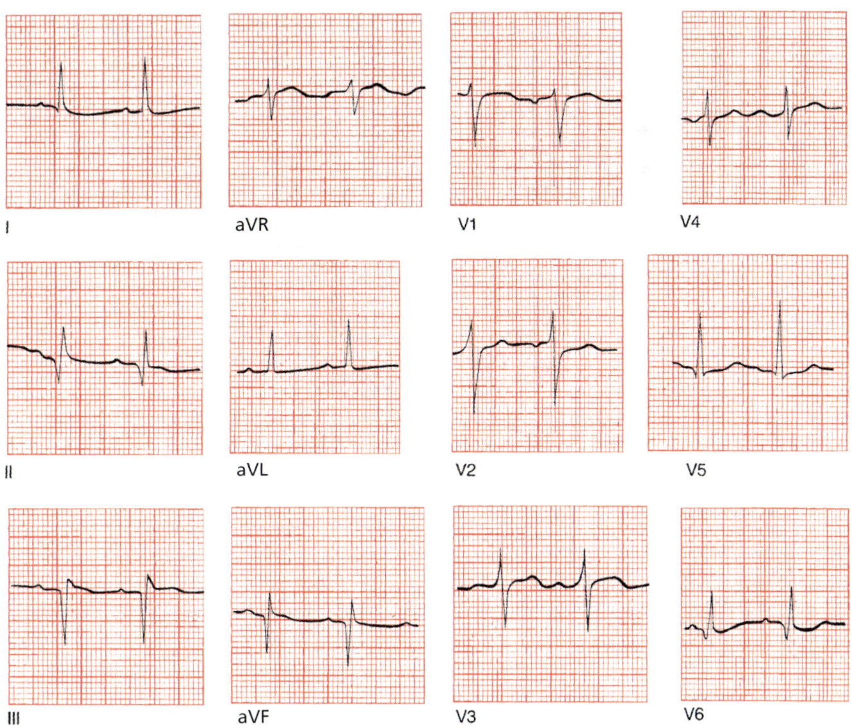

A fully evolved inferior infarction. Deep Q waves can be seen in leads II, III, and aVF.

Lateral Infarction

Lateral infarction usually results from occlusion of the left circumflex artery. Changes may be seen in leads I, aVL, V5, and V6. Reciprocal changes may be seen in the inferior leads.

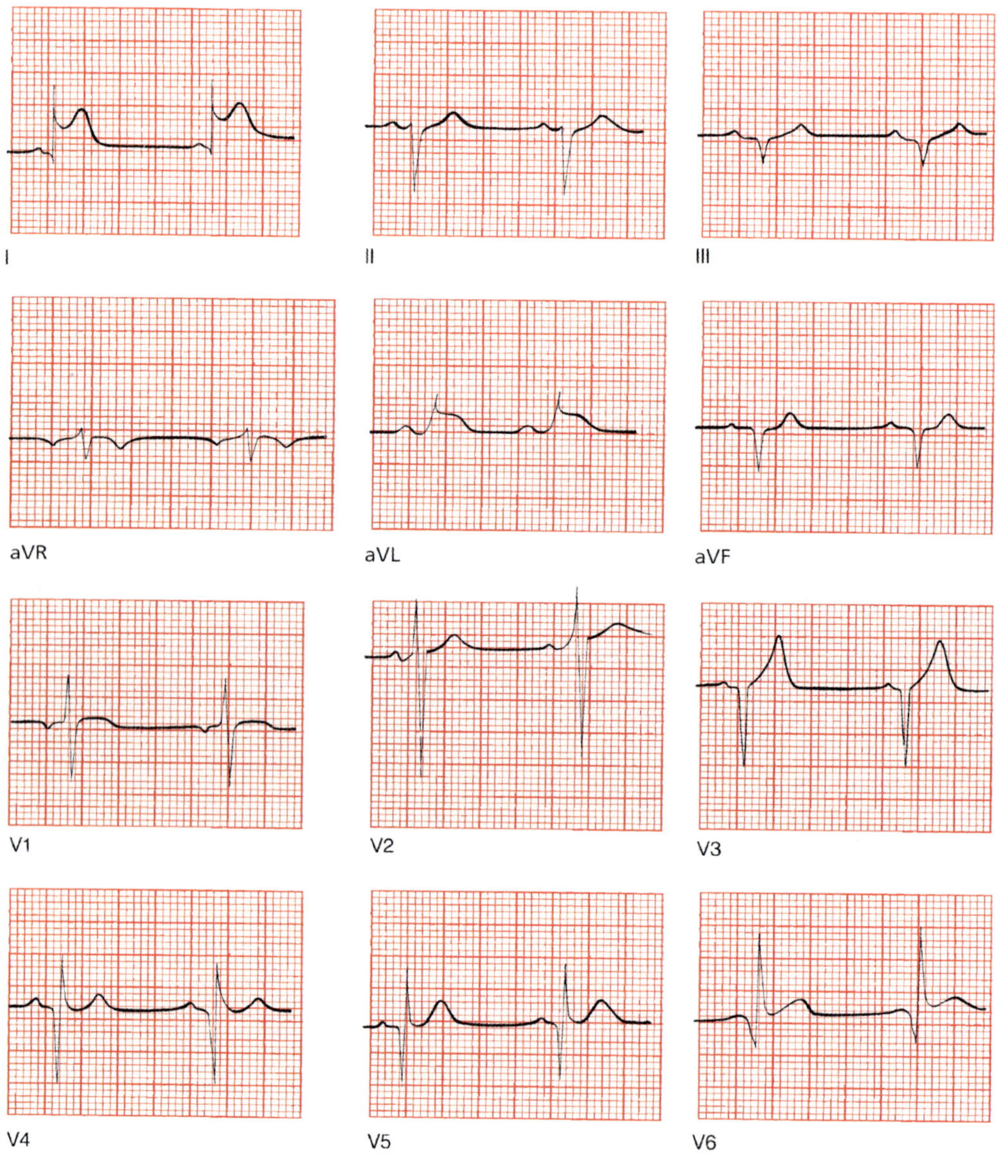

An acute lateral wall infarction. ST elevation can be seen in leads I, aVL, V5, and V6. Note also the deep Q waves in leads II, III, and aVF, signifying a previous inferior infarction. Did you also notice the deep Q waves in leads V3 through V6? These are the result of yet another infarction that occurred years ago, this one affecting the anterior portion of the left ventricle.

Anterior Infarcts

Anterior infarction most often results from occlusion of the LAD. Changes are seen in the precordial leads (V1 through V6). If the left main artery is occluded, an *anterolateral infarction* may result, with changes in the precordial leads and in leads I and aVL. Reciprocal changes, when present, are seen inferiorly.

The loss of anterior electrical forces in anterior STEMI is not always associated with Q-wave formation. In some patients with an anterior STEMI, there may be only a loss or diminishment of the normal pattern of precordial R-wave progression. As you already know, under normal circumstances, the precordial leads show a progressive increase in the height of each successive R wave as you look from lead V1 to V5. In normal hearts, the amplitude of the R waves should increase at least 1 mm per lead as you progress from V1 to V4 (and often V5); the amplitude of the R wave should normally exceed that of the S wave by lead V4. This pattern may vanish with anterior infarction, and the result is called *poor R-wave progression*. One simple criterion for the diagnosis of poor R-wave progression is an R wave in lead V3 that is not larger than 3 mm. Even in the absence of significant Q waves, poor R-wave progression may signify an anterior infarction.

Poor R-wave progression is not specific for the diagnosis of anterior infarction. It can also be seen with right or left ventricular hypertrophy, with left anterior fascicular block, in patients with chronic lung disease, in patients who are obese, in the elderly, and—perhaps most often—with improper placement of the leads on the chest wall. It can even be a normal variant.

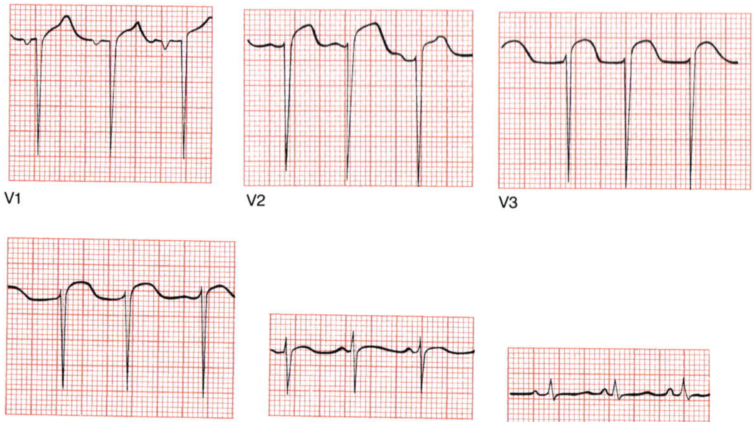

An anterior infarction with poor R-wave progression across the precordium.

Anterior STEMIs can have devastating clinical consequences, since they can compromise the bulk of the left ventricular myocardium. Recognizing them early is critical for your patients. It is therefore important to point out two special types of T-wave abnormalities that can herald occlusion of the left anterior descending (LAD) artery and an anterior myocardial infarction:

1. **de Winter T waves:** In a patient with chest pain, upsloping ST depression leading into tall, symmetric, hyperacute T waves in the precordial leads can be the first sign of an anterior infarction. These peaked T waves are called de Winter T waves and should be considered every bit as concerning for an acute occlusion of the LAD coronary artery as ST-segment elevation. If you see de Winter T waves in a patient with a suspected infarction, move quickly. Approximately 2% of acute LAD occlusions present with de Winter T waves rather than with ST-segment elevation.

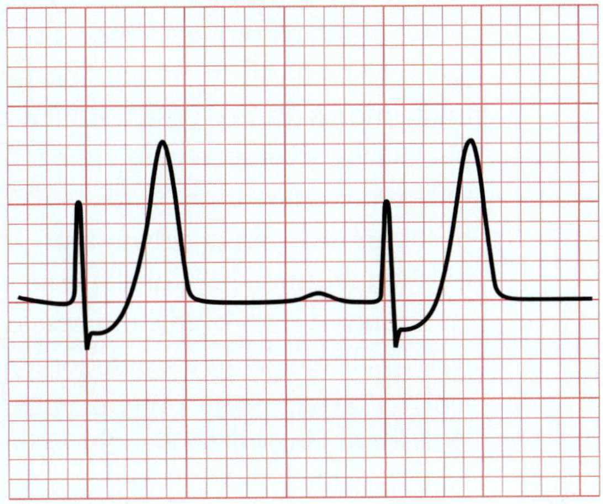

de Winter T waves

2. **Wellens waves:** Deeply inverted or biphasic T waves in leads V2, V3, and sometimes V4 predict a proximal occlusion of the LAD artery and are cause for concern. Patients may or may not have chest pain, and their cardiac enzymes may not be elevated. This is more of a subacute situation than the more acute one associated with de Winter T waves. When you see biphasic T waves in leads V2, V3, or V4, a tip-off that these may be Wellens waves is that the upright portion of the T wave occurs first, followed by inversion of the terminal portion. There may or may not be ST-segment elevation.

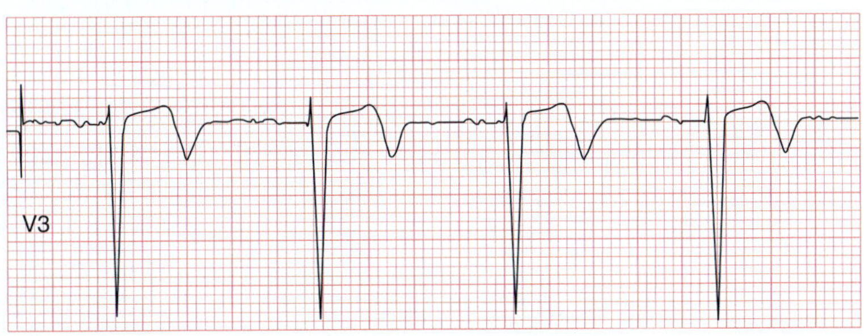

Wellens waves

Posterior Infarction

Posterior infarction typically results from an occlusion of the right coronary artery, the same artery responsible for most inferior infarctions. Therefore, as mentioned earlier, posterior infarction rarely occurs in isolation, but usually accompanies inferior and sometimes lateral infarctions. Of the various types of myocardial infarction, this is the one most often misdiagnosed, particularly in those uncommon cases when it occurs in isolation (at most 10% of all posterior infarctions). Because none of the conventional leads overlie the posterior wall, the diagnosis requires finding reciprocal changes in the anterior leads. In other words, because we can't look for ST-segment elevation and Q waves in nonexistent posterior leads, we have to look for *ST-segment depression* and *tall R waves* in the anterior leads, notably lead V1. In other words, posterior infarctions are the mirror images of anterior infarctions on the EKG (see the EKG on page 284).

The normal QRS complex in lead V1 consists of a small R wave and a deep S wave; therefore, the presence of a tall R wave, particularly with accompanying ST-segment depression, should be easy to spot. In the appropriate clinical setting, the presence of an R wave of greater amplitude than the corresponding S wave in lead V1 is highly suggestive of a posterior infarction.

Because in most posterior infarctions you will also see evidence of an inferior infarction, the complete EKG picture will often show clear-cut evidence of inferior ST elevation.

There is one other way to recognize a posterior infarction. It is a very simple matter to put electrodes on a patient's back to get a good look at the posterior electrical forces. When this is done (and, unfortunately, it is done only rarely), the ability of the EKG to diagnose a posterior myocardial infarction is greatly enhanced. These so-called 15-lead EKGs, which include three V electrodes placed on the back (V7, V8, and V9), can often detect ST-segment elevation in patients with a suspected posterior STEMI in whom the standard 12-lead EKG is not diagnostic.

One caveat before we leave the subject of posterior infarctions. You will recall that the presence of a large R wave exceeding the amplitude of the accompanying S wave in lead V1 is also one criterion for the diagnosis of right ventricular hypertrophy. The diagnosis of right ventricular hypertrophy, however, also requires the presence of right axis deviation, which is not present in posterior infarction.

Right Ventricular Infarctions

Because the left ventricle is so much more powerful than the right ventricle, it demands much more from its blood supply and, therefore, is far more susceptible to infarction when its blood supply is compromised. However, right ventricular infarctions do occur, virtually always accompanying inferior infarctions. What you will typically see are the expected changes of an inferior infarction (ie, ST elevation and so forth in leads II, III, and aVF) along with T-wave changes and ST-segment elevation in the most rightward anterior lead, V1. If there is also ST elevation in lead V2, it will be of smaller magnitude than that in V1, and often V2 will show ST depression. In the limbs leads, one tip-off that an inferior infarction is accompanied by a right ventricular STEMI is that the ST elevation in lead III is greater than that in lead II (why?—because lead III lies far to the right of lead II).

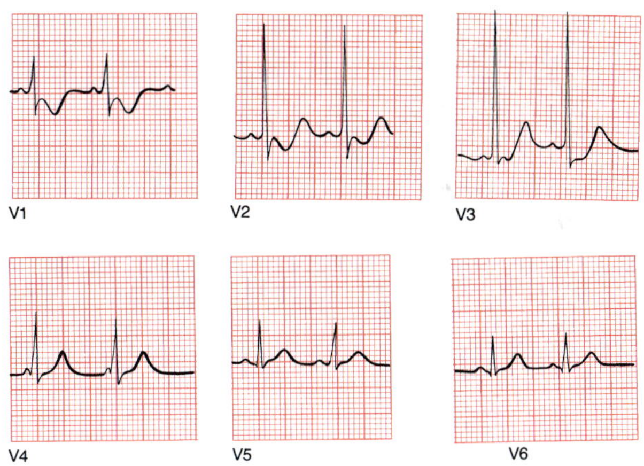

A posterior infarction. In lead V1, the R wave is larger than the S wave. There is also ST depression and T-wave inversion in leads V1 and V2.

Another way to recognize a right ventricular infarction is to place electrodes over the right chest wall, as shown in the picture on the next page. Because these electrodes will then overlie the right heart, they may show the characteristic features of infarction.

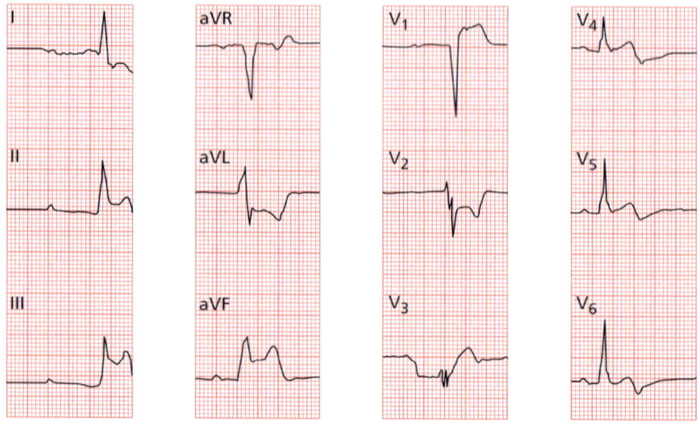

An evolving inferior STEMI with a right ventricular STEMI. Note the inferior changes, with the ST elevation greater in lead III than lead II, plus the ST elevation in lead V1 and ST depression in lead V2.

Does it make any difference clinically whether an infarction of the inferior wall of the left ventricle is accompanied by right ventricular infarction? Yes, indeed, it does. Patients with right ventricular infarctions are "preload sensitive," that is, they require high fluid volumes to maintain an adequate cardiac output and blood pressure, and they can become extremely hypotensive if they are treated with nitrates, such as nitroglycerin, which are vasodilators.

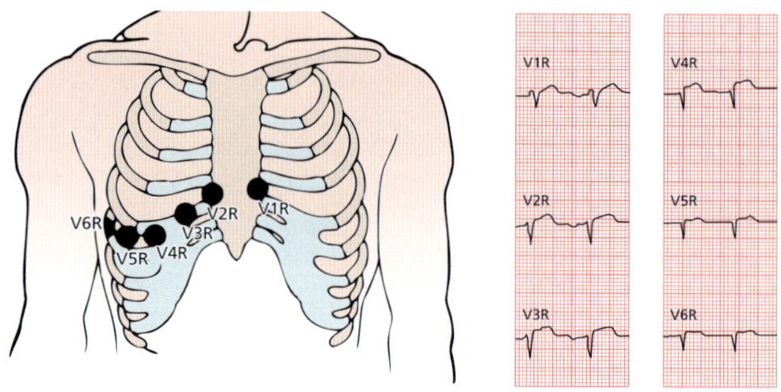

The figure on the *left* shows the proper alignment of right ventricular leads. The tracing on the *right* shows the resultant ECG in a patient with a right ventricular STEMI; ST-segment elevation is most notable in leads V3R through V6R.

Where is the infarct? Is it acute?

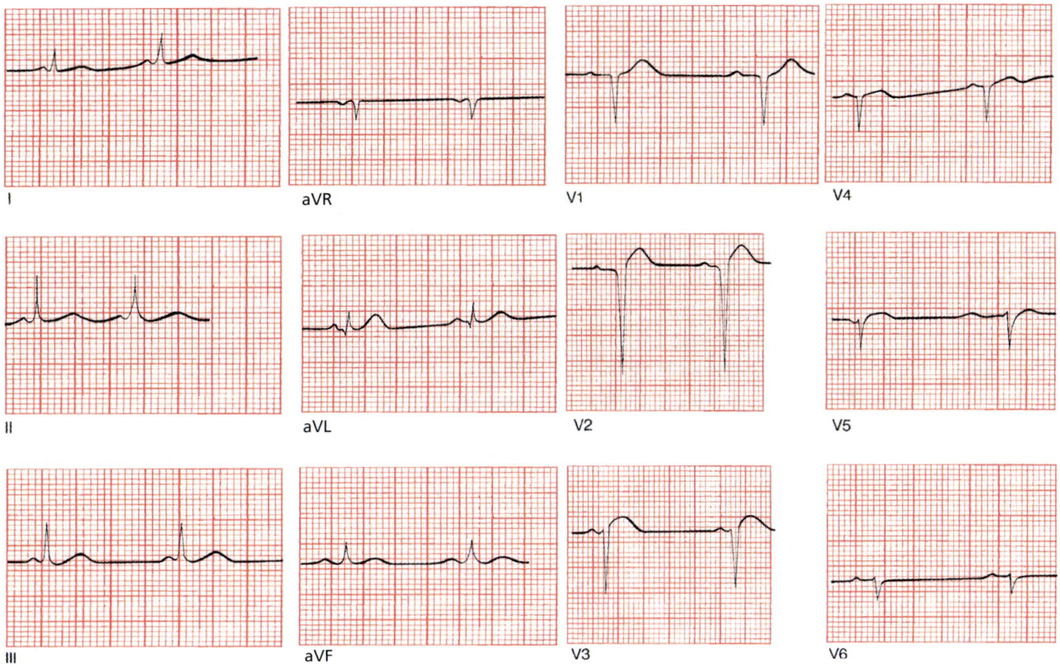

This is an example of an anterior infarction. There is ST-segment elevation in leads V2 and V3 as well as poor R-wave progression.

Where is the infarct? Is it acute?

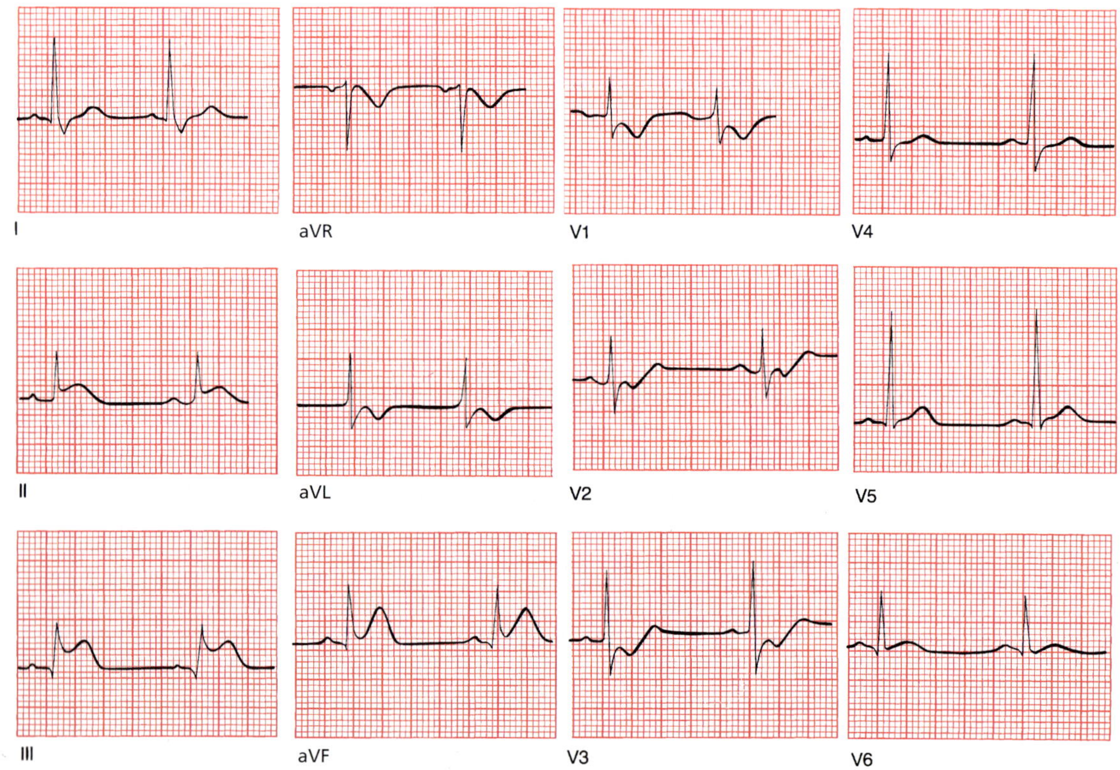

This tracing shows an acute posterior and inferior infarction. (Remember how we said that most posterior infarctions are accompanied by evidence of inferior infarction?) ST-segment elevation can be seen in leads II, III, and aVF, indicating an acute inferior infarction. There is also evidence of posterior wall involvement, with a tall R wave, ST-segment depression, and T-wave inversion in lead V1.

Non–ST-Segment Elevation Myocardial Infarctions

Not all myocardial infarctions are associated with ST-segment elevation. These infarctions, or non-STEMIs, also do not lead to the evolution of deep Q waves. Most often, non-STEMIs are caused by either nonocclusive thrombosis of a major coronary artery or complete occlusion of a small offshoot of one of the major coronary arteries. Unlike STEMIs, they usually cannot be localized to a particular region of the heart supplied by a single coronary vessel. **The only EKG changes seen with non-STEMIs are T-wave inversion and ST-segment depression (*not elevation*).**

Non-STEMIs are actually more common than STEMIs. They behave much like small, incomplete infarctions and have a lower initial mortality rate but a higher risk for further infarction and mortality than STEMIs. Cardiologists usually take an aggressive stance with these patients, in particular those patients at high risk for further infarction and death, often sending them for coronary angiography and proceeding with revascularization right away.

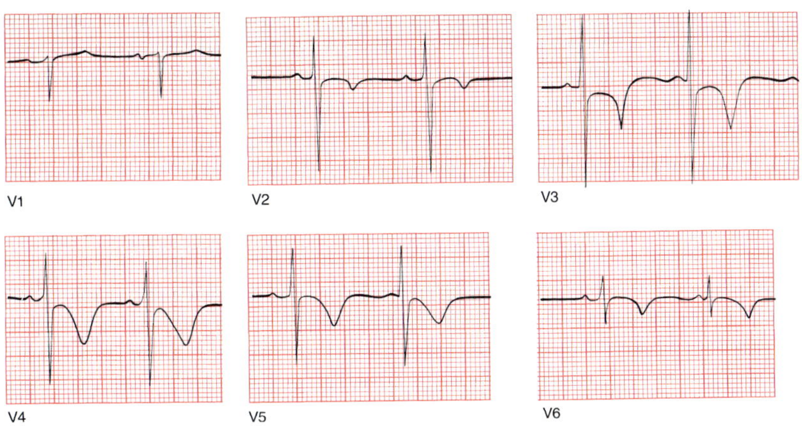

A non-STEMI. ST-segment depression is most prominent in leads V2, V3, and V4, and T-wave inversion can be seen in leads V2 through V6. This patient never evolved Q waves, but his cardiac enzymes soared, confirming occurrence of a true infarction.

Takotsubo Cardiomyopathy

Takotsubo cardiomyopathy is a condition that can closely mimic an acute STEMI on the EKG, complete with T-wave inversions and ST-segment elevations. However, the EKG changes are variable and not always present. As many as 2% of patients, most often postmenopausal women under extreme psychological stress (such as the death of a loved one or watching their grandchild play in a tense—is there any other kind?—soccer match), who have what appears to be an acute infarction on their EKG will prove to have this syndrome instead. The EKG changes reflect ballooning of the left ventricle, and the condition has therefore also been referred to as *apical ballooning syndrome.* It acquired the name "takotsubo" because the bulging ventricle reminded the original investigators of the shape of an octopus trap, for which the Japanese term is takotsubo.

Because the cause is often psychological or emotional stress, yet another name for this syndrome is *broken heart syndrome.** The pathologic mechanism is not fully understood. There may or may not be underlying atherosclerosis, but in any case, it is not responsible for the syndrome. In most patients, the coronary arteries appear perfectly normal. One of the leading theories posits a state of excessive catecholamine (sympathetic) stimulation. Alternatively, because takotsubo cardiomyopathy occurs more commonly in persons with migraine headaches and Raynaud syndrome, generalized vasomotor dysfunction may play a role in its genesis.

Troponin levels can be elevated, although rarely as high as in an acute infarction, and there is no evidence of significant underlying coronary artery disease should the patient be brought to the catheterization lab. As many as 50% of these patients may develop transient heart failure, and rarely can even go into shock. Patients generally improve over several weeks, but recurrences can occur.

There are no electrocardiographic criteria that can reliably distinguish takotsubo cardiomyopathy from a STEMI caused

---

*Actually, physical triggers, such as acute respiratory failure or surgery, are more common precipitants than emotional stresses.

by coronary artery occlusion. The distinction is made in the catheterization lab; patients with takotsubo cardiomyopathy will not show the occluded coronary arteries seen with a STEMI.

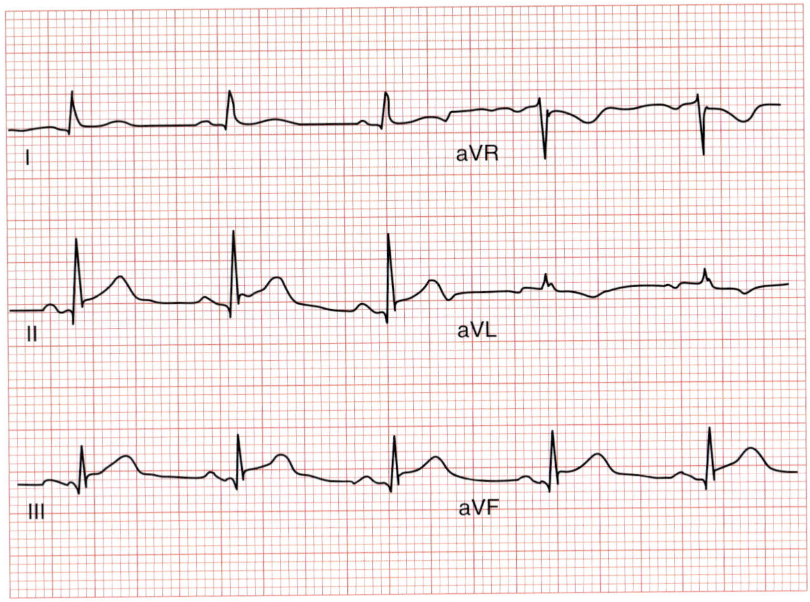

Limb leads in a patient with takotsubo cardiomyopathy. The ST-segment elevation looks for all the world like a typical inferior wall STEMI.

Takotsubo cardiomyopathy is one of several disorders that have been grouped under the heading *myocardial infarction with normal coronary arteries* (MINOCA; of course, there had to be an acronym!). In addition to takotsubo cardiomyopathy, other causes of MINOCA include small vessel coronary artery disease, coronary vasospasm, spontaneous coronary artery dissection, and myocarditis.

Angina Without Infarction

During an attack of angina, the EKGs of patients with both stable and unstable angina may demonstrate T-wave inversion and often ST-segment depression. Between attacks, the EKG is usually normal.

Since the EKGs of patients with non-STEMIs also typically show these changes, how can you determine whether a patient is suffering from an anginal attack without infarction or is in the process of evolving a non-STEMI? The answer is simple: measure the cardiac enzymes. If they are significantly elevated, the patient is having a non-STEMI; if they are normal, infarction is highly unlikely.

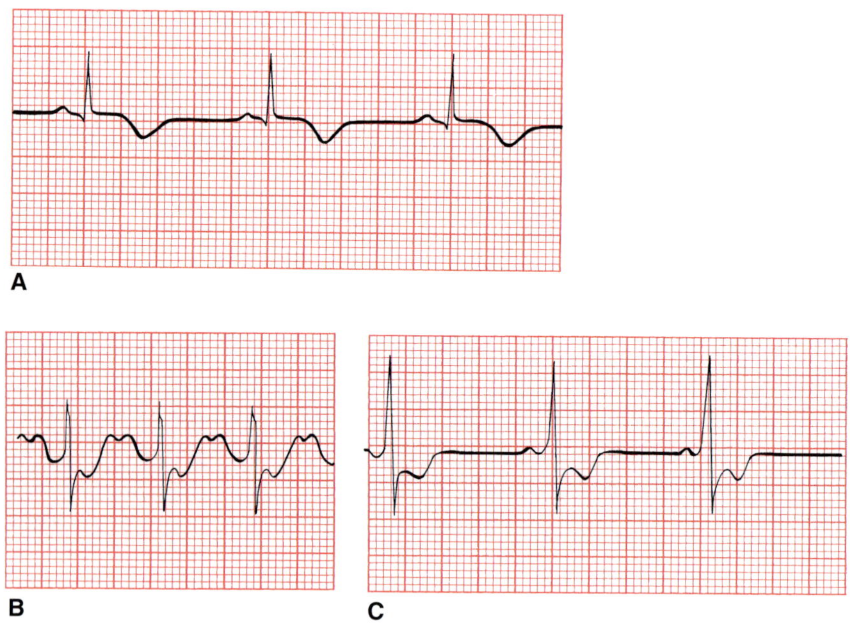

Three examples of the EKG changes that can accompany angina without infarction: (*A*) T-wave inversion, (*B*) ST-segment depression, and (*C*) ST-segment depression with T-wave inversion (the ST segment and T waves merge seamlessly).

Prinzmetal Angina

There is one type of angina that is associated with ST-segment *elevation* (Yes, nothing is ever as easy as it first seems). Whereas typical angina is usually brought on by exertion and is the result of progressive atherosclerotic cardiovascular disease, Prinzmetal angina can occur at any time and results from coronary artery spasm in the absence of significant coronary artery disease. Presumably, the ST-segment elevation reflects reversible transmural injury. Thus, unlike a STEMI, the ST-segment elevation is transient. The contours of the ST segments often will not have the rounded, domed appearance of true infarction.

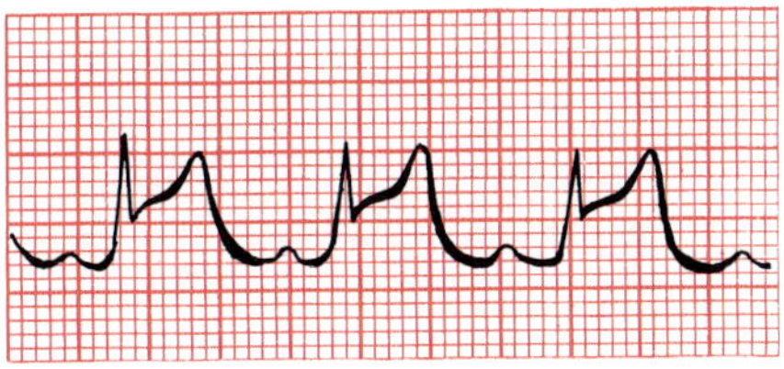

Prinzmetal angina, with ST-segment elevation.

Sorting Out the Different Ischemic Syndromes

Are you having trouble trying to remember what the various ischemic symptoms and syndromes do to the EKG? T-wave changes are not particularly helpful since ischemia of any type can cause T-wave inversion. The key is to focus on the ST segments and to measure the cardiac enzymes. Whether or not Q waves evolve is generally not helpful in the acute setting. The following table should help you get your thoughts in order:

Symptom or Syndrome	ST-Segment Changes	Cardiac Enzymes
Stable angina without infarction	ST depression	Normal[a]
Unstable angina without infarction	ST depression	Normal[a]
STEMI	ST elevation	Elevated
Non-STEMI	ST depression	Elevated
Takotsubo cardiomyopathy	ST elevation	Usually elevated[b]
Prinzmetal angina	ST elevation	Normal

[a]Stable and unstable angina are distinguished by the clinical history as described earlier.

[b]Patients often have to undergo cardiac catheterization to distinguish this from infarction.

Recognizing elevated ST segments is critical to quickly diagnosing a STEMI, but it is important to remember that—as we mentioned when discussing J-point elevation/early repolarization—there are other things that can elevate the ST segment. The clinical context is always helpful in sorting these out, but there are accompanying features on the EKG that can be helpful as well (eg, the presence of reciprocal changes). We will discuss many of the other confounding entities in the next chapter, so don't worry if you don't recognize everything on the following list. For now, just take a good look so you can start to get this differential diagnosis into your head:

Causes of ST-Segment Elevation

- An evolving STEMI
- Prinzmetal angina
- J-point elevation/early repolarization
- Takotsubo cardiomyopathy
- Acute pericarditis
- Acute myocarditis
- Pulmonary embolism
- Brugada pattern
- Hypothermia (Osborne waves)
- Ventricular aneurysm
- CNS catastrophes
- Postcardioversion
- Left bundle-branch block
- Left ventricular hypertrophy
- Paced rhythms

Because virtually all myocardial infarctions affect the left ventricle, lead aVR is of little value in their diagnosis. Although we do not expect to see acute ST-segment elevation in lead aVR during an ischemic episode or infarction, ST elevation can occasionally accompany a massive occlusive event involving the left main or proximal LAD arteries or one involving three vessels at the same time. However, you will not need to identify ST elevation in lead aVR to diagnose such a large infarction since many other leads will also show the characteristic changes. There are numerous other causes of ST elevation in lead aVR, including global cardiac ischemia (eg, from severe anemia or dissection of the thoracic aorta) or a massive pulmonary embolus. You may also see it with left bundle-branch block, left ventricular hypertrophy with repolarization abnormalities, marked hypokalemia, sodium channel blocker toxicity, Brugada syndrome (these last three are discussed in Chapter 7), and accompanying some supraventricular tachycardias. Does anyone expect you to memorize this list? Certainly not, but it is here for your future referral when you do encounter unexpected ST-segment elevation in that right-sided outlier, aVR.

There are also several causes of ST-segment depression, but you will be happy to know that there aren't quite so many of these:

Causes of ST-Segment Depression

- Stable and unstable angina without infarction
- Non-STEMI
- Supraventricular tachycardias—ST depression in this setting does not imply coexisting ischemic disease
- Typically seen in leads V1 to V3 with right bundle-branch block
- Hypokalemia

Limitations of the EKG in Diagnosing an Infarction

Because the electrocardiographic picture of an evolving myocardial infarction typically includes T-wave changes, ST-segment changes, and sometimes Q-wave formation, any underlying cardiac condition that masks these effects by distorting the T wave, ST segment, and QRS complex will render electrocardiographic diagnosis of an infarction extremely difficult. We've already discussed several of these entities, including Wolff–Parkinson–White (WPW), left ventricular hypertrophy, and left bundle-branch block, all of which can distort the EKG in ways that make recognizing an infarction problematic. Right bundle-branch block is generally of less concern because most infarctions involve the left ventricle.

Special mention should be paid to the diagnosis of an infarction in patients with preexisting left bundle-branch block. Several criteria and algorithms have been devised and tested that are helpful in the EKG assessment of myocardial infarction in this setting. We're getting in a bit deep here, but if you are interested, here are the critical points: in a patient with left bundle-branch block the presence of any of the following is strongly suggestive of an evolving infarction: (1) ST-segment elevation of at least 1 mm in any lead with a predominant R wave (ie, the ST elevation is directed in the same direction as the QRS complex—this is referred to as concordance) *or* (2) ST-segment depression of at least 1 mm in leads V1 to V3 if deep S waves are present (again, the ST-segment is concordant with the QRS complex, only this time the direction is downward), or (3) ST-segment elevation in any lead in which the extent of the ST elevation exceeds 25% of the S wave in the same complex.

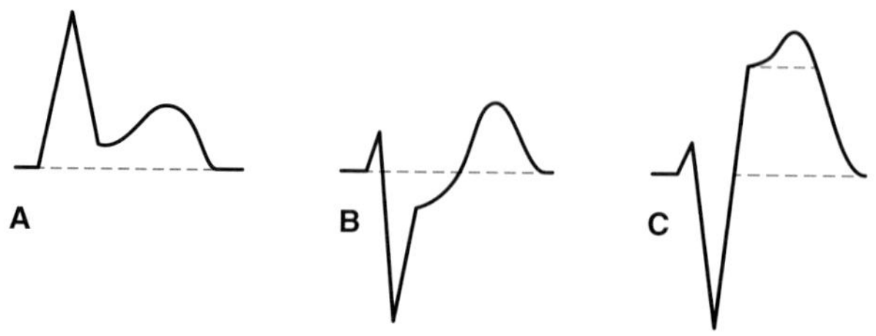

The criteria for diagnosing an infarction in a patient with preexisting left bundle branch are referred to as Sgarbossa Criteria. (*A*) concordant ST elevation of >1 mm in any lead; (*B*) concordant ST depression >1 mm in leads V1, V2, or V3; (*C*) ST elevation >25% of the S wave in the same complex in any lead.

One very important point that you should not overlook: the appearance of a *new left bundle-branch block* may signify infarction and should be treated with the same urgent attention as a STEMI.

Stress Testing

Stress testing is a noninvasive method for assessing the presence and severity of coronary artery disease. It is by no means flawless (false-positive and false-negative results abound), but it can be useful in patients who have or are suspected of having underlying atherosclerosis in order to help determine if their hearts, when stressed, show evidence of inadequate blood flow to parts of their myocardium.

Stress testing is usually done by having the patient ambulate on a treadmill, although stationary bicycles have been used just as effectively. The patient is hooked up to an EKG monitor, and a rhythm strip is monitored throughout the test. A complete 12-lead EKG is taken every minute or so and at the peak of exercise. Every few minutes, the speed and angle of incline of the treadmill are increased until (1) the patient cannot continue for any reason; (2) the patient's maximal heart rate is achieved; (3) symptoms, such as chest pain, supervene; or (4) significant changes are seen on the EKG.

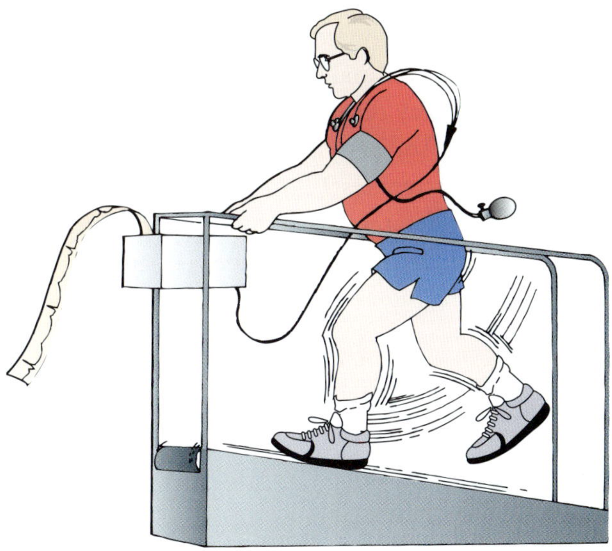

The physiology behind stress testing is simple. The graded exercise protocol causes a safe and gradual increase in the patient's heart rate and systolic blood pressure. The product of the patient's systolic blood pressure multiplied by the heart rate, called the *double product*, is a good measure of myocardial oxygen consumption. If cardiac oxygen demands exceed consumption, electrocardiographic changes and even symptoms of myocardial ischemia may occur.

Significant coronary artery disease of one or several coronary arteries limits blood flow to the myocardium and hence limits oxygen consumption. Although a patient's resting EKG may be normal, the increased demands of exercise may therefore bring out evidence of subclinical coronary artery disease.

With a positive test for coronary artery disease, the EKG will reveal *ST-segment depression*. T-wave changes are too nonspecific to have any meaning in this setting.

There is a wealth of literature looking at precisely what constitutes significant ST-segment depression during an exercise test. It is generally acknowledged that ST-segment depression of >1 mm that is horizontal or downsloping and persists for more than 0.08 seconds after the J point is suggestive of coronary artery disease. If depression of 2 mm is used as the criterion, the number of false-positive results is greatly reduced, but the number of false-negative results increases. Occasionally, upsloping depressed ST segments may signify coronary artery disease, but the number of false-positive results is very high.

You may be wondering: what if I see ST-segment elevation during a stress test? Fortunately, this is a very rare occurrence, because this indicates the high likelihood of an unstable plaque and impending infarction. If you see ST-segment elevation in any lead other than aVR during a stress test, get your patient right to the catheterization lab!

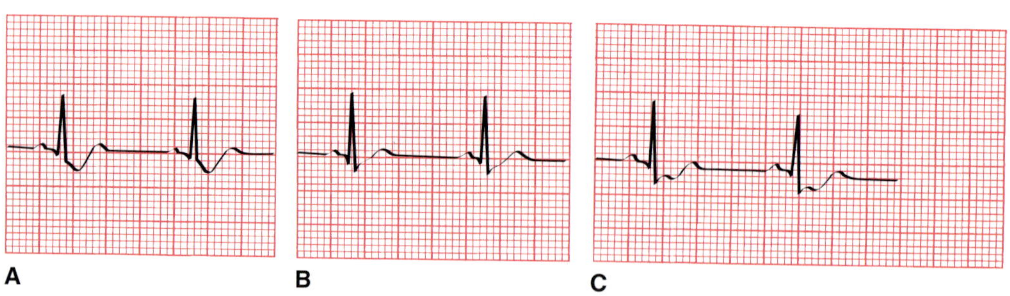

The ST segment during a stress test. (*A*) Downsloping ST depression. (*B*) Upsloping ST depression. (*C*) Horizontal ST depression. Only (*A*) and (*C*) are highly suggestive of coronary artery disease.

The earlier in the test that ST segment depression occurs—particularly, if the changes persist several minutes into the recovery period—the greater the likelihood that coronary artery disease is present and the greater the possibility that the left main coronary artery or several coronary arteries are involved. On the other hand, rapid resolution of ST-segment changes at the conclusion of the test is a hopeful prognostic indicator. The onset of symptoms (eg, chest pain or dizziness) and falling blood pressure are particularly poor prognostic signs, and the test must be stopped immediately and further workup initiated.

The incidence of false-positive and false-negative results is dependent on the patient population that is being tested. A positive test in a young healthy individual with no symptoms and no risk factors for coronary artery disease is likely to be a false test. On the other hand, a positive test in an elderly man with chest pain, a prior infarction, and hypertension is much more likely to be a true-positive result. In no one does a negative test result absolutely exclude the possibility of obstructive coronary artery disease. Here is why:

You may remember from earlier in this chapter that small plaques may be more unstable and liable to rupture than large ones. Many of these plaques are actually not technically "small," but rather grow into the blood vessel wall rather than out into the lumen and therefore do not greatly occlude blood flow. Stress testing will only find plaques that occlude at least 70% of the lumen, that is, the ones large enough to significantly obstruct blood flow. Patients who "rule out" for significant coronary artery disease by stress testing may therefore still be at risk, and this is probably the major reason limiting its utility. A negative stress test in someone with a history worrisome for coronary artery disease therefore mandates additional testing.* One option is CT angiography, which is better at visualizing the plaque in its entirety, at least in the large coronary arteries.

---

*They are also sometimes ordered to evaluate patients for arrhythmias that are provoked by exercise.

The bottom line on stress testing is this: we generally order a stress test only for individuals at risk of harboring coronary artery disease who have symptoms with exertion. But recognize that even in this population, false-negative tests can occur. If you are interested in looking for underlying coronary artery disease to identify plaques that are at risk of causing a myocardial infarction, a coronary CT angiogram is a better test.

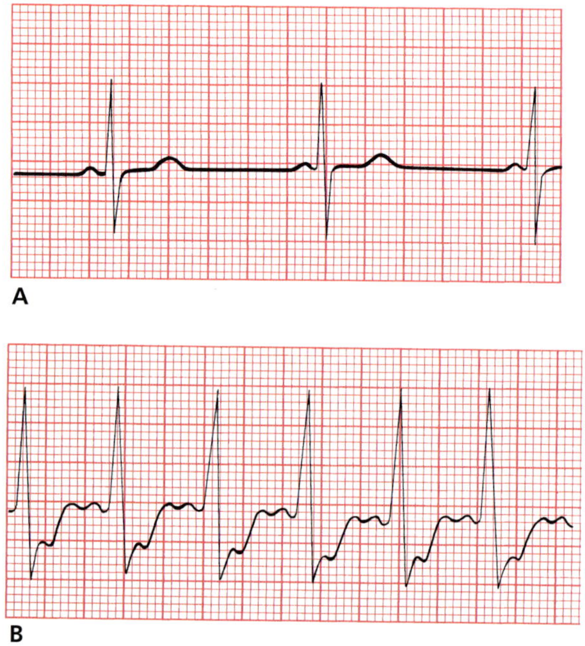

(*A*) A patient's resting EKG. (*B*) The same lead in the same patient 12 minutes into an exercise test. Note the prominent ST-segment depression associated with the increased heart rate.

Both the sensitivity and specificity of the exercise stress test can be increased by (1) doing an **echocardiogram** before and after the procedure, looking for exercise-induced changes in wall motion that might signify myocardium in jeopardy or (2) injecting the patient with **radioactive imaging agents** during the test and then recording images of the heart. In the latter procedure, termed **myocardial scintigraphy**, the myocardium extracts the radiotracer from the coronary circulation, but regions of compromised blood flow will be unable to extract the radiotracer.

In patients who are unable to exercise, there are alternatives to the traditional stress test. These include **adenosine stress testing** and **dobutamine stress testing**.

Adenosine, given intravenously, produces transient coronary vasodilatation, increasing coronary blood flow up to 400%. Vessels with significant stenosis, however, are already maximally vasodilated at rest and are unable to expand any further, so that the territory of the heart they supply will not show increased coronary flow. Typically, there are no diagnostic EKG changes during this test.

A dobutamine stress test mimics the stress of exercise on the heart. Dobutamine is an adrenaline-like agent that is given in incremental doses over several minutes. In patients with coronary artery disease, EKG changes just like those induced by exercise may be seen, and transient wall motion abnormalities will be seen on an accompanying echocardiogram.

CASE 9

Joan L. is a 62-year-old business executive. She is on an important business trip and spends the night at a hotel in the small town she is visiting. Early the next morning, she is awakened with shortness of breath and severe chest pressure that radiates into her jaw and left arm. She gets out of bed and takes an antacid, but the pain does not go away. Feeling dizzy and nauseated, she sits down and phones the front desk. Her symptoms are relayed by phone to the doctor covering the hotel, who immediately orders an ambulance to take her to the local emergency room. She arrives there 2 hours after the onset of her symptoms, which have continued unabated despite three sublingual nitroglycerin tablets given to her during the ambulance ride.

In the emergency room, a 12-lead EKG reveals the following:

Is she having an infarction? If so, can you tell if it is acute and what region of the heart is affected?

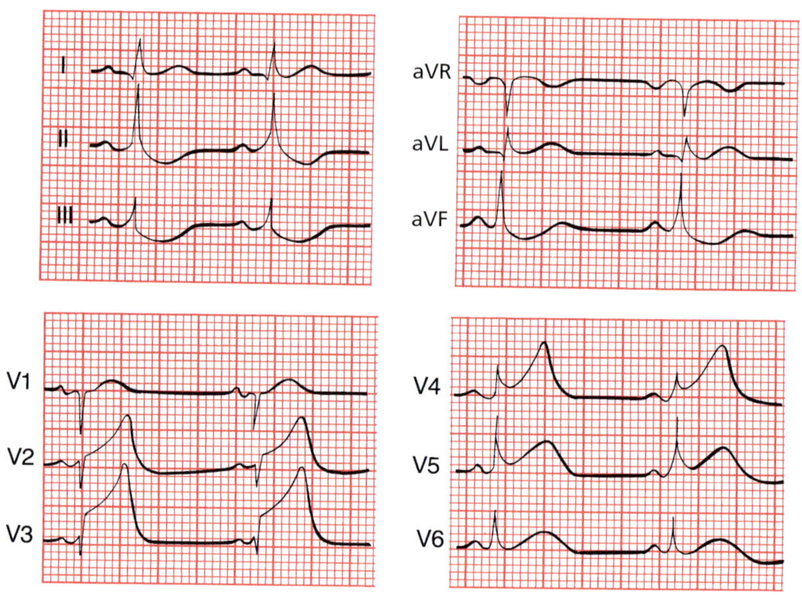

The EKG shows ST-segment elevation in leads V2 through V5. There are no Q waves. Joan is in the throes of an acute anterior STEMI.

Joan's prompt arrival in the emergency room, the elevated ST segments, and the absence of Q waves on the EKG mean that she is an excellent candidate for either thrombolytic therapy or acute coronary angioplasty. Unfortunately, she relates that only 1 month ago, she suffered a mild hemorrhagic stroke, leaving her with some weakness in her left arm and leg, making the risks of thrombolytic therapy prohibitive. In addition, acute angioplasty is not available at this small community hospital, and the nearest large medical center is several hours away. Therefore, doing the best they can under the circumstances, the medical staff have Joan admitted to the cardiac care unit (CCU) to be monitored. Her pain is controlled with morphine and intravenous nitroglycerin. Aspirin is also given, but all other anticoagulant agents are withheld because of her stroke history. Her first troponin level comes back elevated.

Late on the first night of her hospital stay, one of the nurses notices peculiar beats on her EKG:

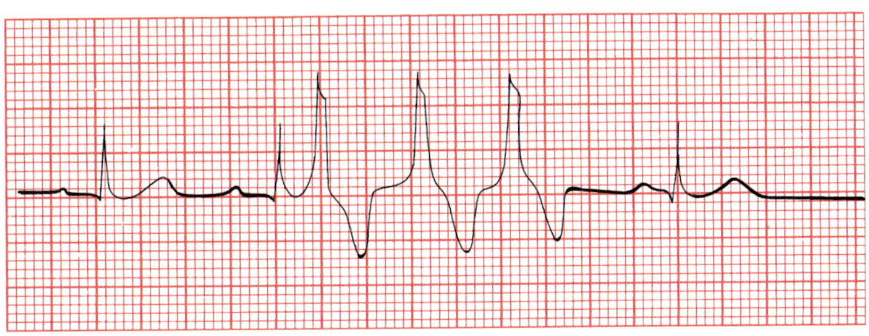

What are they?

The patient's normal sinus rhythm is being interrupted by a run of three consecutive premature ventricular contractions (PVCs). In the setting of an acute infarction, these can be concerning. Her clinicians decided to start her on a beta blocker to lessen sympathetic stimulation to her heart.

The next morning, Joan's EKG looks like this. What has changed?

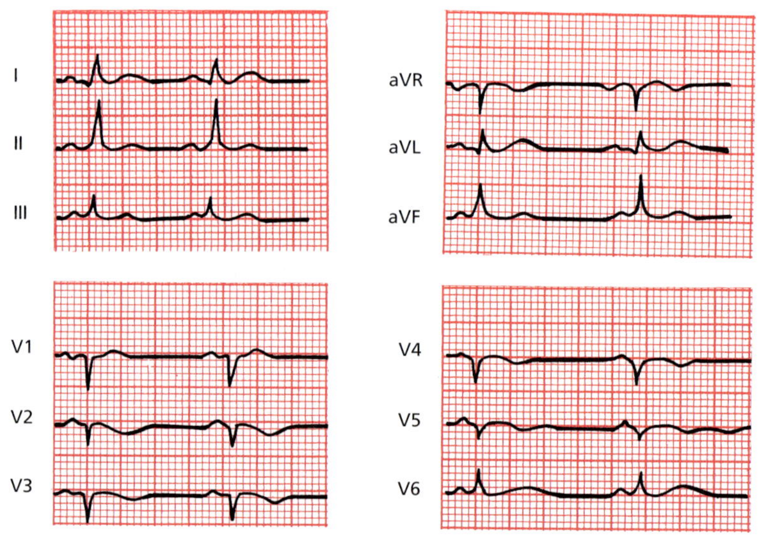

Joan's EKG shows that all ventricular ectopy has been suppressed. It also shows new Q waves in the anterior leads, consistent with full evolution of an anterior infarct.

Later in the afternoon, Joan again begins to experience chest pain. A repeat EKG is taken. What has changed?

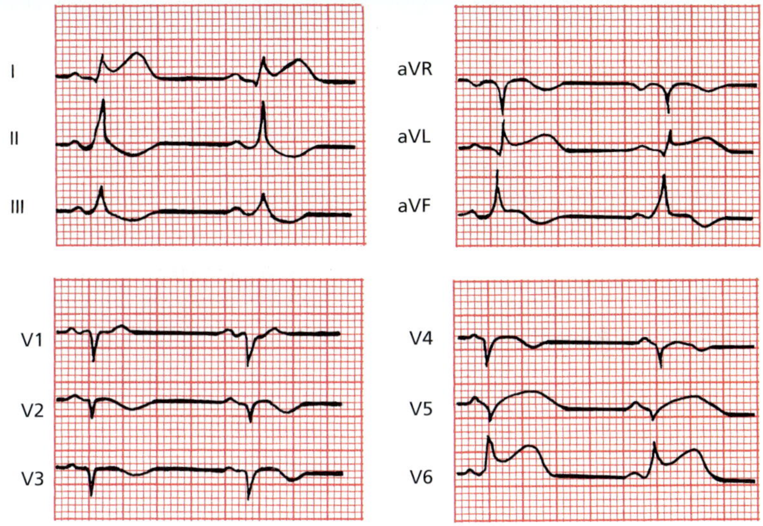

Joan is extending her infarct. New ST elevations can be seen in the left lateral leads.

A few hours later, she complains of lightheadedness, and another EKG is performed. Now what do you see?

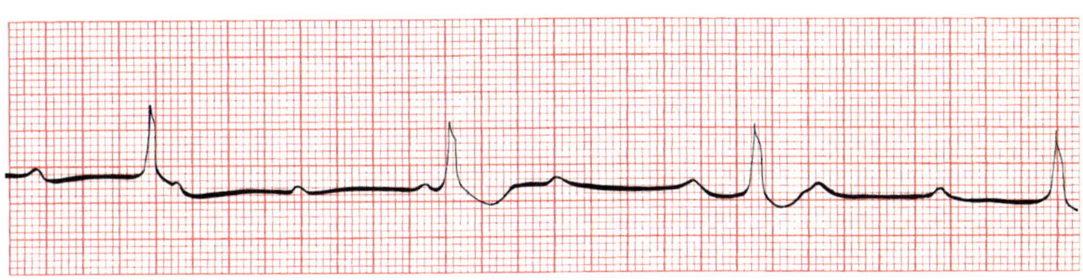

Joan has gone into third-degree AV block. Serious conduction blocks can develop during a myocardial infarction. Her light-headedness is due to inadequate cardiac output in the face of a ventricular escape rhythm of ~35 beats per minute. Pacemaker insertion is mandatory.

A pacemaker is placed without difficulty, and Joan suffers no further complications during her hospital stay. One week later, ambulatory and pain free, she is discharged. The morning after returning home, she again awakens short of breath and is taken to the emergency room. There, she is found to be in congestive heart failure. An echocardiogram reveals markedly diminished left ventricular function as a result of her large myocardial infarction. She is treated in the hospital and is discharged after 3 days. No further problems develop, and she is able to return to her normal life at home and at work.

This case is very typical of the sort of thing you may see over and over again in hospitals across the country. It emphasizes how critical the EKG is in diagnosing and managing patients with acute myocardial infarctions. With Joan, an EKG confirmed the initial suspicion that she was having an infarct. In the CCU, electrocardiographic surveillance permitted the diagnosis of further infarction and accompanying rhythm and conduction disturbances and guided major therapeutic decisions. Finally, we should stress that although Joan was managed successfully at her small local hospital, whenever possible, patients should be treated at hospitals with access to a catheterization laboratory.

CASE 10

Sam S., a 45-year-old florist, is referred to you for a preoperative evaluation prior to an elective cholecystectomy. His medical history is unremarkable, and his physical examination is normal. He is on no medications. The surgeon has requested a preop EKG and lab work. You move on to your next patient, and the technician in your office draws the patient's blood and runs a 12-lead EKG before letting the patient go home.

Later that day, before leaving the office, you check his EKG. Let's look at just the precordial leads. What do you see?

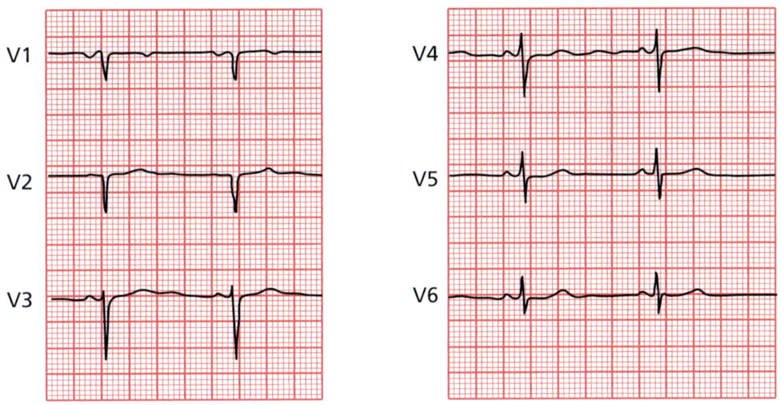

Note the Q wave (actually a QS wave) in lead V2 and poor R-wave progression. It looks like Sam may have had an anterior myocardial infarction sometime in the past.

You call Sam at his flower shop (he keeps very late hours, like you), and he assures you he is fine and has never experienced a moment of chest pain in his life. Nevertheless, you are concerned and ask him to come back the next day. He does, and you repeat the EKG, this time running it yourself. Now what do you see?

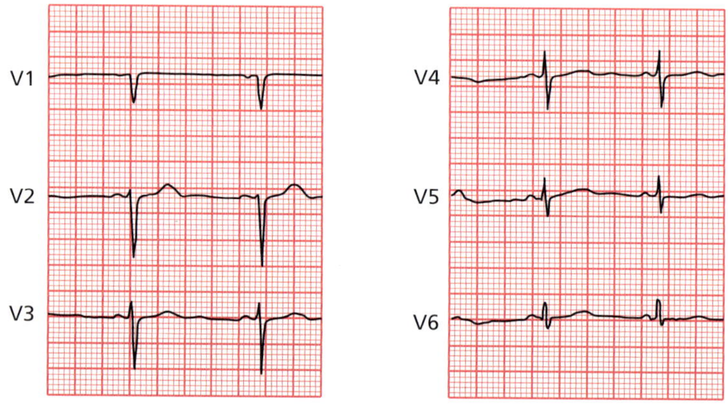

You heave a sigh of relief; the Q wave has magically disappeared; what first looked like a Q wave in lead V2 turns out to be a deep S wave preceded by a small R wave, a normal QRS complex! Or *maybe not so magically*. As you suspected, the first EKG was an error, in this case, a common error of lead placement. Attaching leads V1 and V2 too high on the chest wall (toward the head) is common and can cause precisely this sort of confusion. With this mistake in lead placement, the view of the heart can be altered just enough so that, during the initial stage of ventricular depolarization, the current appears to be moving away from the electrodes, generating Q waves. In the hands of someone less astute, this mistake could have had important repercussions, leading to a delay in the patient's surgery and to unnecessary testing (eg, a stress test or even cardiac catheterization).

Happy ending: Sam had his gallbladder removed without complication and is back at work feeling just fine!

7 Finishing Touches

In this chapter, you will learn:

1 | that the EKG can be changed by and help diagnose a remarkable variety of other cardiac and noncardiac disorders. We will discuss the most important of these as well as several other settings where the role of the EKG is perhaps more controversial:

A. electrolyte disturbances, especially abnormalities in potassium and calcium levels
B. hypothermia
C. digitalis effects, both therapeutic and toxic
D. medications that prolong the QT interval, and a helpful primer on the QT interval in general
E. other cardiac disorders—pericarditis, cardiomyopathy, myocarditis, and atrial septal defect (ASD)
F. pulmonary disorders
G. central nervous system (CNS) diseases
H. sleep disorders
I. eating disorders
J. sudden cardiac death in persons without coronary artery disease
K. the athlete's heart—what are normal EKG findings, and what are cause for concern?
L. screening young athletes before participating in sports—should you get an EKG?
M. common artifacts seen on the EKG
N. the role of the EKG in the preoperative evaluation

2 | about the cases of Amos T., whose EKG proves to be the key to unraveling an emergent, life-threatening noncardiac condition, and Ursula U., almost done in by some very commonly prescribed medications

Many medications, electrolyte disturbances, and a multitude of cardiac and noncardiac disorders can substantially alter the normal pattern of the EKG. It is not always obvious *why* the EKG is so sensitive to such a diffuse array of things, but it is, and you need to know about them.

In some of these instances, the EKG may actually be the most sensitive indicator of an impending catastrophe or at least the first and best clue that something serious may be going on. Many of these conditions will factor into your differential diagnosis when confronting specific abnormalities on the EKG, many of which we have already discussed. So, all things considered, you need to know this stuff. The payoff for you—and especially your patients—can be huge.

We will conclude this chapter by exploring the pros and cons of obtaining a routine 12-lead EKG prior to sports participation and before surgery. The guidelines continue to evolve, but a general consensus is emerging.

Electrolyte Disturbances

Alterations in the serum levels of potassium and calcium, both too high and too low, can profoundly alter the EKG.

Hyperkalemia

Hyperkalemia is the great imitator. It can do almost anything to the EKG. This should not surprise you, since potassium is so critical to the electrical activity of all heart cells.

In its most classic—but by no means only—presentation, hyperkalemia produces a progressive evolution of changes in the EKG that can, if allowed to go uncorrected, culminate in ventricular fibrillation and death. *The presence of any electrocardiographic changes is a better measure of clinically significant potassium toxicity than is the serum potassium level.*

As the potassium begins to rise, the T waves across the entire 12-lead EKG begin to peak. This effect can easily be confused with the peaked T waves of an acute myocardial infarction. One difference is that the changes in an infarction are confined to those leads overlying the area of the infarct, whereas in hyperkalemia, the changes are diffuse, seen in most, if not, all leads.

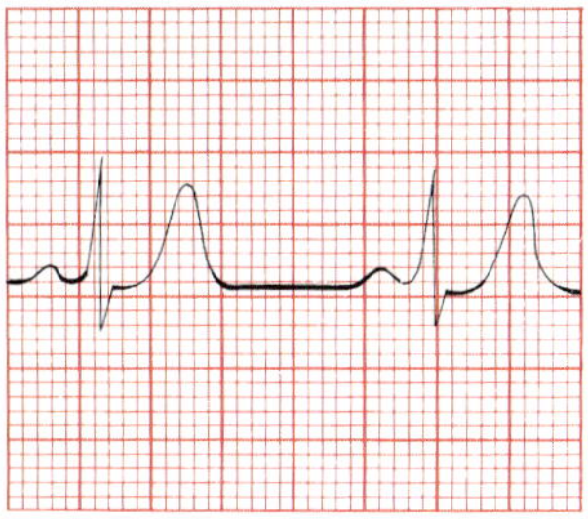

The peaked, symmetric T waves of hyperkalemia.

With a further increase in the serum potassium, the PR interval becomes prolonged, and the P wave gradually flattens and then disappears.

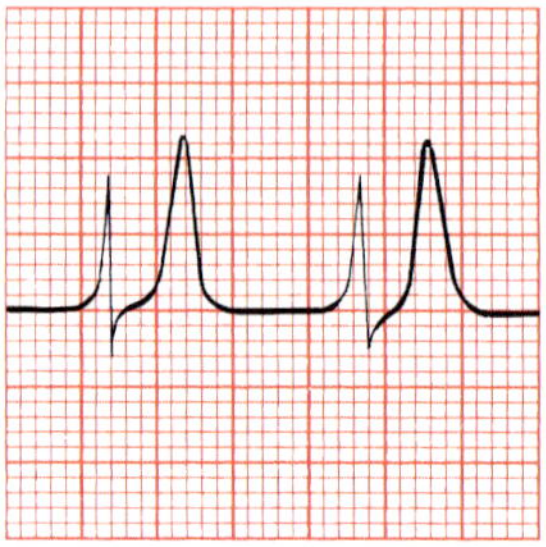

As the potassium level rises, P waves are no longer visible. The T waves are even more peaked.

The third change is that the QRS complex widens, ultimately merging with the T wave to create a sine wave-like pattern (apologies for forcing you to reach back to your high school geometry class). We're already seen several causes of a widened QRS complex, so, to help you sort them out, here is an EKG pearl: the presence of a *rightward axis* (a negative QRS complex in lead I, a positive QRS in aVF) may be an important clue that the wide QRS complexes are the result of hyperkalemia (see the box below).

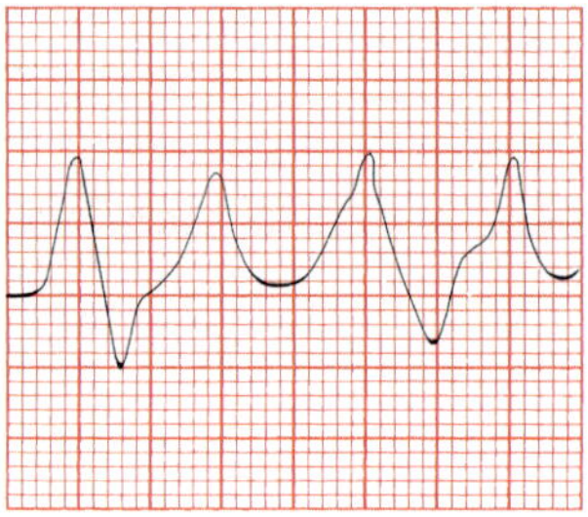

Progressive hyperkalemia leads to the classic sine wave pattern. The widened QRS complexes and peaked T waves are almost indistinguishable.

Hyperkalemia is just one cause of *right axis deviation*; we have seen several others. Here, they are in one handy list that should prove helpful whenever you see right axis deviation and are mulling over the diagnostic possibilities:

- Right ventricular hypertrophy (Chapter 2)
- Left posterior fascicular block (Chapter 4)
- Chronic and acute pulmonary disease (see later in this chapter)
- Hyperkalemia
- Ventricular ectopy/ventricular tachycardia (the axis can be rightward depending on the site of origin of the arrhythmia)
- An old lateral myocardial infarction (you know why—the electrical forces move away from the left lateral wall and therefore point rightward)
- Certain drugs, particularly sodium channel blockers (coming up later in this chapter)
- Misplaced leads (alas, all too common)
- Dextrocardia with situs inversus
- Infants and newborns, in whom it is normal because the right ventricle is able to outcompete the left ventricle for electrical dominance

Conduction blocks—high-degree AV blocks and bundle-branch blocks—can also appear as the serum potassium rises. Asystole or ventricular fibrillation may eventually develop.

It is important to note that, whereas the classic EKG changes often do occur in the order described as the serum potassium rises, they do not *always* do so. Progression to ventricular fibrillation can occur with devastating suddenness. **Any change in the EKG due to hyperkalemia mandates immediate clinical attention**!

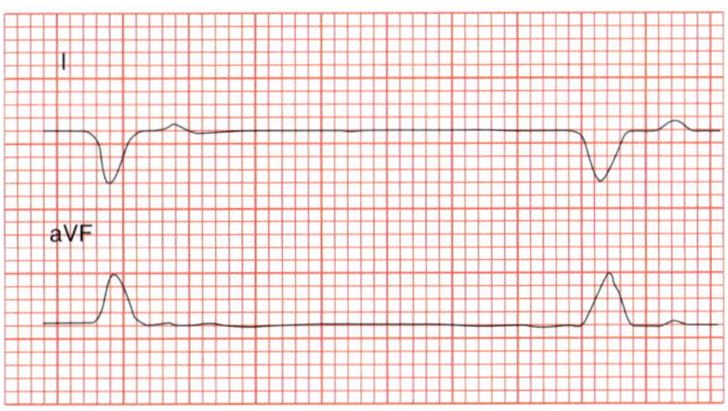

Leads I and aVF in a patient with hyperkalemia. The QRS complexes are wide, and there is a rightward axis. The rhythm is a slow junctional escape rhythm.

Hypokalemia

With hypokalemia, the EKG may again be a better measure of serious toxicity than the serum potassium level. Several changes can be seen, occurring in no particular order:

- ST-segment depression
- Flattening of the T wave with prolongation of the QT interval
- Appearance of a U wave

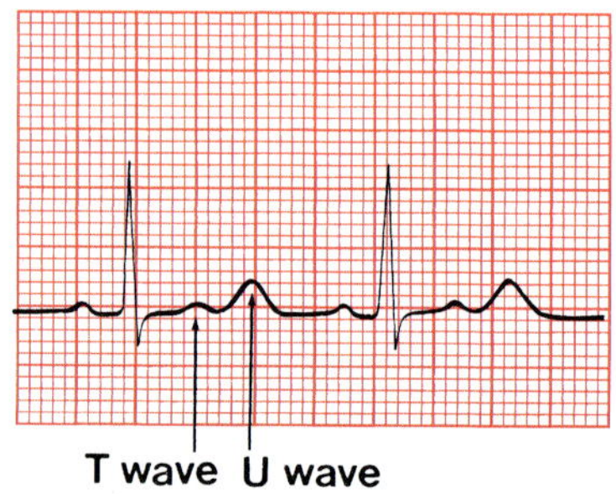

Hypokalemia. The U waves are even more prominent than the T waves. Slight ST-segment depression can also be seen.

We haven't discussed U waves yet. The short but relentless alphabetic progression of EKG waves has this one additional surprise in store for us. The term *U wave* is given to a wave appearing after the T wave in the cardiac cycle. They can be normal or pathologic. A U wave usually has the same axis as the T wave and is often best seen in leads V2 and V3. When seen in healthy hearts with no underlying pathology, their amplitude is usually much less than the T waves in the same leads.

The precise physiologic meaning of U waves is not fully understood. They can sometimes be surprisingly difficult to recognize; at first glance, you may think you are looking at a biphasic T wave. Although U waves are the most characteristic feature of hypokalemia, they are not in and of themselves diagnostic. Other conditions can produce prominent U waves (eg, central nervous system disease [CNS] and certain antiarrhythmic drugs). Inverted U waves (negative in leads with positive T waves) in the anteriolateral leads can be a marker for underlying ischemic, hypertensive or valvular heart disease. The evolution of inverted U waves during a stress test is fairly specific for stenosis of the left anterior descending artery, but has low sensitivity.

Severe hypokalemia can also cause prolongation of the QT interval, although what is perceived as a prolonged QT interval may really be the merging of the T wave with an ensuing U wave. It can also lead to supraventricular and ventricular tachyarrhythmias.

Calcium Disorders

Alterations in the serum calcium primarily affect the QT interval.

Hypocalcemia prolongs it; hypercalcemia shortens it. The former predisposes to that variant of ventricular tachycardia called torsade de pointes (see page 168).

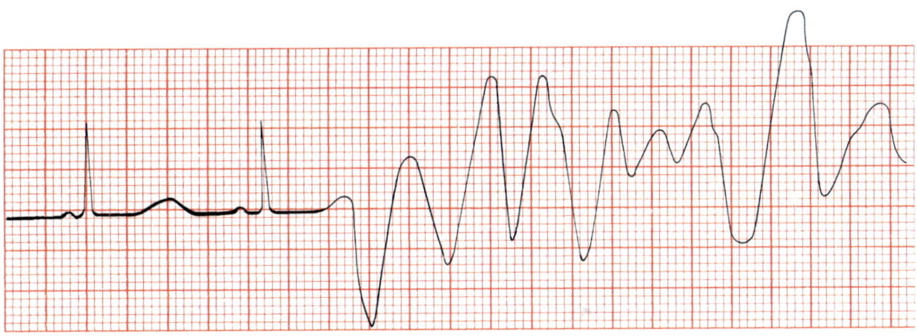

Hypocalcemia. The QT interval is prolonged. A premature ventricular contraction (PVC) falls on the prolonged T wave and sets off a run of torsade de pointes.

Other electrolyte disorders can also prolong the QT interval. These include hypokalemia (just discussed) and hypomagnesemia. We're not done with the QT interval just yet; stay tuned.

Hypothermia

You won't diagnose hypothermia with an EKG, you'll do it with a thermometer. But the changes on the EKG that accompany a very low body temperature can mimic other cardiac conditions, so they are important to recognize.

As the body temperature dips below normal, several things happen on the EKG:

1. Everything slows down. Sinus bradycardia is common, and all the segments and intervals—PR, QRS, QT, etc.—become prolonged.

2. A distinctive and virtually diagnostic type of ST-segment elevation may be seen. It consists of an abrupt ascent right at the J point and then an equally sudden plunge back to baseline. The resultant configuration is called a *J wave* or *Osborn wave.* J waves will disappear as the patient is rewarmed. The ST-segment elevation can be quite dramatic, as shown below, and can sometimes be confused with acute coronary syndrome.

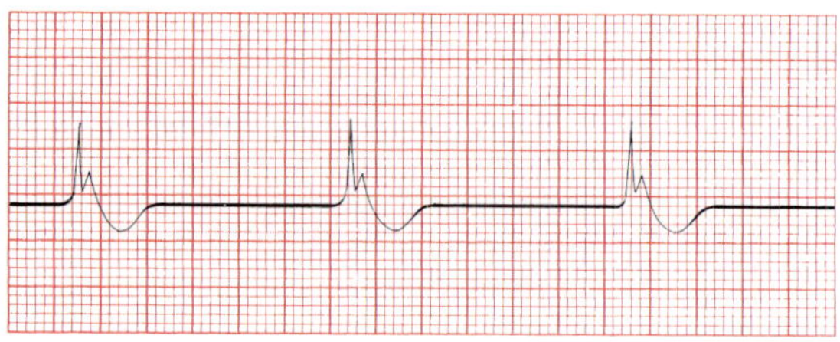

Hypothermia. The Osborn waves are very prominent.

3. Various arrhythmias may appear, not just sinus bradycardia, but also a slow junctional rhythm or slow atrial fibrillation.

4. A muscle tremor artifact due to shivering may complicate the tracing. A similar artifact may be seen in patients with Parkinson disease. As shown on the next page, muscle tremor artifact can mimic atrial fibrillation or atrial flutter.

Tremors occur at different frequencies. Whereas the tremor of hypothermia can occur at almost any frequency, the tremor of Parkinson disease can easily be mistaken for atrial flutter, since both tend to cycle at about 5 Hz, or 300 times per minute.

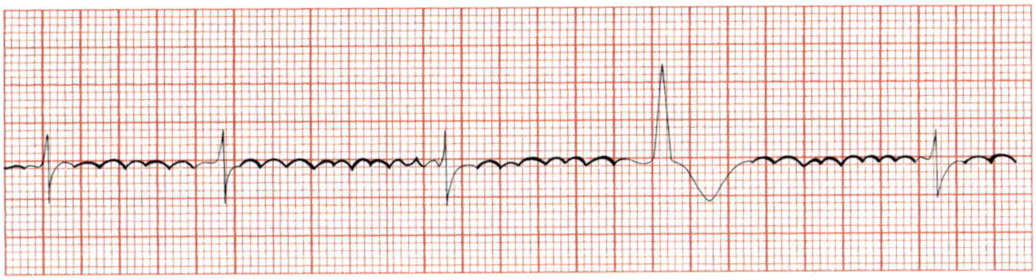

A muscle tremor artifact resembles atrial flutter.

Drugs

Digitalis

We don't use digitalis all that much anymore, but EKG books love the stuff because it can do so many interesting things to the EKG. We will continue in that glorious tradition. There are two distinct categories of electrocardiographic alterations caused by digitalis: those associated with *therapeutic* blood levels of the drug and those seen with *toxic* blood levels.

EKG Changes Associated With Therapeutic Blood Levels

Therapeutic levels of digitalis produce characteristic ST-segment and T-wave changes. These changes are known as the *digitalis effect* and consist of (1) ST-segment depression with (2) flattening or inversion of the T wave. The depressed ST segments have a very gradual downslope, emerging almost imperceptibly from the preceding R wave. This distinctive appearance usually permits differentiation of the digitalis effect from the more symmetric ST-segment depression of ischemia; differentiation from ventricular hypertrophy with repolarization abnormalities can sometimes be more problematic, especially because digitalis is still sometimes used in patients with congestive heart failure who often have left ventricular hypertrophy.

The digitalis effect is usually most prominent in leads with tall R waves. *Remember:* the digitalis effect is normal and predictable and does not necessitate discontinuing the drug.

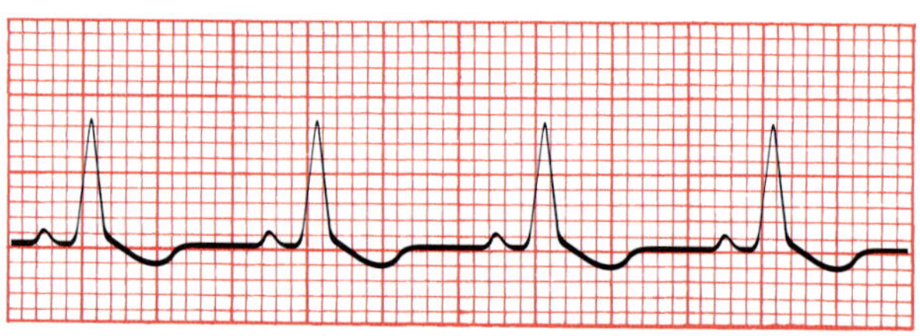

The digitalis effect, with asymmetric ST-segment depression.

EKG Changes Associated With Toxic Blood Levels

The *toxic manifestations* of digitalis, on the other hand, may require clinical intervention. Digitalis intoxication can elicit conduction blocks and tachyarrhythmias, alone or in combination.

Sinus Node Suppression

Even at therapeutic blood levels of digitalis, the sinus node can be slowed, particularly in patients with the sick sinus syndrome (page 189). At toxic blood levels, sinus exit block or complete sinus node suppression can occur.

Conduction Blocks

Digitalis slows conduction through the AV node and can therefore cause first-, second-, and even third-degree AV block.

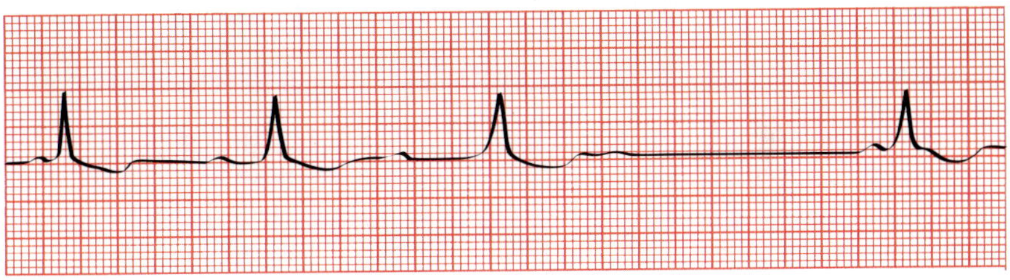

Mobitz type I second-degree AV (Wenckebach) block caused by digitalis intoxication.

The ability of digitalis to slow AV conduction can be useful in the treatment of supraventricular tachycardias. For example, digitalis can slow the ventricular rate in patients with atrial fibrillation; however, the ability of digitalis to slow the heart rate, best seen when patients are sitting or lying quietly for their EKG recording, is commonly lost during exertion. Beta blockers, such as atenolol or metoprolol, also affect AV conduction but may control the rate better when there is increased adrenergic tone (eg, during exercise or stress).

Tachyarrhythmias

Because digitalis enhances the automatic behavior of all cardiac conducting cells, causing them to act more like pacemakers, there is no tachyarrhythmia that digitalis cannot cause. Paroxysmal atrial tachycardia (PAT, see page 156) and premature ventricular contractions (PVCs) are the most common, junctional rhythms are fairly common, and atrial flutter and fibrillation are the least common.

Combinations

The combination of PAT with second-degree AV block is the most characteristic rhythm disturbance of digitalis intoxication. The conduction block is usually 2:1 but may vary unpredictably. Digitalis is the most common, but not the only, cause of PAT with block.

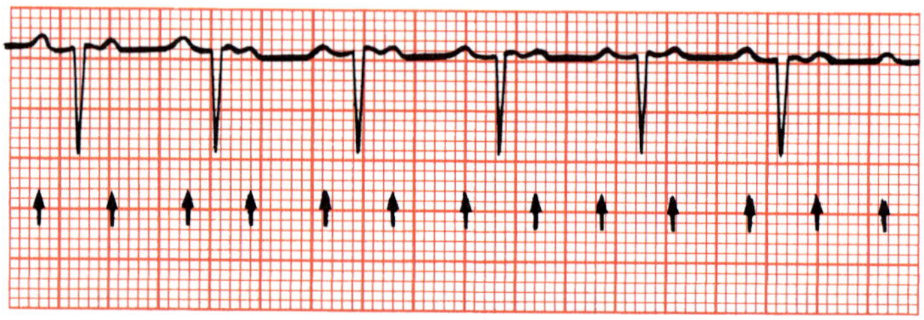

PAT with 2:1 block. The *arrows* point to each P wave.

Sodium Channel Blockers

The sodium ion channels are important in nerve conduction, so anything that interferes with their function can alter the EKG. The most commonly used sodium channel blockers are the tricyclic antidepressants (eg, amitriptyline and nortriptyline), but many antiarrhythmic agents (eg, sotalol, amiodarone, dofetilide, and dronedarone), and hyperkalemia also can block the sodium channels. Cocaine is also a sodium channel blocker. EKG findings can include sinus tachycardia, a wide QRS complex, a right axis with a tall R wave in the most rightward leads (aVR and V1), and a long QT interval.

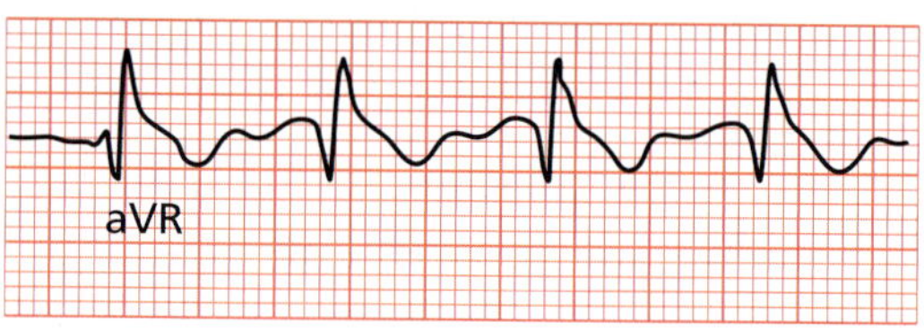

Lead aVR in a patient who overdosed on amitriptyline. Lead aVR normally has a deep negative deflection, whereas here you can see the tall R wave. Note also the widened QRS complex and prolonged QT interval.

Medications That Prolong the QT Interval

We have already seen that hypocalcemia, hypomagnesemia, and severe hypokalemia can prolong the QT interval. Many medications can also prolong the QT interval and increase the risk for a serious ventricular tachyarrhythmia. As we mentioned above, sodium channel blocking medications can prolong the QT interval, including several antidepressants, cocaine, and many antiarrhythmic agents. Antiarrhythmic agents are used to treat arrhythmias, but by increasing the QT interval, some of them (class I and III) can paradoxically increase the risk for serious ventricular tachyarrhythmias. The QT interval must be carefully monitored in all patients taking any of these medications, especially if more than one is being used at the same time, and the drug(s) should be stopped if substantial prolongation occurs.

Other commonly used drugs can also prolong the QT interval. For most of these, especially in conventional doses, the risk of a potentially fatal arrhythmia is very small. Among them are the following:

- Antibiotics: macrolides (eg, erythromycin, clarithromycin, azithromycin) and fluoroquinolones (eg, levofloxacin and ciprofloxacin)
- Antifungals (eg, ketoconazole)
- Nonsedating antihistamines (eg, astemizole, terfenadine)
- Psychotropic agents: antipsychotics (eg, haloperidol, phenothiazines), selective serotonin reuptake inhibitors (eg, citalopram, fluoxetine), opiates and methadone
- Some gastrointestinal medications, antineoplastic agents, and diuretics (the last by causing hypokalemia or hypomagnesemia)

The risk of developing a significantly prolonged QT interval, leading to a high risk of progressing to torsade de pointes, is increased in patients who take more than one of these drugs. It is also enhanced when their metabolism is compromised, leading to higher blood levels. Grapefruit juice, for example, inhibits the activity of the cytochrome P-450 enzyme system, which is responsible for metabolizing many of these drugs, and the resulting higher serum drug levels can lead to QT prolongation.

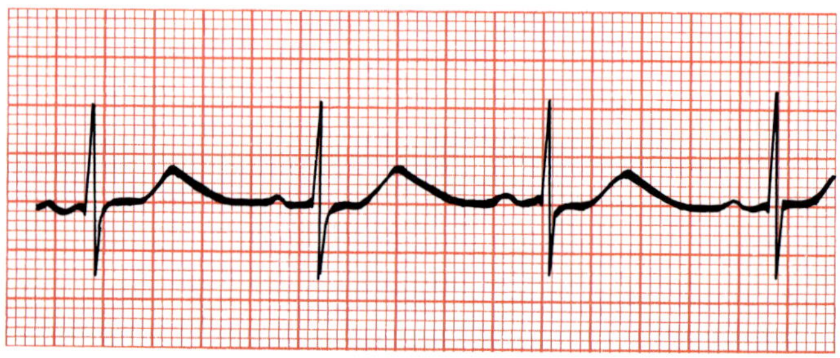

The prolonged QT interval on this tracing mandated reducing the patient's sotalol dosage.

More on the QT Interval

Several *inherited disorders of cardiac repolarization* associated with long QT intervals have been identified and linked to specific chromosomal abnormalities. The cause in almost half of genotyped individuals is one of various mutations in a gene that encodes pore-forming subunits of the membrane channels that generate a slow K^+ current that is adrenergic sensitive. All individuals in these families need to be screened for the presence of the genetic defect with resting and stress EKGs. If the abnormality is found, beta-blocking drugs and sometimes implantable defibrillators are recommended because the risk for sudden death from a lethal arrhythmia is greatly increased, especially during childhood or early adulthood.

How to Measure the QT Interval Accurately

Because the QT interval varies with the heart rate, a *corrected QT interval*, or QTc, is used to assess absolute QT prolongation. The QTc adjusts for differences in the heart rate by dividing the QT interval by the square root of the R-R interval—that is, the square root of one cardiac cycle:

$$QTc = \frac{QT}{\sqrt{RR}}$$

The QTc should not exceed 500 ms during therapy with any medication that can prolong the QT interval (550 ms if there is an underlying bundle-branch block); adhering to this rule will reduce the risk for ventricular arrhythmias. This simple formula for determining the QTc is most accurate at heart rates between 50 and 120 beats per minute; at the extremes of heart rate—really fast or really slow—its usefulness is limited.

Causes of a Prolonged QTc Interval

Hypocalcemia
Hypomagnesemia
Hypokalemia (severe)
Congenital disorders
Medications (discussed above)
Hypothermia
Cardiac ischemia

Can the QT interval ever be too short? The answer is yes. A short QT interval is generally defined—not everyone agrees on the precise number—as a QT interval <360 ms. Congenital short QT syndrome is far less common than its more lengthy compatriot. It can be caused by any number of inherited "channelopathies." Most patients appear to have no complications, but there is an increased risk of atrial and ventricular arrhythmias. The differential diagnosis of a short QT interval includes hyperkalemia and hypercalcemia.

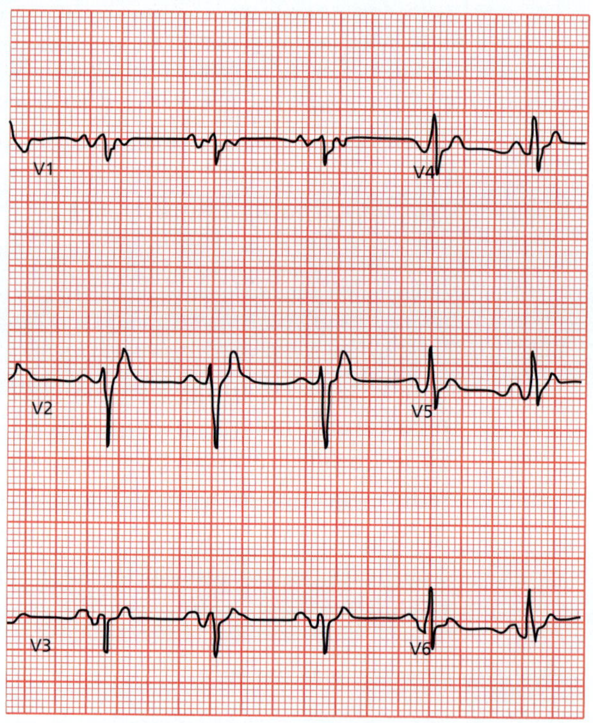

An example of a short QT interval.

Other Cardiac Disorders

Pericarditis

Acute pericarditis—inflammation of the outer lining of the heart—can cause ST-segment elevation and T-wave flattening or inversion. These changes can easily be confused with an evolving infarction, as can the clinical picture. Certain features of the EKG can be helpful in differentiating pericarditis from infarction*:

1. The ST-segment and T-wave changes in pericarditis tend to be diffuse, involving more leads than we would expect to see from the localized effect of an infarction. The ST segment is typically concave upward (saddle shaped), unlike the ST elevation seen with an infarction. With STEMIs, you may also see reciprocal ST depression; you won't see this with pericarditis. And one final point: if the ST-segment elevation is greater in lead III than lead II, you are probably dealing with a STEMI and not acute pericarditis.
2. In pericarditis, T-wave inversion usually occurs only *after* the ST segments have returned to baseline. In infarction, T-wave inversion usually precedes normalization of the ST segments.
3. In pericarditis, Q-wave formation does not occur.
4. The EKG change that everyone seems to harp on is depression of the PR interval, and indeed, the PR interval is often depressed, usually in many leads (aside from aVR). However, do not overrely on this criterion. It is not specific to pericarditis and can sometimes (as much as 12% of the time) be seen with a STEMI. Only once you have convinced yourself that your patient does not have a STEMI should you turn to the PR interval for help in determining if your patient may have pericarditis.

---

*These electrocardiographic changes are not seen in all patients, and some patients with confirmed pericarditis may show no EKG abnormalities at all. Why is this? The pericardium is actually electrically silent, so the electrocardiogram will only be affected when the pericardial inflammation spreads to involve other regions of the heart, notably the myocardium.

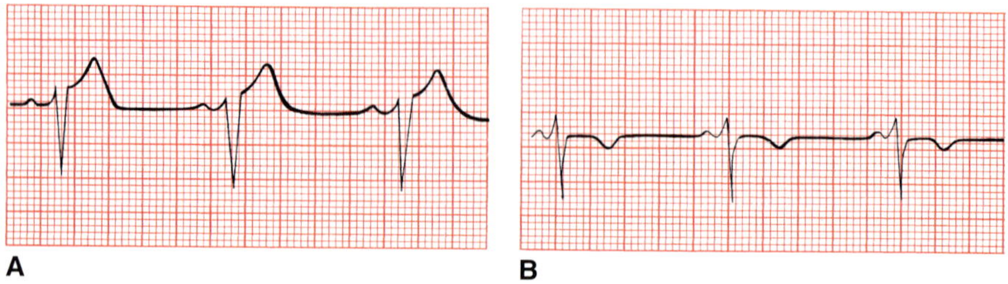

(*A*) Lead V3 shows the ST-segment elevation of acute pericarditis. (*B*) The same lead several days later shows that the ST segments have returned to baseline and the T waves have inverted. There are no Q waves.

One other clue to the presence of pericarditis is what has been termed the *Spodick sign*. This refers to downsloping of the TP segment, extending from the end of the T wave to the start of the P wave. If you see this in a patient whom you suspect may have acute pericarditis *and* you have pretty much ruled out a STEMI, your patient probably has pericarditis. Again, make sure you have ruled out a STEMI; Spodick sign may be present in 5% of STEMIs.

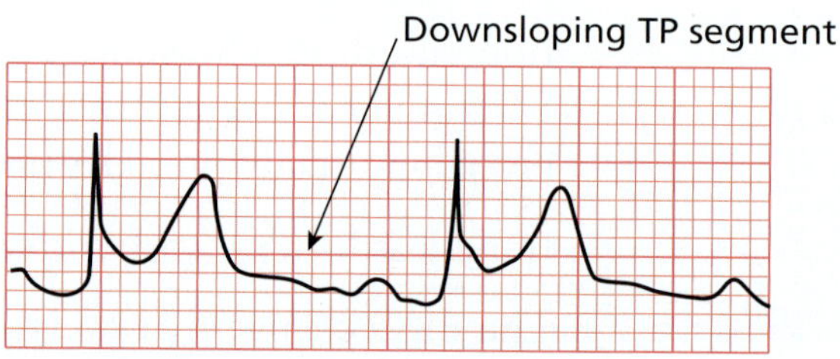

The Spodick sign

The EKG is only one part of the puzzle when differentiating the chest pain of pericarditis from the chest pain of cardiac ischemia. Recognizing the clinical presentation of pericarditis is essential. If your patient is a young adult with no risk factors for ischemic heart disease, then pericarditis is more likely, but be careful—keep in mind that more than 100,000 myocardial infarctions are diagnosed each year in the United States in patients aged 29 to 44 years.

Unlike angina, the pain of acute pericarditis is usually sharp, exacerbated by inspiration and coughing, and felt diffusely across the entire anterior chest wall, often radiating to the upper back. The pain usually eases when the patient sits leaning forward. On examination, you may be able to hear a pericardial friction rub over the left sternal border.

Some patients with pericarditis will develop a *pericardial effusion*. There are numerous other causes as well, such as chest trauma, malignancy, autoimmune diseases, renal failure, and hypothyroidism. Formation of a substantial pericardial effusion dampens the electrical output of the heart, resulting in low voltage in all leads. The ST-segment and T-wave changes of pericarditis may still be evident.

How do we define low voltage? By now, this should come as no surprise, but there are definitive criteria. The most sensitive are:

1. the sum of the total QRS voltage in leads I, II, and III is <15 mm or
2. the sum of the total QRS voltage in leads V1, V2, and V3 is <30 mm.

More specific criteria are

1. the QRS voltage in all limb leads is <5 mm or
2. the QRS voltage in all precordial leads is <10 mm.

A pericardial effusion is not the only cause of low voltage. Anything that dampens the ability of the surface electrodes to detect the electricity generated by the heart can be responsible, such as the expanded, air-filled lungs of chronic lung disease; a pneumothorax; a large pleural effusion; or the marked adiposity of someone who is very obese. Also, anything that reduces the heart's ability to generate normal voltage can be the culprit, for example, infiltrative diseases of the heart (such as amyloidosis), severe hypothyroidism, and end-stage cardiomyopathy caused by multiple infarctions.

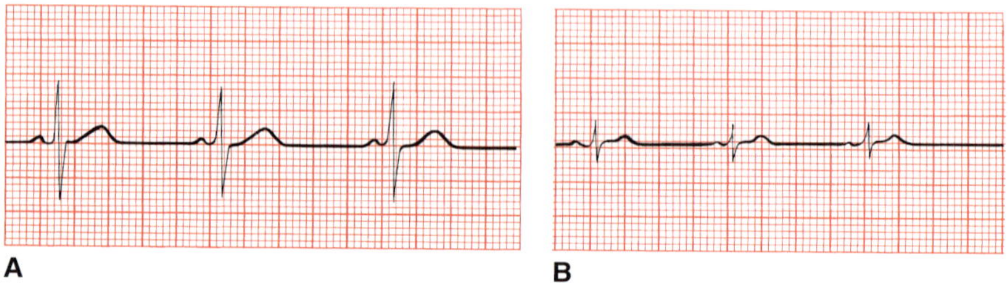

Lead I before (*A*) and after (*B*) the development of a pericardial effusion. Decreased voltage is the only significant change.

If an effusion is sufficiently large, the heart may actually rotate freely within the fluid-filled sac. This produces the phenomenon of *electrical alternans* in which the electrical axis of the heart varies with each beat. This can affect not only the axis of the QRS complex but also that of the P and T waves. A varying axis is most easily recognized on the EKG by the varying amplitude of each waveform from beat to beat.

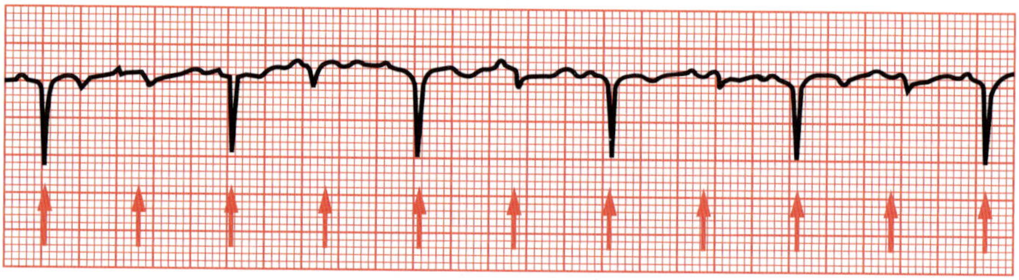

Electrical alternans. The *arrows* point to each QRS complex.

Hypertrophic Obstructive Cardiomyopathy

We have already discussed hypertrophic obstructive cardiomyopathy, also known as idiopathic hypertrophic subaortic stenosis, in the case of Tom L. (page 106). Some patients with hypertrophic obstructive cardiomyopathy have normal EKGs, but left ventricular hypertrophy and left axis deviation are common. Deep, narrow, dagger-like Q waves may also be seen laterally and inferiorly. These do not represent infarction.

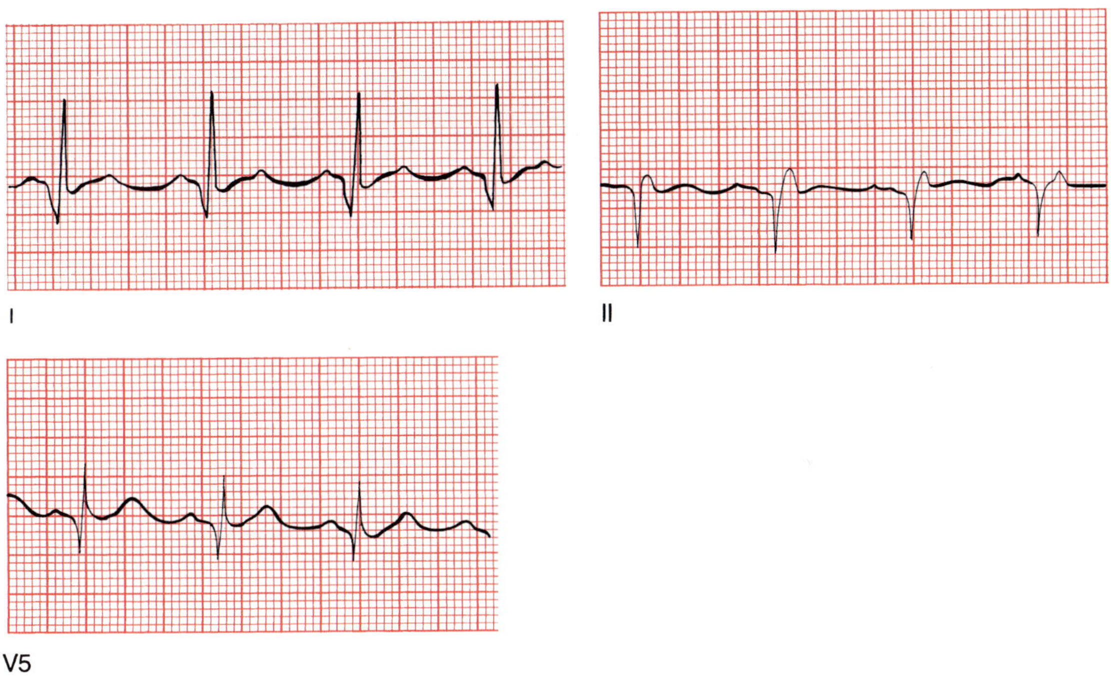

Hypertrophic obstructive cardiomyopathy. Deep Q waves can be seen in both lateral and inferior leads.

Myocarditis

Any diffuse inflammatory process involving the myocardium can produce a number of changes on the EKG. Infections—think COVID, but also many other viruses, bacteria, parasites and even vaccines (very rarely)—and many drugs and toxins can be responsible. As with pericarditis, ST-segment elevation can occur that is usually but not always diffuse. Also common are conduction blocks, including bundle-branch blocks and AV blocks of any degree.

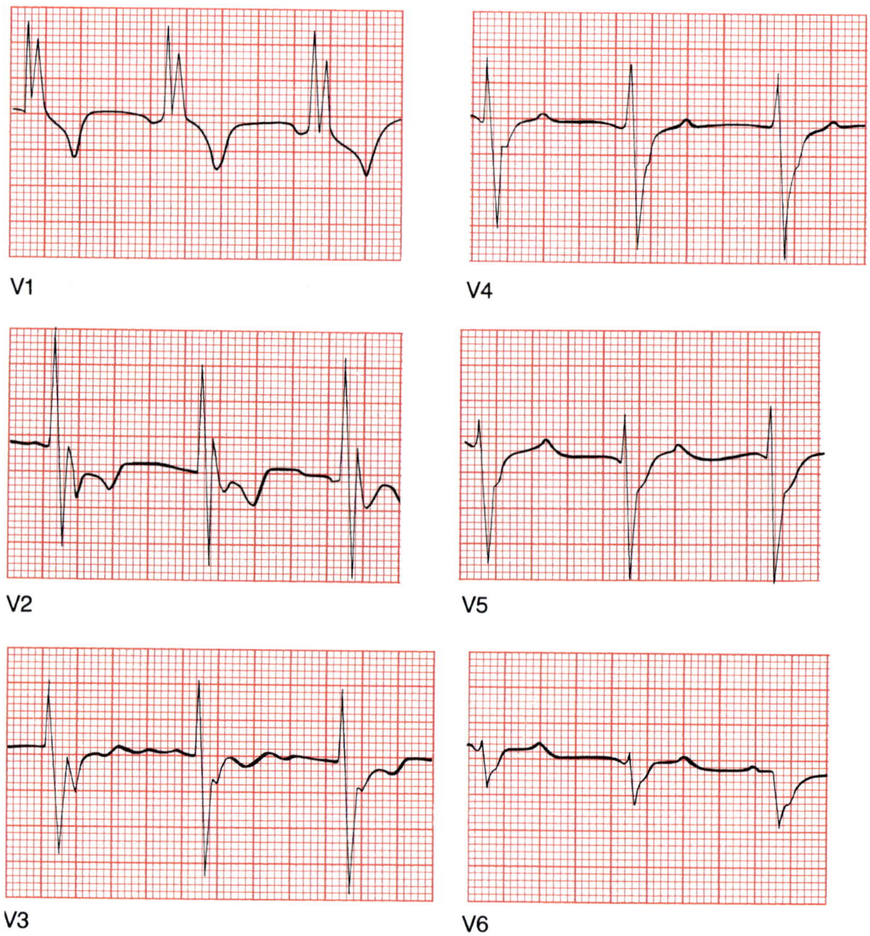

Right bundle-branch block in a patient with active myocarditis following a viral infection.

Atrial Septal Defect

An atrial septal defect (ASD) is a small opening between the left and right atria. It is often first diagnosed in adulthood. Symptoms arise from the prolonged shunting of blood from the high-pressure left atrium into the right atrium, and typically include fatigue and shortness of breath. Complications can include atrial arrhythmias, pulmonary hypertension, and paradoxical embolization, in which an embolus from a deep venous thrombosis in the extremities travels to the heart, is shunted to the left side of the heart through the ASD, and enters the systemic circulation, where it can cause a stroke. Closure of the ASD is indicated for patients with symptoms or evidence of right heart enlargement.

The EKG may be normal. With enlargement of the right atrium and right ventricle, however, you can see first-degree AV block, atrial tachyarrhythmias, incomplete right bundle-branch block, and, with the more common secundum ASD, right axis deviation (you may see left axis deviation with a primum ASD). The most characteristic finding, however, is what has been termed the *crochetage pattern*, a small notch in the QRS complexes in the inferior leads. It can occur early or late in the QRS complex. Interestingly, the size of the notch is proportional to the size of the ASD and the size of the shunt. Crochetage can also be seen in patients with a patent foramen ovale and sometimes in perfectly normal hearts.

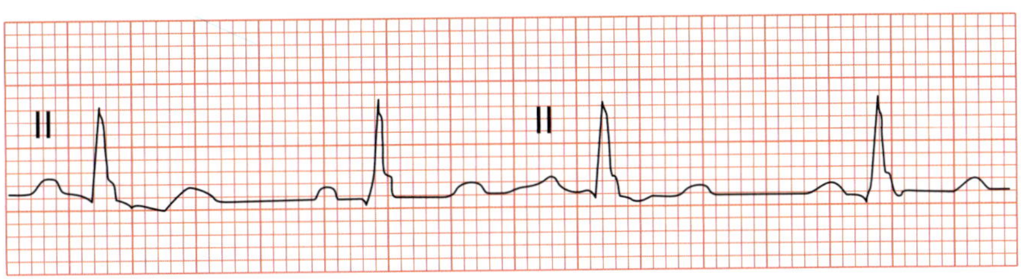

The small notch in the terminal portion of these QRS complexes is the crochetage pattern of an ASD.

Pulmonary Disorders

Chronic Obstructive Pulmonary Disease

The EKG of a patient with long-standing emphysema may show low voltage, right axis deviation, and poor R-wave progression in the precordial leads. The low voltage is caused by the dampening effects of the large residual volume of air trapped in the lungs. Right axis deviation is caused by the expanded lungs forcing the heart into a vertical or even rightward-oriented position, as well as by the pressure overload hypertrophy from pulmonary hypertension.

Chronic obstructive pulmonary disease can lead to chronic cor pulmonale and right-sided congestive heart failure. The EKG may then show right atrial enlargement (P pulmonale) and right ventricular hypertrophy with repolarization abnormalities.

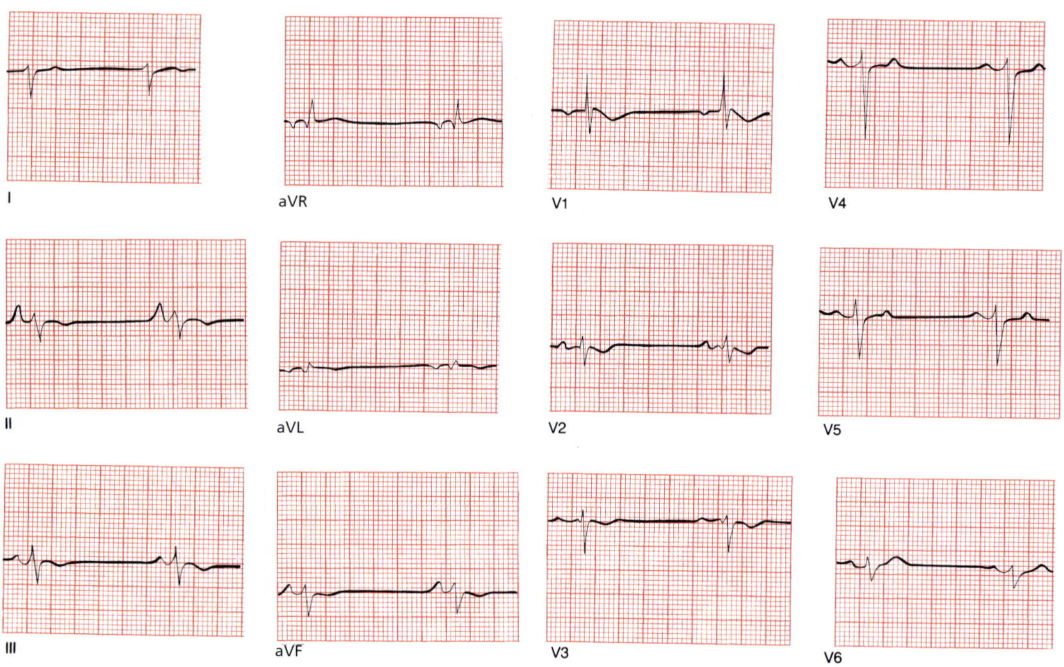

Chronic obstructive pulmonary disease. Note the low voltage, extreme right axis deviation, right atrial enlargement (in lead II), and precordial criteria for right ventricular hypertrophy.

Acute Pulmonary Embolism

A sudden massive pulmonary embolus can profoundly alter the EKG. Findings may include the following:

1. A pattern of right ventricular hypertrophy with repolarization changes, presumably due to right ventricular dilatation, although it takes time for the right ventricle to enlarge, so criteria for right ventricular hypertrophy may not be seen acutely.
2. Right bundle-branch block.
3. A large S wave in lead I and a deep Q wave in lead III. This is called the *S1Q3 pattern*. The T wave in lead III may also be inverted (S1Q3T3 pattern). Unlike an inferior infarction, in which Q waves are usually seen in at least two of the inferior leads, the Q waves in an acute pulmonary embolus are generally limited to lead III. Note: Although this is the finding that everyone talks about when discussing the EKG changes associated with a pulmonary embolus, it is actually quite uncommon. It is neither sensitive nor specific for an embolus, but if you see it in someone in whom an embolism is in the differential diagnosis, it should at least prick up your ears to the possibility and should factor into your evaluation.
4. T-wave inversion or flattening may be seen over the inferior and right precordial leads. This is actually the most common EKG abnormality associated with a pulmonary embolism, present in about one-third of patients.
5. A number of arrhythmias may be produced; the most common is sinus tachycardia.

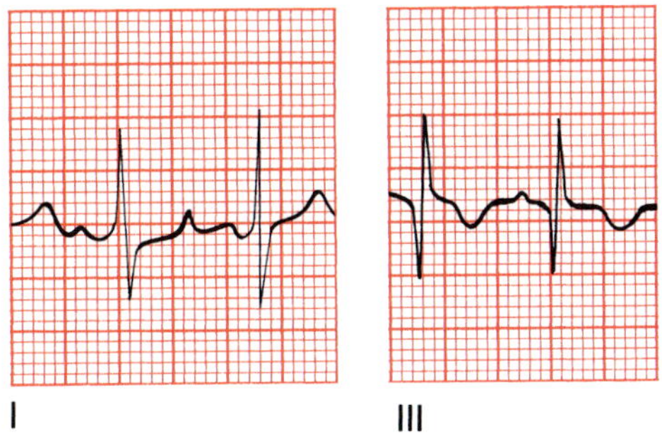

The S1Q3T3 pattern of a massive pulmonary embolus.

The EKG in a nonmassive pulmonary embolism is normal in most patients, or it may show only a sinus tachycardia.

Central Nervous System Disease

CNS catastrophes, such as a subarachnoid bleed or cerebral infarction, when associated with altered mental status and increased intracranial pressure, can produce diffuse T-wave inversion and prominent U waves. The T waves are typically very deep and very wide, and their contour is usually symmetrical (unlike the asymmetrical inverted T waves of secondary repolarization associated with ventricular hypertrophy). These changes are believed to be due to enhanced activity of the sympathetic and parasympathetic nervous systems affecting the heart.

Prolongation of the QTc interval is also common. Sinus bradycardia—and less often various tachyarrhythnias—can occur, as can ST-segment elevation and depression mimicking primary cardiac disease.

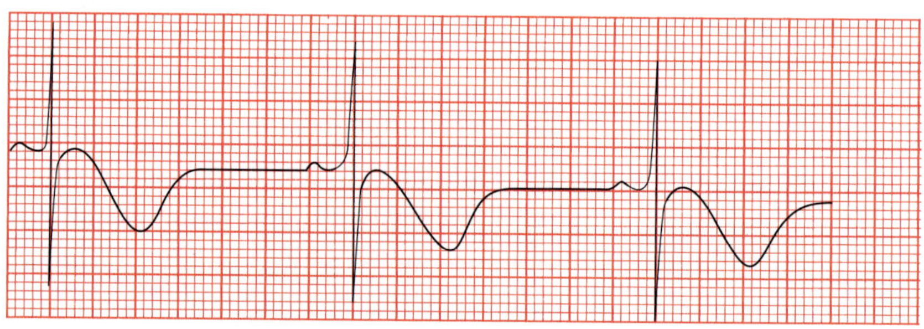

V4

Deeply inverted, wide T waves in lead V4 in a patient with a central nervous system bleed.

Sleep Disorders

Many of us are tired during the day, and most often the cause is obvious—we just don't get enough sleep. However, some people with daytime sleepiness have one of various sleep disorders, such as sleep apnea or restless legs syndrome.

Patients with sleep apnea are at increased risk of atrial and ventricular arrhythmias (it is a leading cause of atrial fibrillation) and heart block, as well as nocturnal angina, myocardial infarction, systemic and pulmonary hypertension, and right heart failure. Disrupted sleep causes transient hypoxia and altered autonomic function that probably underlie these problems.

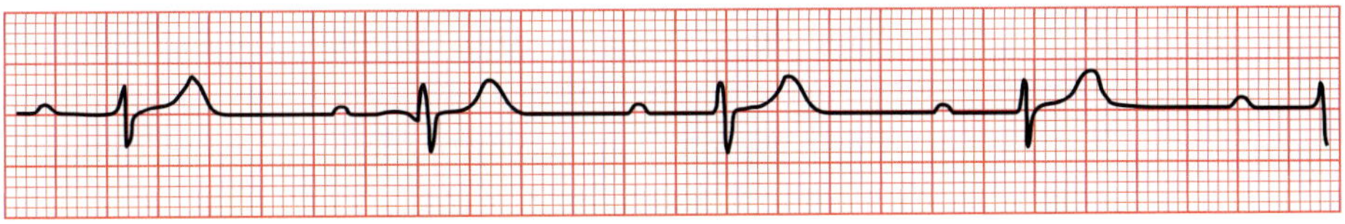

Part of a rhythm strip obtained during sleep in a patient with sleep apnea. Note the sinus bradycardia (~50 beats per minute) and first-degree AV block (prolonged PR interval).

Eating Disorders

Of the three most common eating disorders—binge eating, bulimia and anorexia nervosa—only the last has been shown to be consistently associated with abnormalities on the EKG. The EKG changes may be correlated with a low body mass index (BMI).

By far the most common finding is bradycardia, in some reports present in the majority of patients with anorexia nervosa. Other features, far less common, include low voltage, a right axis, and conduction abnormalities (especially junctional rhythms). Of most concern, though, are changes in the QTc interval. Reports differ on the prevalence of QTc abnormalities, and QTc prolongation with the attendant risk of ventricular tachycardia and sudden cardiac death appears to occur primarily in those patients with electrolyte abnormalities—hypokalemia, hypomagnesemia and hypophosphatemia accompanied by severe hypocalcemia—due, presumably, to malnutrition.

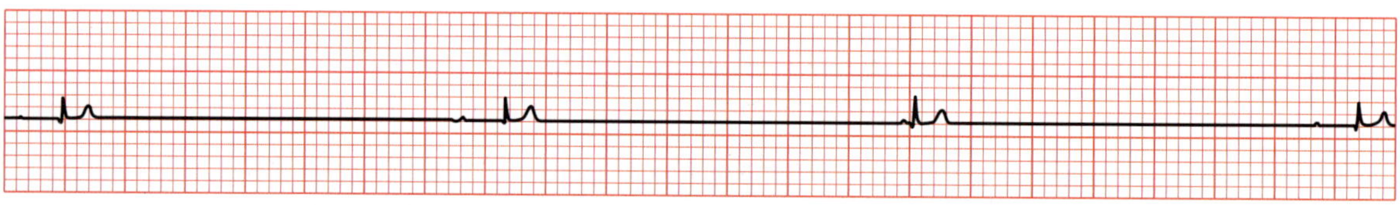

Severe bradycardia (heart rate in the twenties!) in a young patient with anorexia nervosa

Sudden Cardiac Death

By far, the most common cause of sudden cardiac death is underlying atherosclerosis (coronary artery disease), triggering infarction and/or arrhythmia. However, there are many other causes as well, some of which we have discussed. These include the following:

- *Hypertrophic cardiomyopathy*
- *Long QT interval syndrome*, acquired or congenital (and very rarely, short QT syndrome)
- *Wolff–Parkinson–White syndrome*
- *Viral myocarditis*
- *Infiltrative diseases of the myocardium* (eg, amyloidosis and sarcoidosis)
- *Valvular heart disease*
- *Drug abuse* (especially stimulants such as cocaine and amphetamines)
- *Commotio cordis*, in which blunt force to the chest causes ventricular fibrillation
- *Anomalous origin of the coronary arteries*, in which constriction of a coronary artery by surrounding tissue—exacerbating by the increased myocardial contractions of exercise—can cause ventricular fibrillation
- *Brugada syndrome*
- *Arrhythmogenic right ventricular cardiomyopathy (ARVC)*

We need to discuss the last two of these, as they are increasingly being recognized as important and not uncommon causes of syncope and sudden cardiac death.

Brugada pattern (it is called **Brugada syndrome** when the EKG changes are accompanied by symptoms) occurs in structurally normal hearts and, in this way, resembles the long QT syndromes. It is inherited as an autosomal dominant trait, and the average age of symptoms is 41, although the age range runs the gamut from early childhood to the extremes of old age. The cause appears to be a genetic mutation affecting voltage-dependent sodium channels during repolarization.

Brugada pattern can be identified by a specific set of abnormalities on the EKG: (1) a pattern resembling right bundle-branch block with a slow, prolonged downslope of the R′ component of the QRS complex, (2) T-wave inversion in leads V1 and/or V2, and (3) ST-segment elevation in leads V1, V2, and V3. The ST-segment elevation is often concave and descends into an inverted T wave, a pattern referred to as coving. A second pattern, in which the ST segment has a saddle-backed appearance, is less common and less specific for the diagnosis. The EKG abnormalities can come and go, but are usually present at the time of an arrhythmic event.

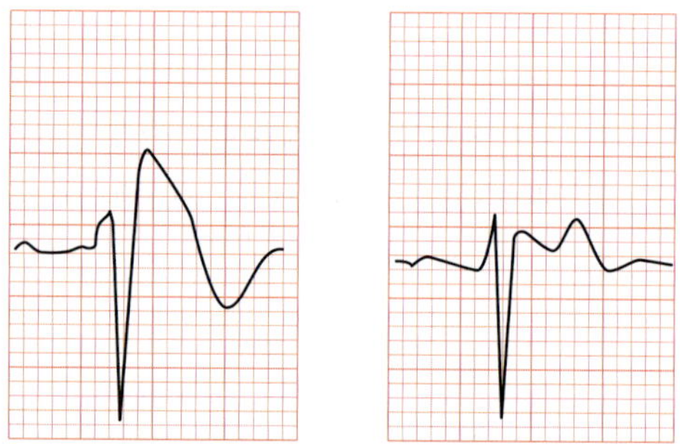

Two examples of Brugada pattern in lead V1. Note the right bundle-branch appearance and the inverted T wave in V1. The ST-segment elevation can appear coved (first figure) or saddle backed (second figure).

The importance of Brugada pattern lies in its propensity to cause ventricular arrhythmias that can lead to sudden death. Patients with the coved ST-segment morphology are at the greatest risk. The most typical arrhythmia is a fast polymorphic ventricular tachycardia that looks just like torsade de pointes. Sudden death is most likely to occur during sleep or when the patient has a fever or is exposed to high ambient temperatures. Sodium channel blocking drugs can also be responsible. Implantable cardiac defibrillators are a critical component of management, as is prompt treatment of any fever. All family members of an affected patient must be screened for this condition.

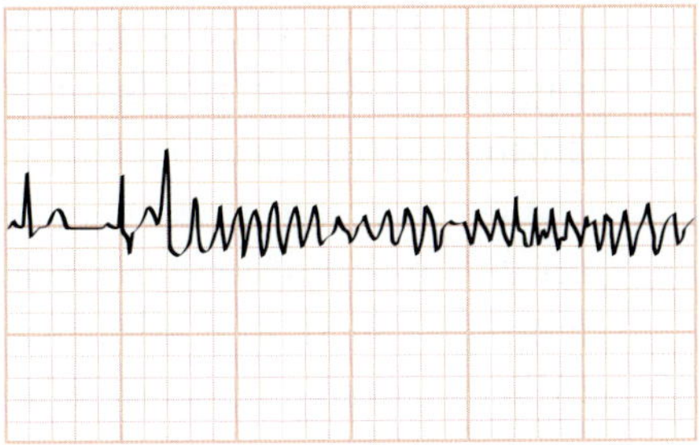

Polymorphous ventricular tachycardia with unusually narrow QRS complexes in a patient with Brugada syndrome.

Arrhythmogenic right ventricular cardiomyopathy (ARVC) is a heritable disorder characterized by fibrofatty infiltration of the right ventricular myocardium.*

It has been increasingly recognized as an important cause of ventricular arrhythmias and sudden death, particularly in young athletes. The genetic mutations that cause ARVC affect desmosomal proteins that are involved in cell-to-cell adhesion and thereby compromise the flow of electric current between cells.

---

*Increasingly, it is being recognized that the pathology need not be limited to the right ventricle, and the term ARVC is gradually being supplanted with the more general one of *arrthymogenic cardiomyopathy*. We'll stick with ARVC for now, but suspect that future editions of this book will gracefully transition to the more general term.

The most common feature on the EKG is T-wave inversion in leads V1 through V3, but this finding—as with most things T-wave related—is not very specific. The most characteristic feature on the EKG—although present in only about 30% of patients with this condition—is a small positive deflection at the end of the QRS complex called an epsilon wave (Why? It looks like the Greek letter epsilon—ε—lying on its side).

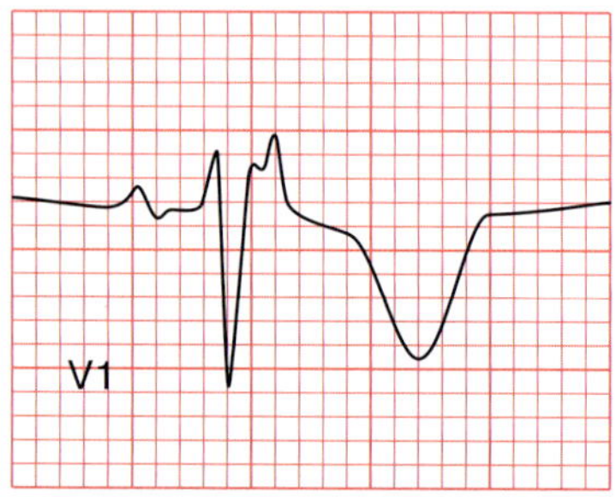

The epsilon wave is the small notch at the terminal portion of the QRS complex in lead V1.

The EKG is a critical tool in evaluating any young person following an unexplained episode of sudden cardiac arrest (from which, of course, they were successfully resuscitated) or loss of consciousness (syncope). You may get lucky and capture an underlying arrhythmia, but even if the EKG shows normal sinus rhythm, you may see evidence of a congenital, drug-induced, or other type of heart condition that predisposes to a potentially lethal arrhythmia. The most common congenital predisposing conditions that you might see on the EKG are hypertrophic cardiomyopathy, a long QT interval, Wolff–Parkinson–White, Brugada pattern, and ARVC.

The Athlete's Heart

Long-distance runners and other athletes involved in endurance training that demands maximal aerobic capacity can develop alterations in their EKGs that can be quite unnerving if you are unfamiliar with them, but are in fact benign. These changes may include the following:

1. A resting sinus bradycardia, sometimes even below 30 beats per minute! Rather than a cause for concern, this profound sinus bradycardia is a testimony to the efficiency of their cardiovascular system.
2. Nonspecific ST-segment and T-wave changes. Typically, these consist of ST-segment elevation in the precordial leads with T-wave flattening or inversion. T-wave inversion in leads V1 through V4 is especially common in self-identified African American athletes.
3. Criteria for left ventricular hypertrophy and sometimes right ventricular hypertrophy.
4. Incomplete right bundle-branch block.
5. Various arrhythmias, including junctional rhythms and a wandering atrial pacemaker.
6. First-degree or Wenckebach AV block.
7. A notched QRS complex in lead V1.

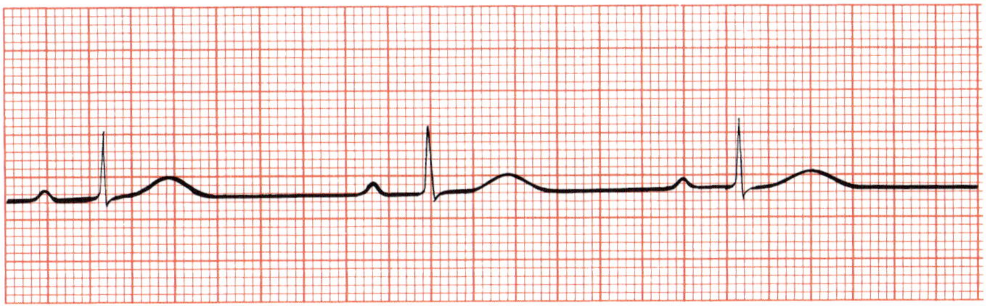

Sinus bradycardia and first-degree AV block in a triathlete.

None of these conditions is cause for concern, nor do they require treatment. More than one endurance athlete, undergoing a routine EKG, has been admitted to the cardiac care unit because of unfamiliarity with these changes.

Preparticipation Screening for Athletes

During exercise, athletes are at an increased risk of sudden death compared to age-matched populations of nonathletes. Fortunately, the number of cases of sudden death in young athletes is very low, estimated as 1 out of 50,000 to 300,000 athletes. The risk increases with age.

The most common causes of sudden death in athletes are disorders of the heart muscle and sudden ventricular arrhythmias. This raises the obvious question: Should young athletes be screened for congenital abnormalities of the heart before participating in sports?

This is a controversial area fraught with heated debate and disagreement. For young individuals with worrisome symptoms—dizziness, syncope, chest pain, shortness of breath, and palpitations—or a family history of congenital heart disease, a complete evaluation with a history, physical, EKG, and additional testing (eg, an echocardiogram, stress test, or ambulatory monitor) is mandatory. But most young athletes have no family history of problems and feel just fine. In these youngsters, there is little evidence that preparticipation screening makes much difference. False positives are common; as we discussed in the preceding section, EKG abnormalities are common among athletes and can be perfectly normal. The presence of an insignificant abnormality may, if interpreted incorrectly in the context of a young athlete, lead to costly, unnecessary testing; anxiety in the patient and family members; and pointless disqualification from further athletic activities. The majority of false positives, however, have been found to stem from EKGs that are read and interpreted by inadequately trained health care personnel, a problem that you have solved by reading this book!

There are EKG findings that do mandate further evaluation:

- T-wave inversion beyond lead V2 in White athletes or beyond V4 in African American or Caribbean athletes
- T-wave inversion in the lateral leads
- ST-segment depression in any lead
- Any of the findings we described in the section on sudden cardiac death, such as evidence of hypertrophic cardiomyopathy, long QT syndrome, Wolff–Parkinson–White, Brugada pattern, or ARVC.

Evaluation starts with a careful history, family history, physical examination, and echocardiogram, and may include genetic testing and a cardiac MRI, which can detect some abnormalities that the echocardiogram may miss.

The Preoperative Evaluation

The overall risk of a surgical procedure depends upon the particular procedure, the type of anesthesia, the experience of the surgeon and the hospital staff, and the patient's overall health. Most serious perioperative complications are either cardiac or pulmonary in nature; the former include ischemic episodes and arrhythmias. In an effort to reduce the risks, many surgeons request preoperative assessments from a patient's primary health care provider. However, for most patients, there is little evidence to support this practice.

All patients, no matter how tenuous their cardiac status, can proceed to low-risk surgical procedures (eg, cataract surgery, dermatologic surgery, and ambulatory procedures such as many arthroscopic procedures) without any evaluation. At the other extreme, patients who require urgent surgery should go right to the operating room without any pause for preoperative evaluation.

What, though, about patients who may have one or more risk factors for a cardiac complication (eg, a history of ischemic heart disease or diabetes) who are undergoing a procedure with intermediate (eg, abdominal surgery) or high (cardiac or vascular surgery) risk? In general, a 12-lead EKG is recommended for (1) anyone undergoing intermediate- or high-risk surgery, (2) who has any significant underlying cardiac risk factor, or (3) who has a history of coronary artery disease, arrhythmia, or other underlying cardiovascular disorder.

A stress test may be appropriate for high-risk patients undergoing high-risk procedures, but only if testing will lead to a change in management. Who is considered to be at high risk? These would include patients with limited functional capacity (<4 METS, which is the threshold for climbing a flight of stairs or doing vigorous housework) or who have multiple cardiovascular risk factors. However, for everyone else, the information gleaned from stress testing has not been consistently proven to lead to preoperative interventions that improve surgical outcomes.

Remember that no patient has zero surgical risk. It is therefore never appropriate to "clear" a patient for surgery; instead, one should state that, based on whatever evaluation has been carried out, *there are no contraindications to the planned procedure and the cardiovascular status is optimized* (meaning that the blood pressure, respiratory status, and heart rate and rhythm are as stabilized as possible).

Artifacts

We've come at last to the final section of new material. So, expert that you now are, what's going on in the tracing below?

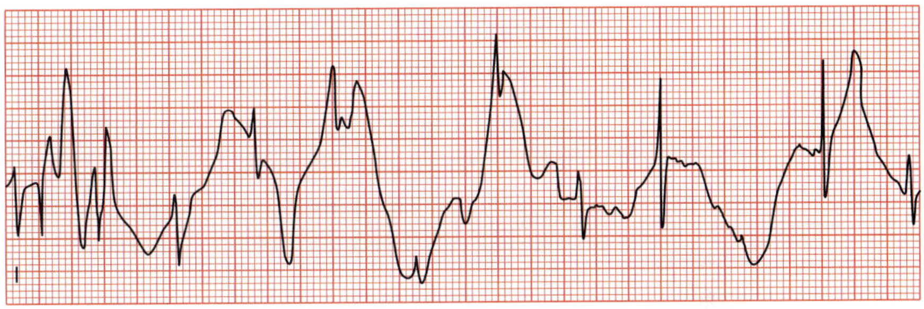

This tracing from lead I certainly looks bizarre

Of course the title of this section gives it away—what you are seeing is a common artifact, in this case caused by a loose electrode, that is, one that is not making proper contact with the skin. Which electrode is causing the problem? Well, here is the tracing from lead III on the same EKG:

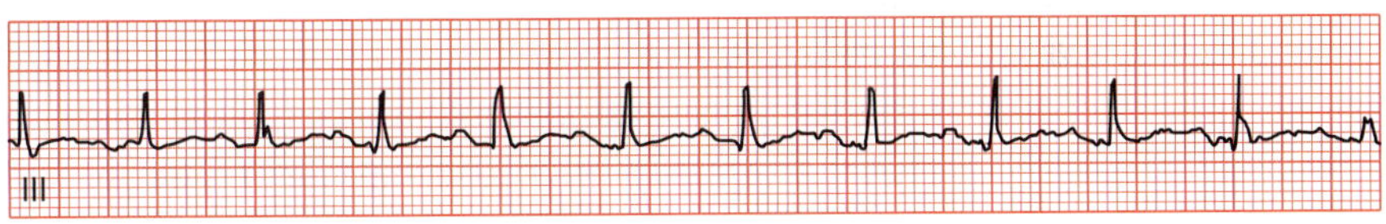

Lead III from the same EKG

Lead III looks perfectly normal, yes? Lead III is created by making the electrodes on the legs positive and the left arm negative. Lead I is created by making the electrode on the left arm positive and the right arm negative. So, by a process of simple—even by the standards of this book—logic, the electrode on the left arm must be correctly attached, so the problem has to lie with the electrode on the right arm. Case solved! Repeat the EKG, paying special attention to attaching that lead firmly to the skin.

There are many other possible EKG artifacts you will encounter. We've already seen some, such as the tremor artifacts of Parkinson Disease and hypothermia. The list is almost endless, but here are some to consider when you see stuff on the EKG that just doesn't make sense:

- Body movement
- Coughing, sneezing, snoring, or even just taking a deep breath
- Electrical interference from nearby electrical devices (cellular phones and electrical toothbrushes, if you keep one in your office) or power lines
- Electrical interference from implanted electrical devices such as left ventricular assist devices (used to treat refractory heart failure), deep brain stimulators (used in Parkinson Disease), or spinal cord stimulators (used, eg, for chronic pain)
- Nearby arterial pulsations (eg, when a limb lead electrode is placed over the radial pulse)
- Compressions during cardiopulmonary resuscitation (CPR)

This is only a partial list. The crucial point is to keep in mind that if you see electrical activity on an EKG that doesn't correspond to anything you are familiar with, or that closely mimics a familiar pattern but doesn't quite fit the clinical setting (hyperkalemia, as we have discussed, can do weird things to the EKG, so always keep that in your differential diagnosis of bizarre EKGs), check your leads, look for potential internal and external sources of interference, and repeat the study once you have corrected for all potential sources of confusion.

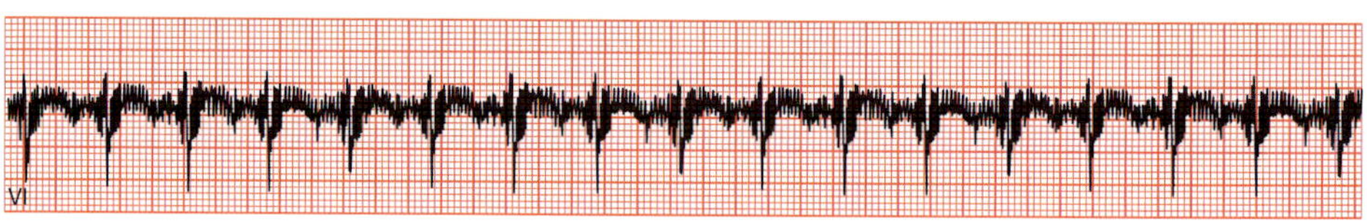

High-frequency electrical interference from a left ventricular assist device

SUMMARY

Miscellaneous Conditions

Electrolyte Disturbances

- *Hyperkalemia:* The great imitator. Evolution of (1) peaked T waves, (2) PR prolongation and P-wave flattening, and (3) QRS widening. Ultimately, the QRS complexes and T waves merge to form a sine wave, and ventricular fibrillation may develop. Right axis deviation is common.
- *Hypokalemia:* ST depression, T-wave flattening, U waves. When severe, prolonged QT interval.
- *Hypocalcemia:* Prolonged QT interval.
- *Hypercalcemia:* Shortened QT interval.

Differential Diagnosis of a Prolonged QT Interval

- Hypocalcemia
- Hypomagnesemia
- Severe hypokalemia
- Congenital heart disorders
- Many medications
- Hypothermia

Differential Diagnosis of a Shortened QT Interval

- Hypercalcemia
- Hyperkalemia
- Congenital heart disorders

Hypothermia

- Osborn waves, prolonged intervals, sinus bradycardia, slow junctional rhythms, and slow atrial fibrillation. Beware of muscle tremor artifact.

Drugs

- *Digitalis: Therapeutic levels* are associated with ST-segment and T-wave changes in leads with tall R waves; *toxic levels* are associated with tachyarrhythmias and conduction blocks; PAT with block is most characteristic.
- *Sodium channel blockers:* Tachycardia, wide QRS complex, right axis, and long QT interval
- *Many antiarrhythmic agents and numerous other drugs:* Prolonged QT interval.

Other Cardiac Disorders

- *Pericarditis:* Diffuse ST-segment and T-wave changes, PR depression. A large effusion can cause low voltage and electrical alternans. Rule out a STEMI before relying on PR depression for your diagnosis.
- *Hypertrophic cardiomyopathy:* Ventricular hypertrophy, left axis deviation, inferior and lateral Q waves.
- *Myocarditis:* Conduction blocks, ST-segment elevation
- *Atrial septal defect:* First-degree AV block, atrial tachyarrhythmias, incomplete right bundle-branch block, right axis deviation, QRS complex crochetage.

Pulmonary Disorders

- *COPD:* Low voltage, right axis deviation, and poor R-wave progression. Chronic cor pulmonale can produce P pulmonale and right ventricular hypertrophy with repolarization abnormalities.
- *Acute pulmonary embolism:* Right ventricular hypertrophy with repolarization abnormalities, T-wave inversions, right bundle-branch block; S1Q3 or S1Q3T3 are neither specific nor sensitive. Sinus tachycardia and atrial fibrillation are the most common arrhythmias.

CNS Disease

Diffuse T-wave inversion, with T waves typically wide and deep; U waves, prolonged QT interval.

Sleep Disorders

- Sleep apnea predisposes to arrhythmias (especially atrial fibrillation), heart block, ischemic heart disease, systemic and pulmonary hypertension, and right heart failure.

Eating Disorders

- Sinus bradycardia is very common; may also see long QTc, low voltage, right axis, conduction abnormalities

Causes of Sudden Cardiac Arrest or Death

- Coronary artery disease
- Hypertrophic cardiomyopathy
- Long QT syndrome
- Wolff–Parkinson–White syndrome
- Viral pericarditis/myocarditis
- Infiltrative diseases of the myocardium
- Valvular heart disease
- Drug abuse (especially stimulants)
- Trauma (commotio cordis)
- Anomalous origin of the coronary arteries
- Brugada syndrome—right bundle-branch pattern with ST elevation in V1–V3
- ARVC—may see an epsilon wave in terminal portion of QRS

The Athlete's Heart

Nonpathologic findings can include sinus bradycardia, junctional rhythms, and a wandering atrial pacemaker, nonspecific ST-segment and T-wave changes, left and right ventricular hypertrophy, incomplete right bundle-branch block, first-degree or Wenckebach AV block, and a notched QRS complex in lead V1.

Preparticipation Screening for Athletes

Findings that require further evaluation:

- T-wave inversion beyond lead V2 in White athletes or beyond V4 in African American or Caribbean athletes
- T-wave inversion in the lateral leads
- ST-segment depression in any lead
- Evidence of a congenital heart condition such as hypertrophic cardiomyopathy, long QT syndrome, Wolff–Parkinson–White syndrome, Brugada syndrome, or ARVC

CASE 11

Amos T., a 25-year-old graduate student, is brought by ambulance to the emergency room, clutching his chest and looking not at all well. Vital signs show a blood pressure of 90/40 mm Hg and an irregular pulse. His rhythm strip looks like this.

Do you recognize the arrhythmia?

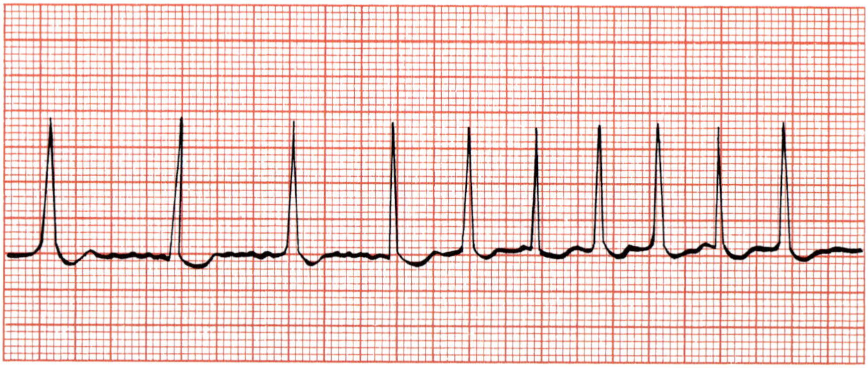

The patient is in atrial fibrillation. There are no P waves, the baseline undulates, and the QRS complexes appear irregularly and are narrow.

Appropriate measures are taken, and Amos is converted back to sinus rhythm, although his rate remains fast at around 100 beats per minute. His blood pressure rises to 130/60 mm Hg. Despite successful conversion of his rhythm, he still complains of severe chest pain and shortness of breath. The emergency room physician wants to send him to the catheterization lab to evaluate him for acute coronary syndrome, but you insist on a 12-lead EKG first—not an unreasonable request because, except for his tachycardia, his vital signs are stable. The EKG shown on the next page was obtained.

Do you now agree with the emergency room physician's assessment?

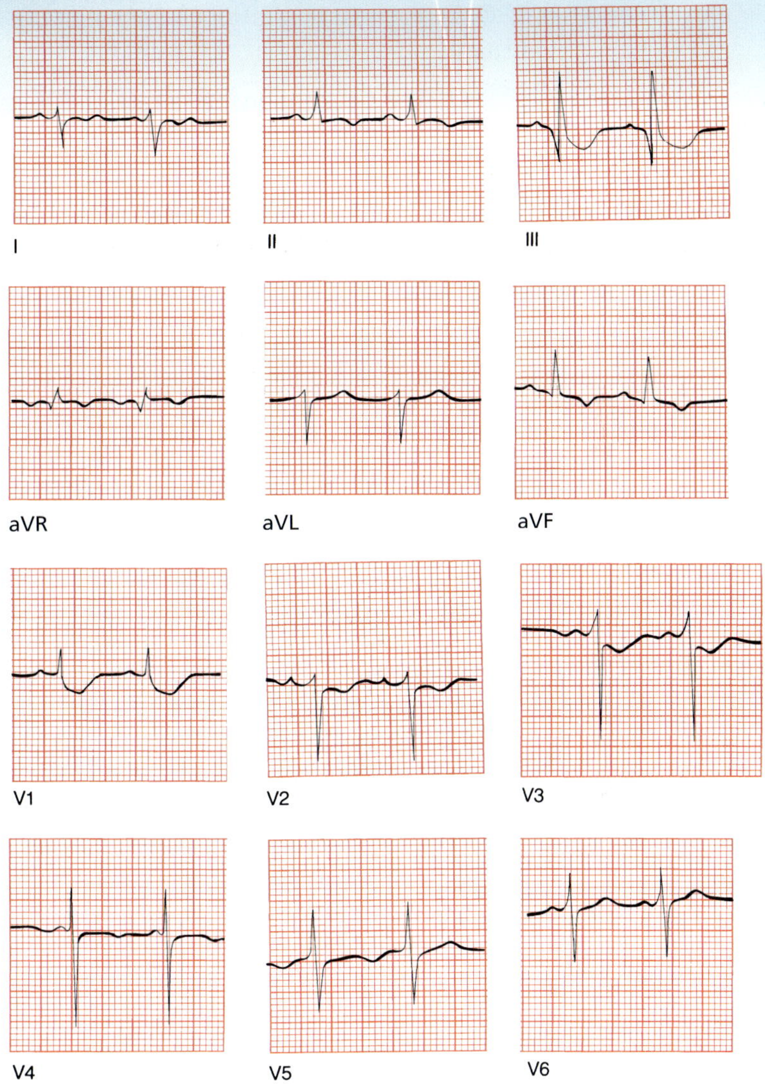
I
II
III
aVR
aVL
aVF
V1
V2
V3
V4
V5
V6

Of course you don't. Hopefully, you noticed some of the following features:

1. The patient now has a rate of 100 beats per minute.
2. A pattern of right ventricular hypertrophy with repolarization abnormalities is present.
3. A deep Q wave is seen in lead III along with an inverted T wave, and there is a deep S wave in lead I, the S1Q3T3 pattern suggestive of an acute pulmonary embolus.

Do you now start jumping up and down and scream that the patient has an acute pulmonary embolus? No. You start jumping up and down and scream that the patient *may* have a pulmonary embolus. These EKG findings are suggestive but hardly conclusive. The sensitivity and specificity of the S2Q3T3 for an acute pulmonary embolism are extremely low, and the right axis and T-wave inversions, although more common with an acute pulmonary embolism, can be seen in other conditions as well. But you have done your job well just by raising the issue; appropriate diagnostic steps can now be taken.

Amos is placed on heparin while awaiting his chest CT scan. This is done within the hour, and the diagnosis of a pulmonary embolism is confirmed. Amos remains in the hospital for several days on heparin therapy and is discharged home on oral anticoagulant therapy. There is no recurrence of his pulmonary embolism.

CASE 12

Ursula U. was recently seen at your local hospital for pyelonephritis (a urinary tract infection involving the kidneys) and discharged home on the antibiotic, trimethoprim-sulfamethoxazole. She seeks routine follow-up care with you. She is fairly new in town and new to your practice. Her infection seems to be responding well to the antibiotic, but you note that her blood pressure is a little elevated at 145/95 mm Hg. She tells you that she is currently taking the blood pressure medication, lisinopril, an angiotensin-converting enzyme inhibitor, but has not seen a physician since the drug was prescribed. Something clicks in your head, and you obtain an EKG. Here are the tracings from just her augmented limb leads. What do you see?

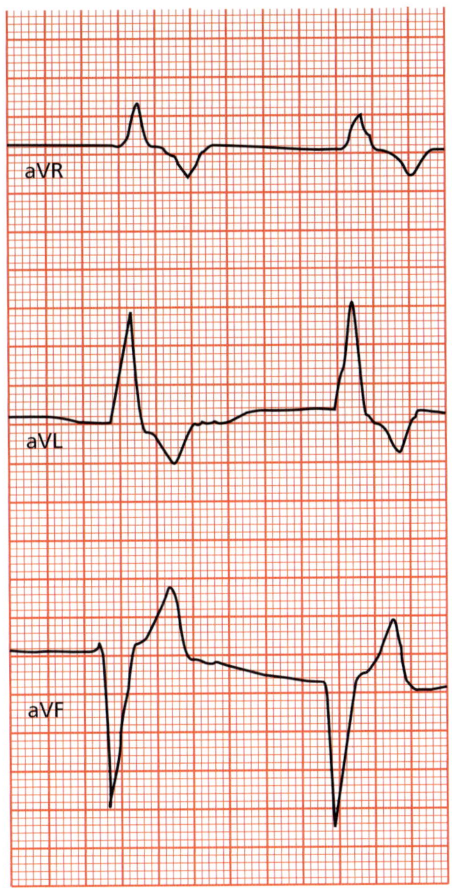

This looks like pretty wild stuff. But analyze this slowly: the QRS complexes are clearly very wide, and there are no visible P waves. Although the QRS complexes and T waves are distinct, they certainly seem to be merging into a single configuration (note particularly lead aVR). Could this be some kind of idioventricular rhythm (see page 170)? Well, perhaps, but the clinical context argues for another interpretation. Both trimethoprim-methoxazole and lisinopril can cause hyperkalemia that is usually mild, but when combined, they can cause severe, even life-threatening elevations in the serum potassium. And that's what you are seeing here—EKG manifestations of hyperkalemia.

Because of the risk of ventricular fibrillation in this setting, you send Ursula right to the emergency room, where she is treated aggressively for hyperkalemia, taken off her medications, and monitored in the cardiac care unit until her EKG returns to normal. Eventually, she is discharged on a different antibiotic and a different class of medication for her blood pressure. She does very well and declares—justifiably—that you are the finest clinician she has ever met and will recommend you to all her new friends.

8 Putting It All Together

In this chapter, you will learn:

1 | a simple method to incorporate everything you have learned into a step-by-step analysis of any EKG

2 | that all good things must come to an end, and we bid you a reluctant and fond farewell!

And that is really all there is to it.

Well, perhaps not quite all. What we need now is a way to organize all of this information, a simple, methodical approach that can be applied to each and every EKG. It is important that every EKG be approached in an orderly fashion, particularly while you are still new at this, so that nothing important is missed. As you read more and more cardiograms, what initially may seem forced and mechanical will pay big dividends and will soon feel like second nature.

Two important pieces of advice:

1. *Know your patient.* It is true that EKGs can be read with fair accuracy in a little gloomy back room in complete seclusion, but the power of this amazing tool only really emerges when it is integrated into a total clinical assessment of your patient.
2. *Read EKGs.* Then, read some more. Read them wherever you can find them—in books, in papers, in patients' charts, on bathroom walls—and please read other books; this may be the only EKG book you will ever need, but it should not be the only one you will ever *want* to read. There are many outstanding textbooks, each with something special to offer.

There are as many approaches to reading EKGs as there are cardiologists. Everyone ultimately arrives at a method that works best for him or her. The following 9-Step Method is probably no better and no worse than most others.

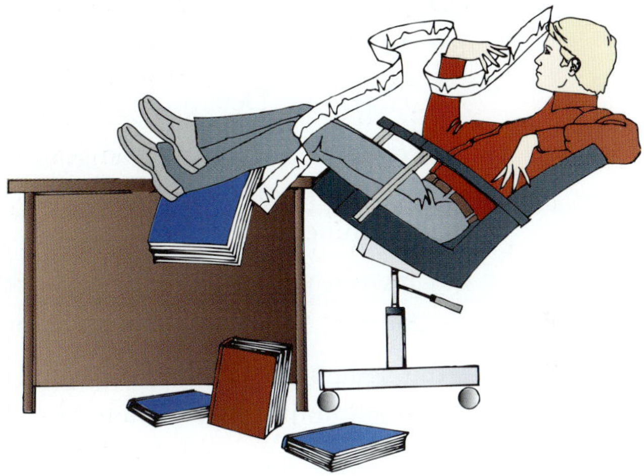

The 9-Step Method for Reading EKGs

Before you start, make sure that the standardization mark on the EKG paper is 10 mm high so that 10 mm = 1 mV. Also, make sure that the paper speed is correct.

1. *Heart rate:* Determine the heart rate.
2. *Intervals:* Measure the length of the PR and QT intervals and the width of the QRS complexes. This is one thing your EKG machine does for you with reasonable accuracy.
3. *Axis:* Is the axis of the P waves, QRS complexes, and T waves normal, or is there axis deviation?

Once these first three items have been accomplished, look for abnormalities in the following:

1. *Rhythm:* Always ask The Four Questions:
   - Are there *normal* P waves present?
   - Are the QRS complexes wide or narrow?
   - What is the relationship between the P waves and QRS complexes?
   - Is the rhythm regular or irregular?
2. *Conduction blocks:*
   - Atrioventricular (AV) block. Apply the criteria in Chapter 4.
   - Bundle-branch block or hemiblock. Apply the criteria in Chapter 4.
3. *Preexcitation:* Apply the criteria in Chapter 5.
4. *Enlargement and hypertrophy:* Apply the criteria for both atrial enlargement and ventricular hypertrophy in Chapter 3.
5. *Coronary artery disease:* Look for Q waves and the ST-segment and T-wave changes described in Chapter 6. Remember that not all such changes reflect coronary artery disease; know your differential diagnoses.
6. *Other conditions:* Is there anything on the EKG that suggests one of the other cardiac or noncardiac conditions discussed in Chapter 7? Are you totally lost? Never hesitate to ask for assistance.

The following pages are memory joggers. In earlier editions of this book, we are going way back in time now, I suggested you cut these pages out and stick them in that little black book of medical pearls that everyone seemed to be toting around. But who carries a little black book anymore? Therefore—if you haven't thought of this already—take a photo of these pages with your smartphone and file them away for easy access, or better yet, download the electronic version of this book. On the other hand, now that I think about it some more, maybe you should cut these pages out anyway; the exercise will do you good after sitting and staring bleary-eyed at this book for so long.

The final chapter contains some sample EKGs with which to test yourself. Some are easy; some not so much. And if you are still thinking, "Is this really all there is to it?" The answer—reminding you that information only becomes knowledge with wisdom and experience—is, "Yes!"

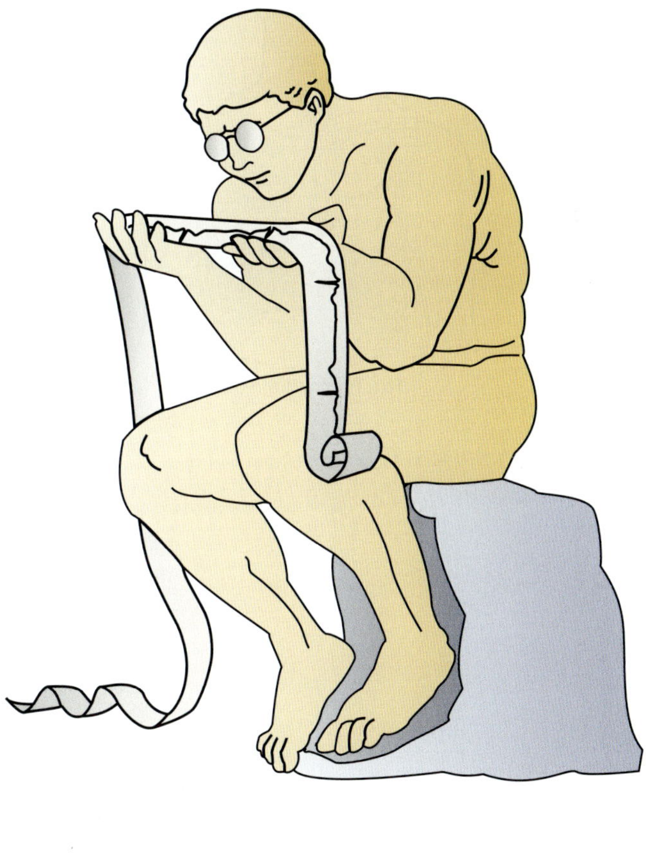

Review Charts

- **The 12 Leads**
- Anterior leads: V2, V3, and V4
- Inferior leads: II, III, and AVF
- Left lateral leads: I, AVL, V5, and V6
- Right leads: aVR and V1

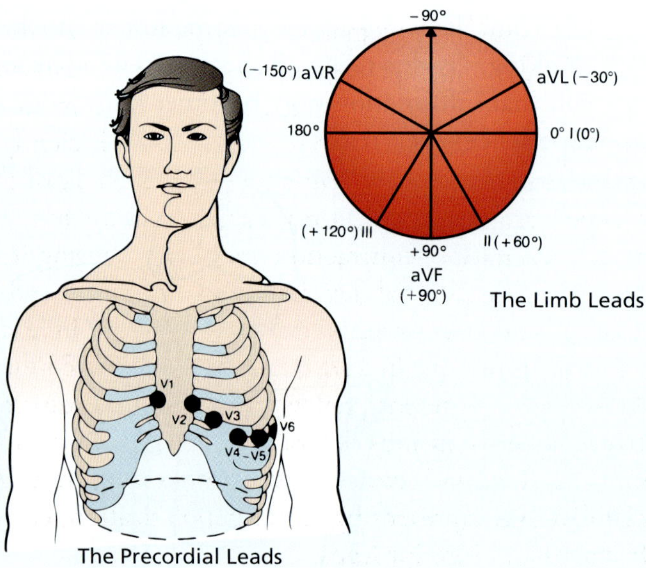

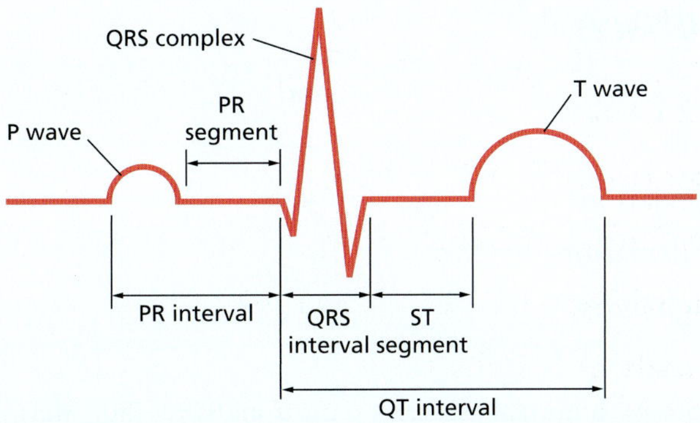

The heart is composed of pacemaker cells, electrical conducting cells, and myocardial cells. *Pacemaker* cells depolarize spontaneously and initiate each wave of depolarization. The SA node is usually the dominant pacemaker. *Electrical conducting cells* carry current rapidly and efficiently to distant regions of the heart. *Myocardial cells* constitute the bulk of the heart. When a wave of depolarization reaches a myocardial cell, calcium is released within the cell (excitation–contraction coupling), causing it to contract.

The *P wave* represents atrial depolarization. It is small and usually positive in the left lateral and inferior leads. It is often biphasic in leads III and V1. Typically, it is most positive in lead II and most negative in lead aVR.

The *QRS complex* represents ventricular depolarization. It is usually predominantly positive in most lateral and inferior leads. Across the precordium, the R waves increase in size, progressing from V1 to V5. A small initial Q wave, representing septal depolarization, can often be seen in the left lateral and inferior leads.

The *T wave* represents ventricular repolarization. It is the most variable waveform, but it is usually positive in leads with tall R waves.

The *PR interval* represents the time from the start of atrial depolarization to the start of ventricular depolarization.

The *PR segment* is the time from the end of atrial depolarization to the start of ventricular depolarization.

The *QRS interval* represents the duration of the QRS complex.

The *ST segment* represents the time from the end of ventricular depolarization to the start of ventricular repolarization.

The *QT interval* represents the time from the start of ventricular depolarization to the end of ventricular repolarization.

Calculating the Axis

	Lead I	Lead aVF
Normal axis[a]	+	+
Left axis deviation[a]	+	–
Right axis deviation	–	+
Extreme right axis deviation	–	–

[a]To be more precise, a normal axis can extent from 0° to –30°; thus, lead I and lead II should both be positive, and aVF can be negative by this criterion.

Atrial Enlargement

Look at the P wave in leads II and V1.

Right atrial enlargement is characterized by the following:

1. Increased amplitude of the first portion of the P wave
2. No change in the duration of the P wave
3. Possible right axis deviation of the P wave

Left atrial enlargement is characterized by the following:

1. Occasionally, increased amplitude of the terminal component of the P wave
2. More consistently, increased P wave duration
3. No significant axis deviation

Ventricular Hypertrophy

Look at the QRS complexes in all leads.

Right ventricular hypertrophy is characterized by the following:

1. Right axis deviation of >100°
2. Ratio of R-wave amplitude to S-wave amplitude >1 in V1 and <1 in V6

Left ventricular hypertrophy is characterized by many criteria. The more that are present, the greater the likelihood that left ventricular hypertrophy is present.

Precordial criteria include the following:

1. The R-wave amplitude in V5 or V6 plus the S-wave amplitude in V1 or V2 exceeds 35 mm.
2. The R-wave amplitude in V5 exceeds 26 mm.
3. The R-wave amplitude in V6 exceeds 18 mm.

Limb lead criteria include the following:

1. The R-wave amplitude in aVL exceeds 11 mm.
2. The R-wave amplitude in aVF exceeds 20 mm.
3. The R-wave amplitude in I exceeds 13 mm.
4. The R-wave amplitude in I *plus* the S-wave amplitude in III exceeds 25 mm.

Perhaps the most accurate single criterion: the R-wave amplitude in aVL plus the S-wave amplitude in V3 exceeds 20 for women and 28 for men.

The presence of repolarization abnormalities (asymmetric ST-segment depression and T-wave inversion) indicates clinically significant hypertrophy, is most often seen in those leads with tall R waves, and may herald ventricular dilatation and failure.

The five basic types of arrhythmias are as follows:

1. Arrhythmias of sinus origin
2. Ectopic rhythms
3. Reentrant rhythms
4. Conduction blocks
5. Preexcitation syndromes

Whenever you are interpreting the heart's rhythm, ask The Four Questions:

1. Are normal P waves present?
2. Are the QRS complexes narrow (<0.12 seconds in duration) or wide (>0.12 seconds)?
3. What is the relationship between the P waves and the QRS complexes?
4. Is the rhythm regular or irregular?

The answers for normal sinus rhythm are the following:

1. Yes, P waves are present.
2. The QRS complexes are narrow.
3. There is one P wave for every QRS complex.
4. The rhythm is regular.

Why Arrhythmias Happen

- Hypoxia
- Ischemia and irritability
- Sympathetic stimulation
- Bradycardia
- Electrolyte imbalances
- Drugs
- Stretch

Rhythms of Sinus Origin

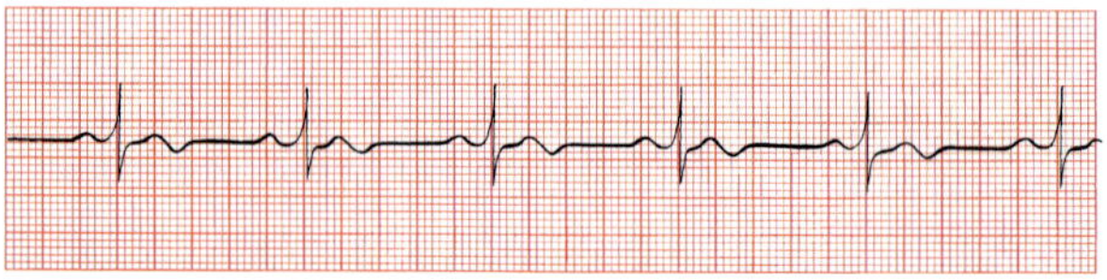

A Normal sinus rhythm.

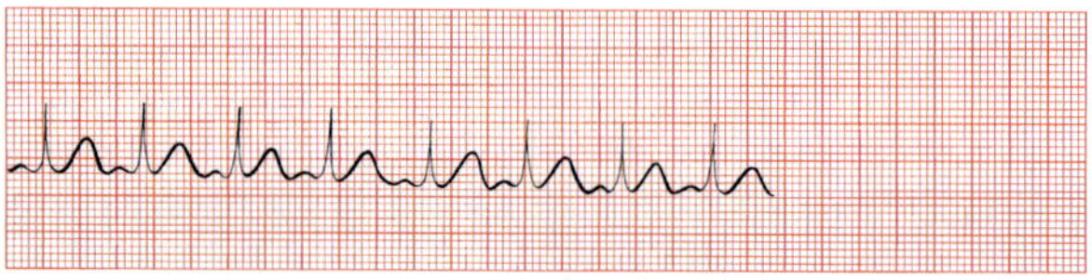

B Sinus tachycardia.

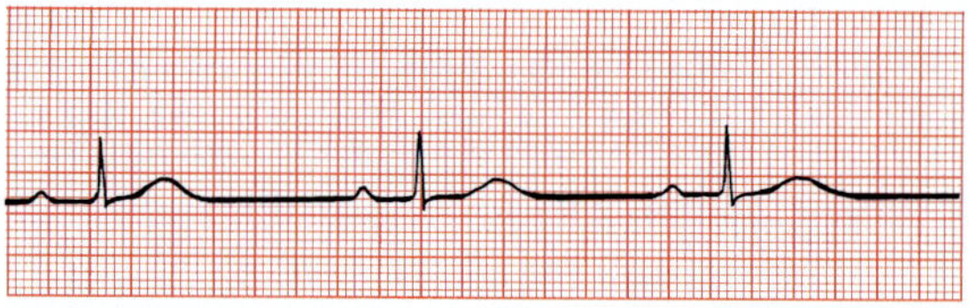

C Sinus bradycardia.

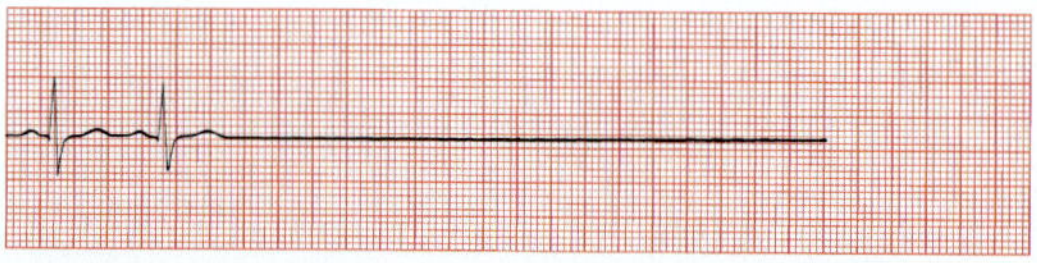

D Sinus arrest or exit block.

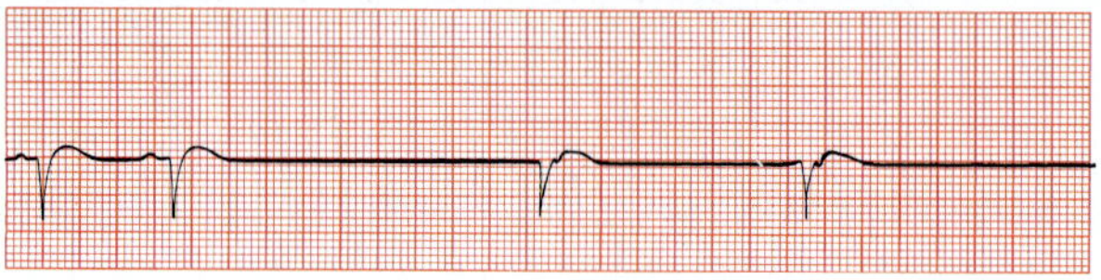

E Sinus arrest or exit block with junctional escape.

Supraventricular Arrhythmias

	Characteristics	EKG
AV nodal reentrant tachycardia (AVNRT)	• Regular • P waves are retrograde if visible • Rate: 150–250 beats per minute • Carotid massage: slows or terminates	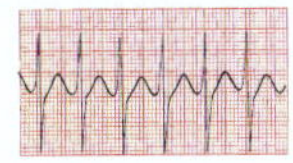
Atrial flutter	• Regular, saw-toothed • 2:1, 3:1, 4:1, etc., block • Atrial rate: 250–350 beats per minute • Ventricular rate: one-half, one-third, one-fourth, etc., of the atrial rate • Carotid massage: increases block	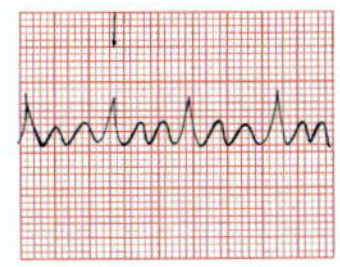
Atrial fibrillation	• Irregular • Undulating baseline • Atrial rate: 350–500 beats per minute • Ventricular rate: variable, typically 120–180 bpm • Carotid massage: may slow ventricular rate	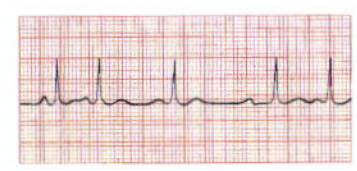
Multifocal atrial tachycardia *(MAT)*	• Irregular • At least three different P-wave morphologies • Rate: usually 100–200 beats per minute; if <100 beats per minute, it is called a wandering atrial pacemaker • Carotid massage: no effect	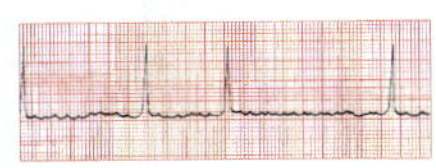
Paroxysmal atrial tachycardia *(PAT)*	• Regular • Rate: 100–200 beats per minute • Characteristic warm-up period in the automatic form • Carotid massage: no effect or only mild slowing	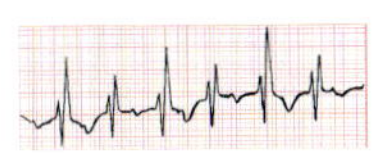

	Characteristics	EKG
AV reciprocating tachycardia	• Regular or irregular • Can be very fast • QRS complexes can be wide or narrow • Seen in WPW	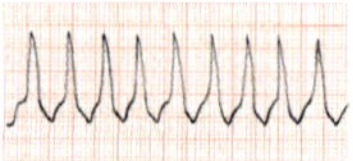

Ventricular Arrhythmias

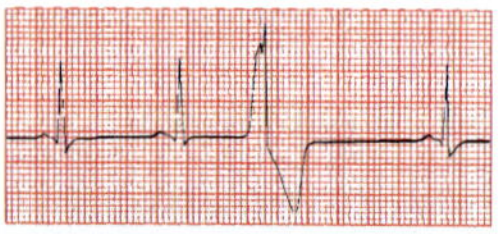

A Premature ventricular contractions (PVCs).

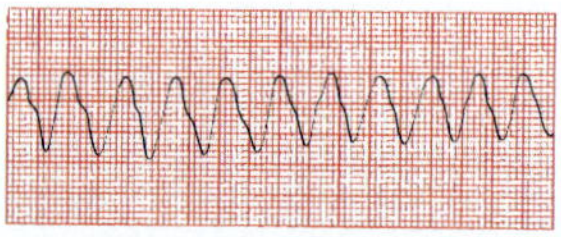

B Ventricular tachycardia.

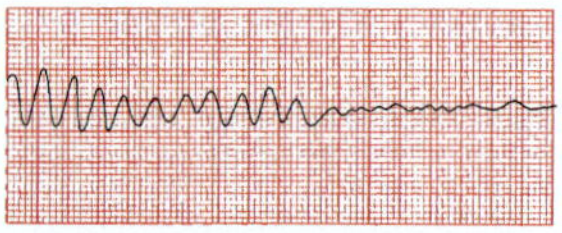

C Ventricular fibrillation.

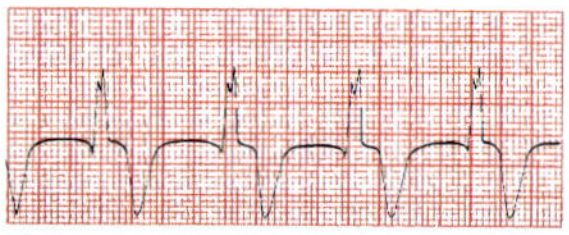

D Accelerated idioventricular rhythm.

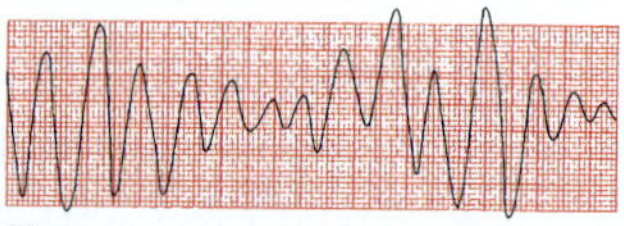

E Torsades de pointes.

Differential Diagnosis of a Wide Complex Tachycardia

1. Ventricular tachycardia
2. SVT with aberrant conduction (eg, with bundle-branch block)
3. SVT in a patient with preexcitation
4. Paced rhythms

Distinguishing Ventricular Tachycardia From Supraventricular Tachycardia With Aberrant Conduction

	Ventricular Tachycardia	Supraventricular Tachycardias With Aberrant Conduction
Clinical clues		
Clinical history	Diseased heart	Usually normal heart
Carotid massage	No response	May terminate
Cannon A waves	May be present	Not seen
EKG clues		
AV dissociation	May be seen	Not seen
Regularity	Slightly irregular	Very regular
Fusion beats	May be seen	Not seen
Initial QRS deflection	May differ from normal QRS complex	Same as normal QRS complex

AV Blocks

AV block is diagnosed by examining the relationship of the P waves to the QRS complexes.

1. *First degree:* The PR interval is >0.2 seconds; all beats are conducted through to the ventricles.
2. *Second degree:* Only *some* beats are conducted through to the ventricles.
   a. Wenckebach block: Progressive prolongation of the PR interval until one P wave fails to conduct.
   b. Mobitz type II block: Normal conduction until one P wave fails to conduct; progressive lengthening of the PR interval does not occur.
3. *Third degree:* No beats are conducted through to the ventricles. There is complete heart block with AV dissociation in which the atria and ventricles are driven by independent pacemakers.

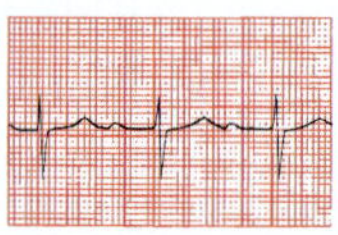

A First-degree AV block.

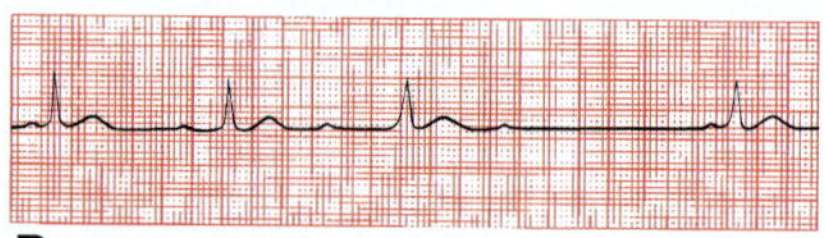

B Mobitz type I second-degree AV block (Wenckebach block).

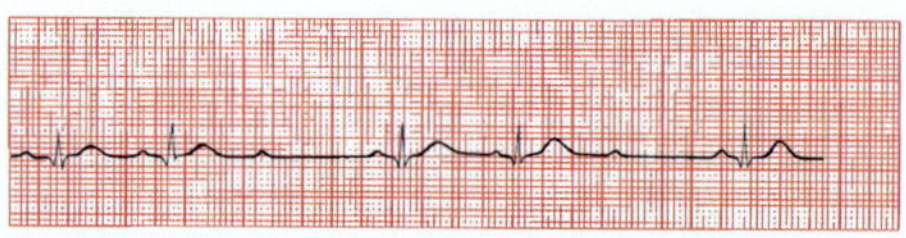

C Mobitz type II second-degree AV block.

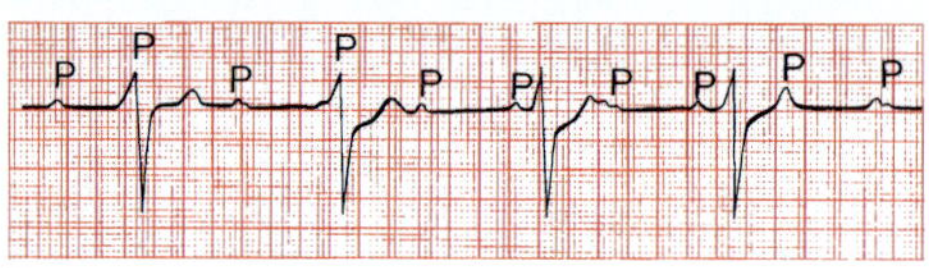

D Third-degree AV block.

Bundle-Branch Blocks

Bundle-branch block is diagnosed by looking at the width and configuration of the QRS complexes.

Criteria for Right Bundle-Branch Block

1. QRS complex widened to >0.12 seconds.
2. RSR′ in leads V1 and V2 (rabbit ears) or a tall, broad R wave; there is also ST-segment depression and T-wave inversion.
3. Reciprocal changes in leads V5, V6, I, and aVL.

Criteria for Left Bundle-Branch Block

1. QRS complex widened to >0.12 seconds.
2. Broad or notched R wave with prolonged upstroke in leads V5, V6, I, and aVL with ST-segment depression and T-wave inversion.
3. Reciprocal changes in V1 and V2.
4. Left axis deviation may be present.

Hemiblocks

Hemiblock is diagnosed by looking for left or right axis deviation.

Left Anterior Hemiblock

1. Normal QRS duration and no ST-segment or T-wave changes.
2. Left axis deviation >–30°.
3. No other cause of left axis deviation is present.

Left Posterior Hemiblock

1. Normal QRS duration and no ST-segment or T-wave changes.
2. Right axis deviation.
3. No other cause of right axis deviation is present.

Bifascicular Block

The features of a right bundle-branch block combined with the left anterior hemiblock are as follows:

Right Bundle-Branch Block

1. QRS wider than 0.12 seconds
2. RSR′ in V1 and V2

Left Anterior Hemiblock

- Left axis deviation

The features of a right bundle-branch block combined with the left posterior hemiblock are as follows:

Right Bundle-Branch Block

- RS wider than 0.12 seconds
- RSR′ in V1 and V2

Left Posterior Hemiblock

Right axis deviation

Preexcitation

Criteria for Wolff–Parkinson–White

1. PR interval <0.12 seconds
2. Wide QRS complexes
3. Delta wave seen in some leads

Criteria for Short PR Without a Delta Wave

1. PR interval <0.12 seconds
2. Normal QRS width
3. No delta wave

Arrhythmias seen with preexcitation include the following:

1. AV reciprocating tachycardia—narrow QRS complexes are more common than wide ones.
2. Atrial fibrillation—can be very rapid and can lead to ventricular fibrillation.

Myocardial Infarction

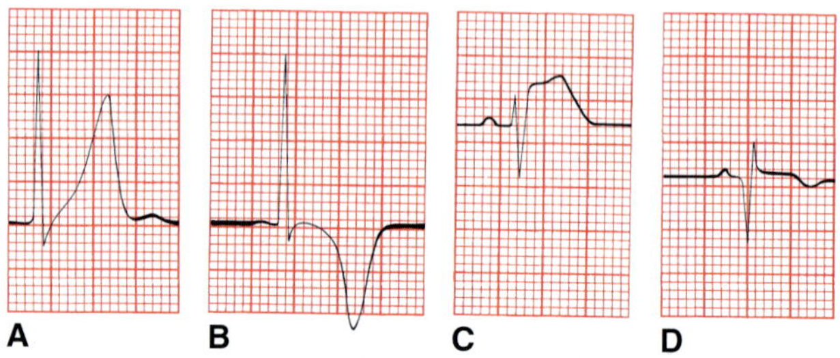

The diagnosis of a myocardial infarction is made by history, physical examination, serial cardiac enzyme determinations, and serial EKGs. During an acute STEMI, the EKG may evolve through three stages:

1. The T wave peaks (*A*) and then inverts (*B*).

   Inverted T waves can be normal in leads V1 through V3 in children and can persist into adulthood in some patients; an isolated inverted T wave in lead III or lead V1 is also a common normal variant.

2. The ST segment elevates (*C*). The ST segment is bowed upward (picture a frown)

3. Q waves appear (*D*).

   Ischemic Q waves are almost never isolated to a single lead.

Criteria for Significant Q Waves

1. The Q wave must be >0.04 seconds in duration.
2. The depth of the Q wave must be at least 25% the height of the R wave in the same QRS complex.
3. Q waves in aVR don't count!

Criteria for Non–Q-Wave Infarctions

1. T-wave inversion
2. ST-segment depression persisting for more than 48 hours in the appropriate setting

Localizing the Infarct

- Inferior infarction: leads II, III, and aVF
    - Often caused by occlusion of the right coronary artery or its descending branch.
    - Reciprocal changes in anterior and left lateral leads. T-wave inversion in aVL is the most common reciprocal change and may appear before ST elevation and T-wave inversion in the inferior leads.
- Lateral infarction: leads I, aVL, V5, and V6
    - Often caused by occlusion of the left circumflex artery
    - Reciprocal changes in inferior leads
- Anterior infarction: any of the precordial leads (V1 through V6)
    - Often caused by occlusion of the left anterior descending artery
    - Reciprocal changes in inferior leads
    - Important T-wave changes not to be missed:
        - de Winter T waves—In a patient with chest pain, upsloping ST depression leading into a tall symmetric T wave can be the first sign of an anterior infarction.
        - Wellens waves—Biphasic T waves in V2 or V3 (sometimes V4) may predict an impending proximal LAD occlusion and an anterior infarction.

- Posterior infarction: reciprocal changes in lead V1 (ST-segment depression, tall R wave that is often greater than the S wave in magnitude)
  - Often caused by occlusion of the right coronary artery.
  - Usually seen in concert with inferior infarctions.
  - Use posterior chest wall leads to confirm.
- Right ventricular infarction: ST elevation in lead V1, often ST depression in V2
  - Virtually always in concert with inferior infarction. Suspect right ventricular infarction if ST elevation in lead III is greater in magnitude than that in lead II.
  - Confirm with right chest wall leads.

Symptom or Syndrome	ST-Segment Changes	Cardiac Enzymes
Stable angina[a] without infarction	ST depression	Normal[a]
Unstable angina[a] without infarction	ST depression	Normal[a]
STEMI	ST elevation	Elevated
Non-STEMI	ST depression	Elevated
Takotsubo cardiomyopathy	ST elevation	Elevated[b]
Prinzmetal angina	ST elevation	Normal

[a]Stable and unstable angina are distinguished by the clinical history.

[b]Patients often have to undergo cardiac catheterization to distinguish this from infarction.

Note: Appearance of a new left bundle-branch block may signify infarction and should be treated with the same urgency as a STEMI.

The ST Segment

Causes of ST-segment *elevation:*

1. An evolving STEMI
2. Prinzmetal angina
3. J-point elevation/early repolarization
4. Takotsubo cardiomyopathy
5. Acute pericarditis
6. Acute myocarditis
7. Pulmonary embolism
8. Brugada pattern
9. Hypothermia
10. Ventricular aneurysm
11. CNS catastrophes
12. Postcardioversion
13. Left bundle-branch block (uncommonly)
14. Left ventricular hypertrophy (uncommonly)
15. Paced rhythms

Causes of ST-segment *depression:*

1. Angina without infarction
2. Non-STEMI
3. During supraventricular tachycardias
4. Typically seen with bundle-branch blocks
5. Hypokalemia

ST *depression* is also one indicator of a positive stress test.

Miscellaneous EKG Changes

Electrolyte Disturbances

- *Hyperkalemia:* The great imitator; evolution of peaked T waves, PR prolongation, P-wave flattening, and QRS widening. Ultimately, the QRS complexes and T waves merge to form a sine wave (a rightward axis in a patient with wide QRS complexes suggests possible hyperkalemia as the cause); conduction blocks can develop; ultimately, asystole and ventricular fibrillation may occur.
- *Hypokalemia:* ST depression, T-wave flattening, U waves; may cause supraventricular and ventricular tachycardias; when severe can prolong the QT interval.
- *Hypocalcemia:* Prolonged QT interval.
- *Hypercalcemia:* Shortened QT interval.
- *Hypomagnesemia:* Prolonged QT interval.

Hypothermia

Osborn waves, prolonged intervals, sinus bradycardia, slow junctional rhythm, and atrial fibrillation. Beware of muscle tremor artifact.

Drugs

- *Digitalis:* Therapeutic levels associated with ST-segment and T-wave changes in leads with tall R waves; toxic levels associated with tachyarrhythmias and conduction blocks. PAT with block is most characteristic.
- *Drugs that can prolong the QT interval:* Sotalol, quinidine, procainamide, disopyramide, amiodarone, dofetilide, dronedarone, tricyclic antidepressants, macrolides, quinolones, psychotropic drugs including selective serotonin reuptake inhibitors, various antifungal medications, some nonsedating antihistamines, and others. Grapefruit juice inhibits cytochrome P-450 and can cause higher serum drug levels and QT prolongation.

Causes of a Prolonged QT Interval

- Hypocalcemia
- Hypomagnesemia
- Hypokalemia (severe)
- Congenital disorders
- Medications
- Hypothermia

Causes of Shortened QT Interval

- Hypercalcemia
- Hyperkalemia

Other Cardiac Disorders

- *Pericarditis:* Diffuse ST-segment and T-wave changes; no Q waves; PR depression. A large effusion can cause low voltage and electrical alternans.
- *Hypertrophic cardiomyopathy:* Ventricular hypertrophy, left axis deviation, deep, narrow Q waves laterally and inferiorly.
- *Myocarditis:* Conduction blocks.
- *Atrial septal defect:* First-degree AV block, atrial tachyarrhythmias, incomplete right bundle-branch block, and right axis deviation; crochetage (small notch in QRS of the inferior leads).

Pulmonary Disorders

- *Chronic obstructive pulmonary disease:* Low voltage, right axis deviation, and poor R-wave progression. Chronic cor pulmonale can produce P pulmonale and right ventricular hypertrophy with repolarization abnormalities.
- *Acute pulmonary embolism:* Right ventricular hypertrophy with strain (although not acutely), right bundle-branch block, and T-wave inversion in right precordial leads. Sinus tachycardia and atrial fibrillation are the most common arrhythmias. S1Q3T3 pattern has poor sensitivity and specificity.

Central Nervous System Disease

Diffuse T-wave inversion, with T waves typically wide and deep; U waves; prolonged QT interval

Sleep Disorders

Suspect with unexplained atrial fibrillation

Eating Disorders

Bradycardia related to low body mass index; less common low voltage, prolonged QTc, right axis, conduction blocks

Causes of Lethal Arrhythmias and Sudden Cardiac Death

- Ischemia
- Hypertrophic cardiomyopathy
- Long QT syndrome
- Wolff–Parkinson–White
- Viral myocarditis
- Infiltrative diseases of the myocardium
- Valvular heart disease
- Drug abuse (notably stimulants)
- Commotio cordis (trauma to the heart)
- Anomalous origin of the coronary arteries
- Brugada syndrome
- Arrhythmogenic right ventricular cardiomyopathy

The Athlete's Heart

- Normal findings can include sinus bradycardia, nonspecific ST-segment and T-wave changes, left and right ventricular hypertrophy, incomplete right bundle-branch block, first-degree or Wenckebach AV block, and occasional supraventricular arrhythmias, notched QRS complex in lead V1
- Findings that require further evaluation: T-wave inversion beyond lead V2 in White athletes and beyond V4 in African American or Caribbean athletes; T-wave inversion in the lateral leads; ST-segment depression in any lead; findings consistent with congenital heart disorders

9 How Do You Get to Carnegie Hall?*

The following EKGs will allow you to try out your new skills. Use the method we outlined in the previous chapter. Don't overlook anything. Take your time. Ready? Here we go!

EKG 1:
A 24-year-old ballet dancer with palpitations, shortness of breath, and anxiety.

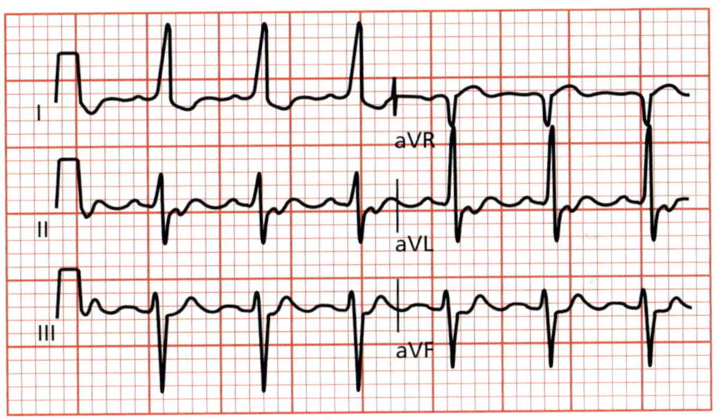

*Practice, practice, practice! A tired, very old joke—I am truly sorry.

- Answer to EKG 1: Sinus tachycardia. Note also the presence of left axis deviation.

EKG 2:

A 70-year-old patient with a prior history of coronary artery disease.

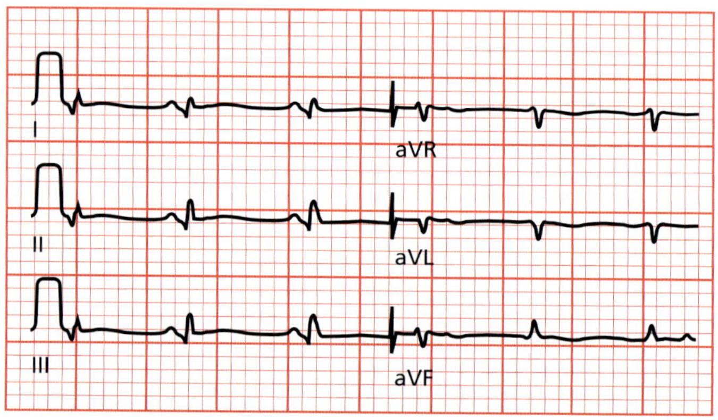

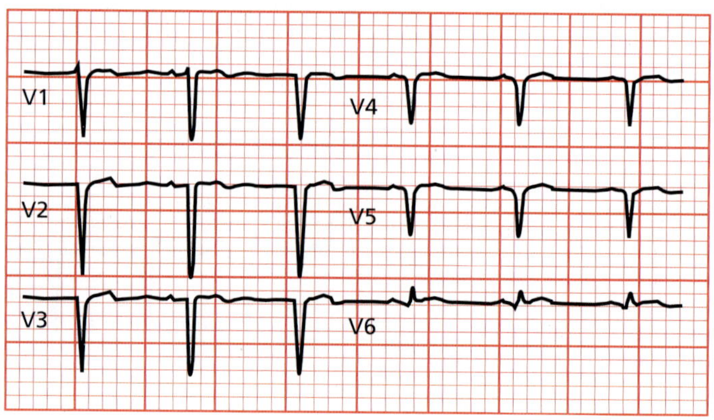

- Answer to EKG 2: The rhythm is sinus tachycardia. Deep anterior Q waves and less prominent, but significant lateral Q waves indicate an anterolateral myocardial infarction.

EKG 3:

A 68-year-old patient with a history of hypertension is presenting for a preoperative evaluation.

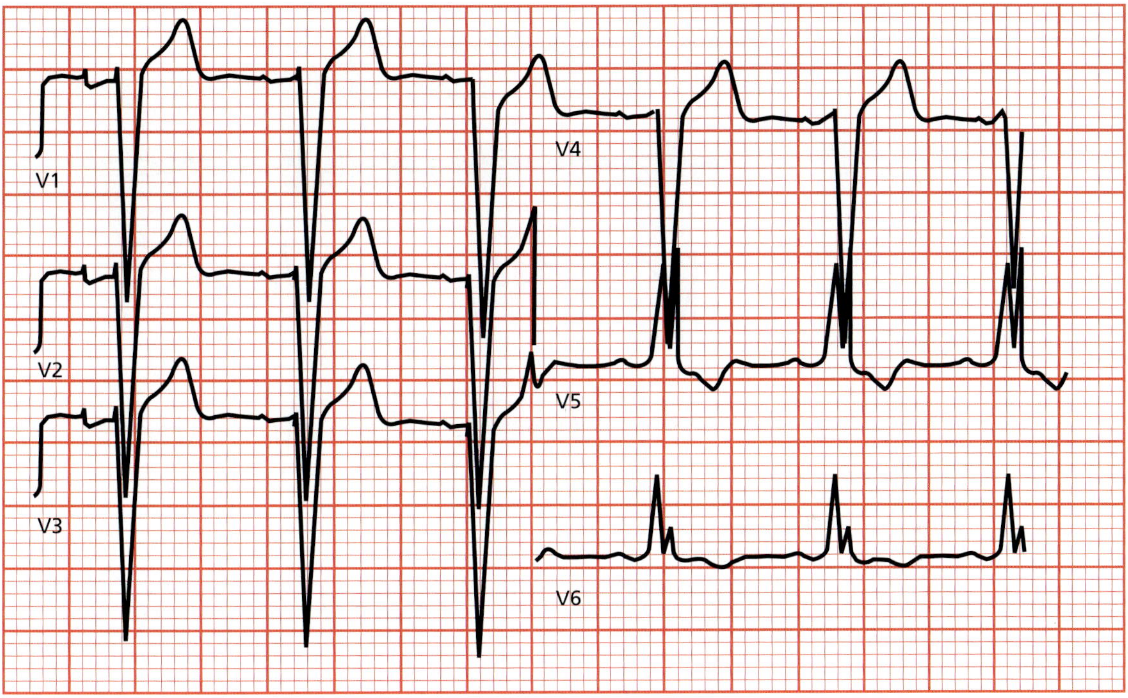

- Answer to EKG 3: The QRS complexes are wide and distorted. In leads V5 and V6, the QRS complexes are notched, and there is ST-segment depression and T-wave inversion. This patient has left bundle-branch block. The rabbit ear configurations in the QRS complexes in leads V5 and V6 are unusual for left bundle-branch block.

EKG 4:

A 58-year-old patient, new to your practice, brings in this recent EKG, which you review even before your office visit.

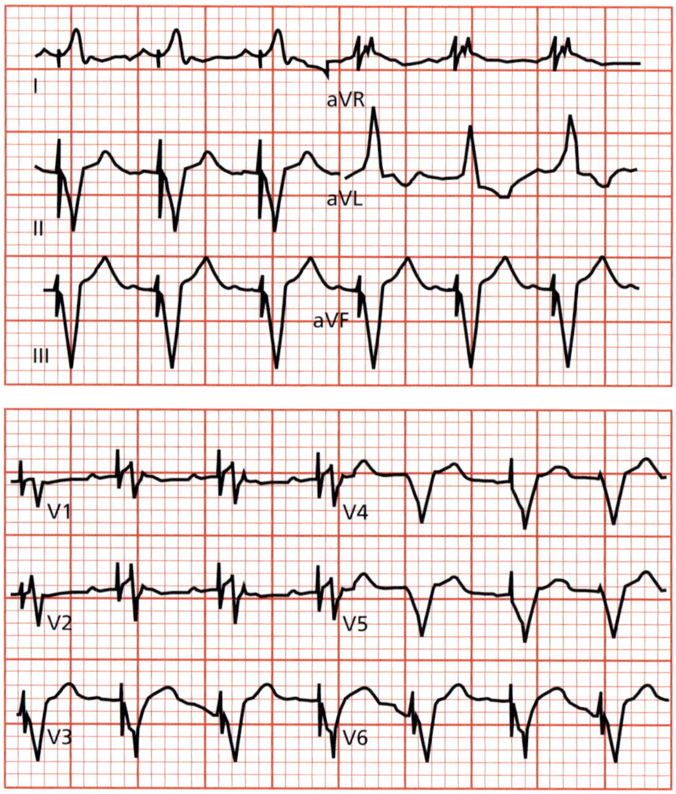

- Answer to EKG 4: The broad, abnormal QRS complexes may immediately attract your attention, but notice the pacer spikes before each one. The spikes are preceded by a P wave (look at leads II, III, aVF, V1, and V2). This pacemaker fires whenever it senses a P wave, ensuring ventricular contraction.

EKG 5:

A 66-year-old patient with a history of occasional chest pain, hyperlipidemia, and diabetes. A week ago, she had a prolonged episode of chest pain associated with nausea and diaphoresis, but did not seek medical care.

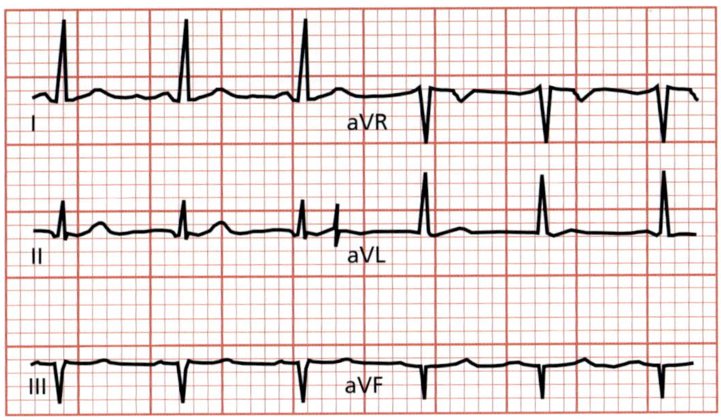

- Answer to EKG 5: There are deep Q waves in leads III and aVF. This tracing shows an inferior infarct.

EKG 6:

A 31-year-old competitive swimmer whose school requires an EKG before the new season begins.

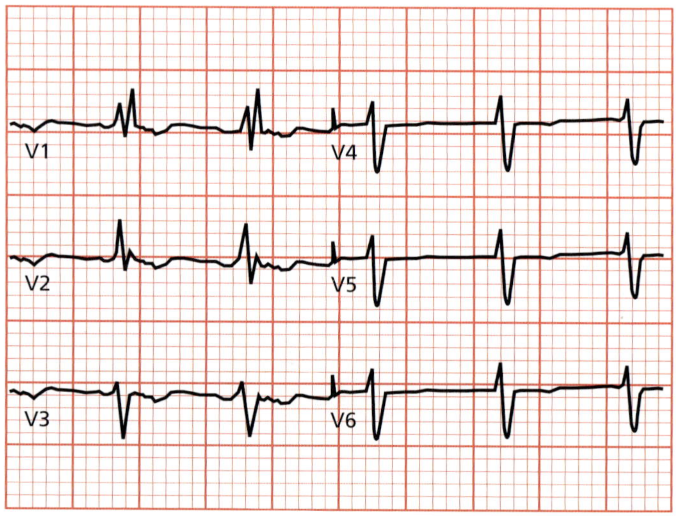

- Answer to EKG 6: The QRS complexes are widened, with beautiful rabbit ears in lead V1. This patient has right bundle-branch block.

EKG 7:
A 41-year-old patient who developed tachycardia an hour ago after trying cocaine for the first time.

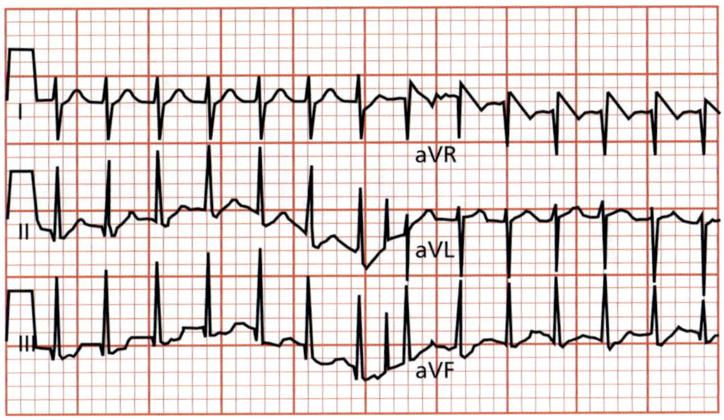

- Answer to EKG 7: The rate is very fast and regular, and the QRS complexes are narrow. Retrograde P waves can be seen in lead III if you look carefully. This patient has AV nodal reentrant tachycardia.

EKG 8:
A 60-year-old marathon runner who intermittently gets episodes of hypotension and tachycardia that last 1 to 2 hours. He has one now as he enters your office.

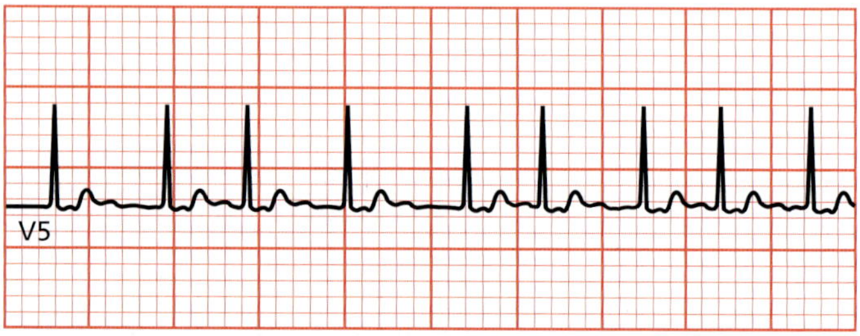

- Answer to EKG 8: The rhythm is irregularly irregular, and the QRS complexes are narrow. This patient is in atrial fibrillation.

EKG 9:

A healthy 39-year-old patient with no symptoms and no cardiac history.

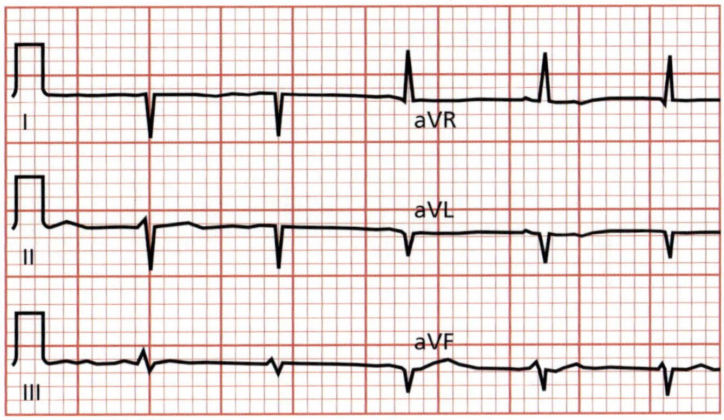

- Answer to EKG 9: Are you confused by what appears to be extreme right axis deviation? Actually, in this instance, the EKG electrodes were accidentally reversed—the right arm and left arm electrodes were placed on the wrong arms. When you see a tall R wave in lead aVR and a deep S wave in lead I, check your electrodes.

EKG 10:

This patient of undetermined age (she appears to be in her sixties or seventies) was successfully resuscitated from an episode of sudden cardiac arrest at home. This EKG was obtained in the emergency department.

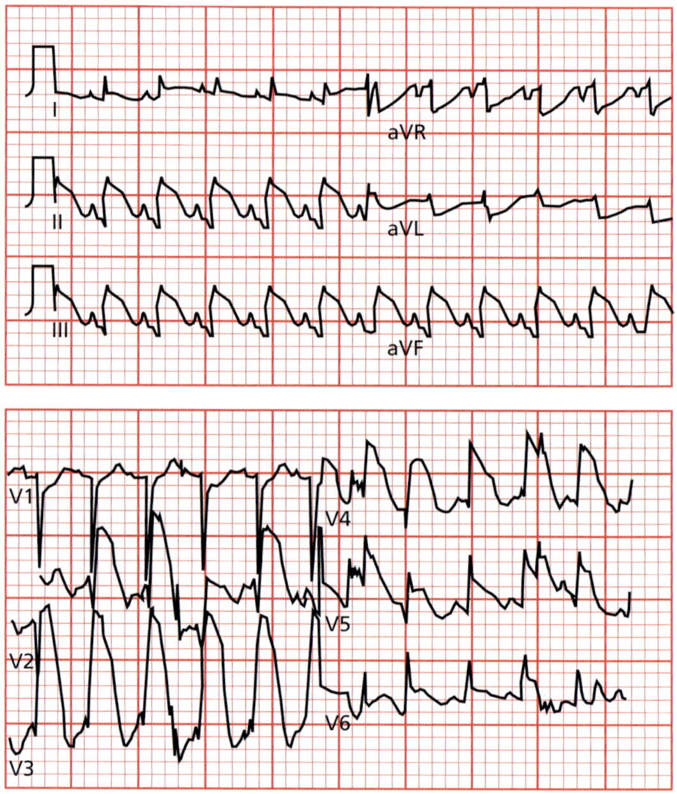

- Answer to EKG 10: Everywhere you look, you see dramatic ST-segment elevation. This EKG shows an evolving infarct affecting the entire heart!

EKG 11:
A 50-year-old patient with palpitations that have persisted for a couple of hours.

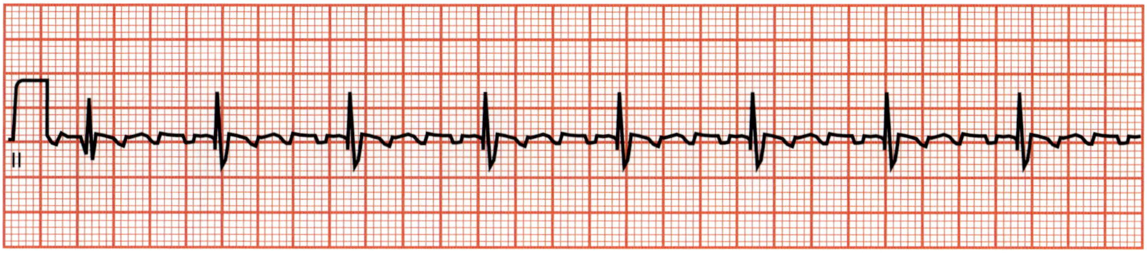

- Answer to EKG 11: You are looking at the classic saw-toothed pattern of atrial flutter.

EKG 12:
A 47-year-old patient with a long history of poorly controlled hypertension.

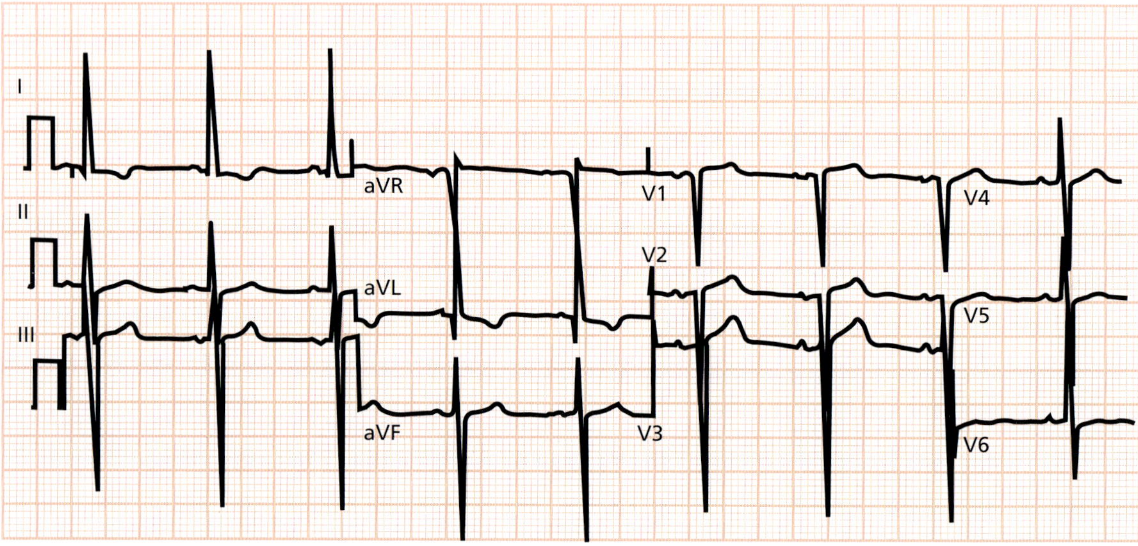

- Answer to EKG 12: Left ventricular hypertrophy satisfying many criteria.

EKG 13:

A 19-year-old patient who had one episode of rapid palpitations last week. He feels fine now.

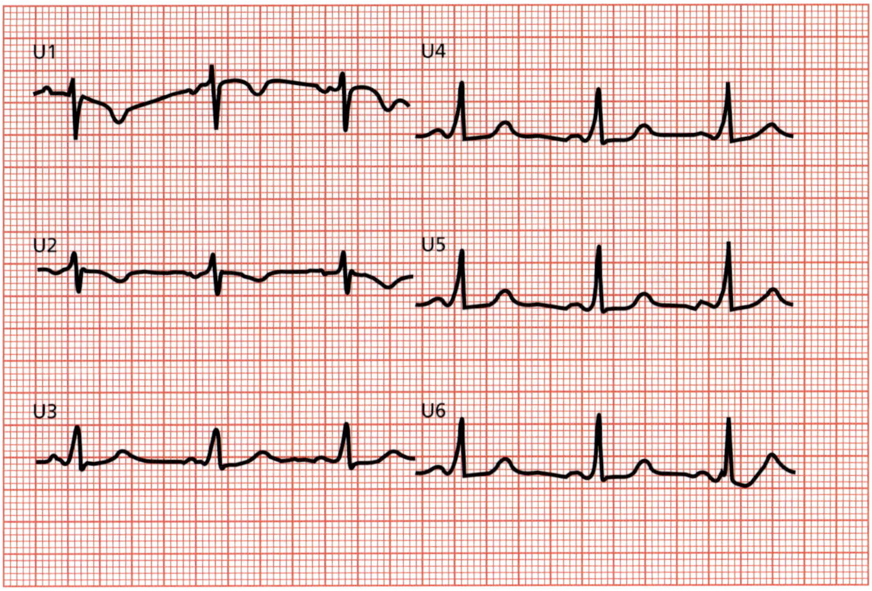

- Answer to EKG 13: Wolff–Parkinson–White syndrome with delta waves and a short PR interval.

EKG 14:
This tracing was taken at night during a sleep study for suspected sleep apnea.

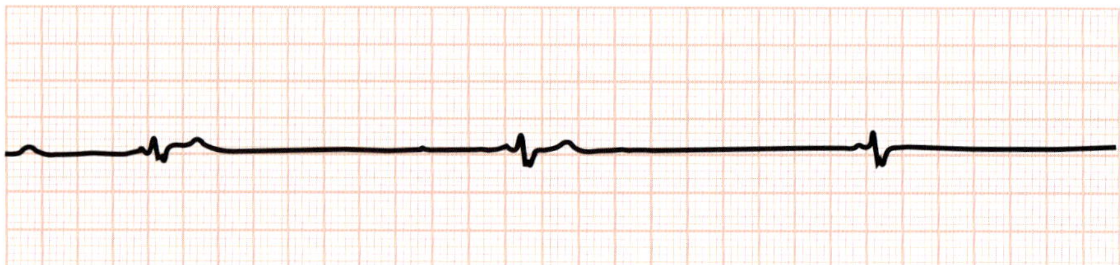

- Answer to EKG 14: Extreme bradycardia resulting from hypoxemia in a patient with sleep apnea.

EKG 15:

An 81-year-old patient who experienced an episode of syncope yesterday but did not seek medical attention. She has been experiencing palpitations and light-headedness for the past few days.

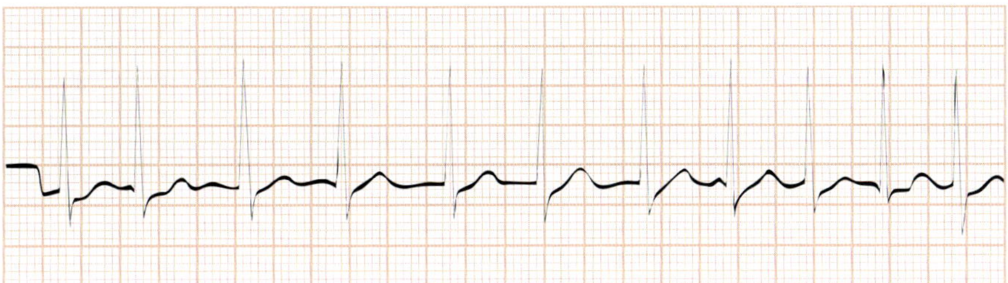

- Answer to EKG 15: Atrial fibrillation with a rapid ventricular response. You can't see the fibrillating baseline, but the rhythm is clearly irregularly irregular.

EKG 16:
This tracing was obtained on a patient in the ICU who suddenly became hypotensive.

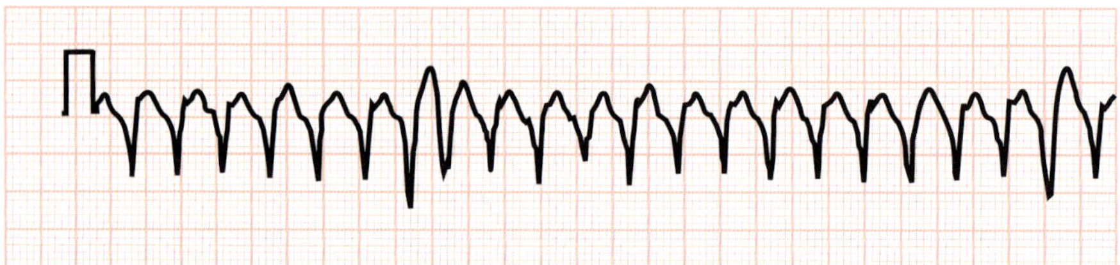

- Answer to EKG 16: Ventricular tachycardia.

EKG 17:

This tracing was the first one obtained on an elderly patient brought by ambulance after an episode of syncope at home.

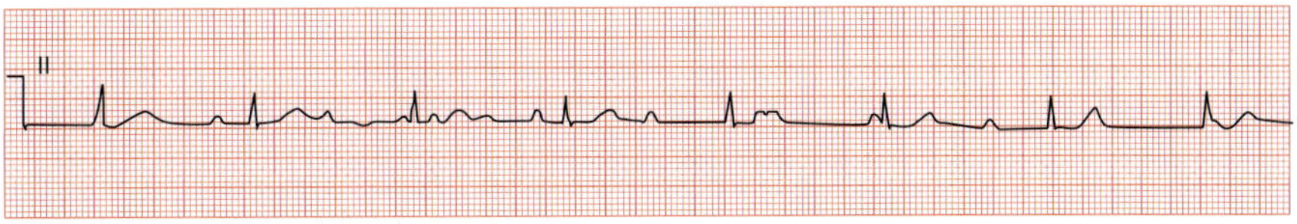

- Answer to EKG 17: How do the P waves and QRS complexes relate to each other? They don't—this is third-degree heart block.

EKG 18:

A 68-year-old patient who is complaining of light-headedness for the past 24 hours.

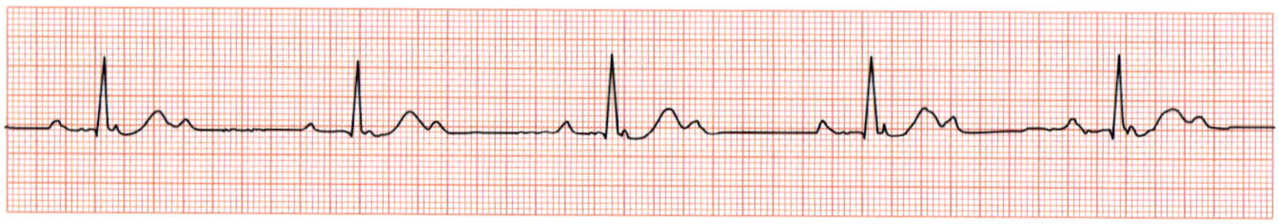

- Answer to EKG 18: Again, look at the relationship of the P waves to the QRS complexes. There are two P waves for every QRS complex—this is 2:1 AV block.

EKG 19:

A 54-year-old patient who presents to the emergency department with shortness of breath and neck pain.

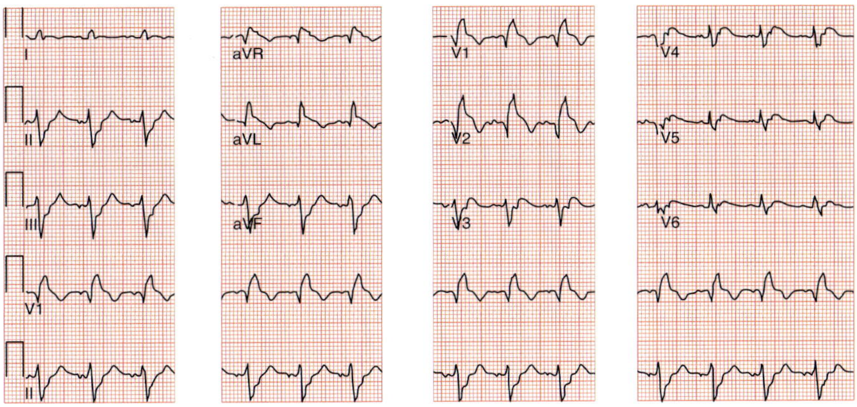

- Answer to EKG 19: The rhythm is normal sinus. The key finding is ST-segment elevation in V1, V2, and aVR with reciprocal changes in the inferior leads and aVL—this patient is having an STEMI.

EKG 20:

A 23-year-old patient who has noted that his pulse has been irregular lately. He otherwise has no symptoms.

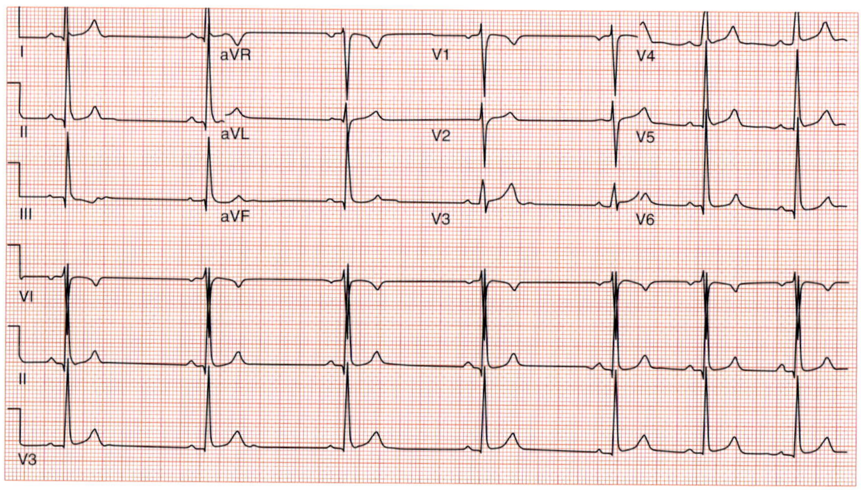

- Answer to EKG 20: What is the rhythm that you see? It is irregular with one P wave for every QRS complex. This is a normal EKG, and what you are seeing is a sinus arrhythmia.

EKG 21:
A 30-year-old patient with sharp, pleuritic chest pain and mild shortness of breath. She tells you that she had a cough and fever the preceding week.

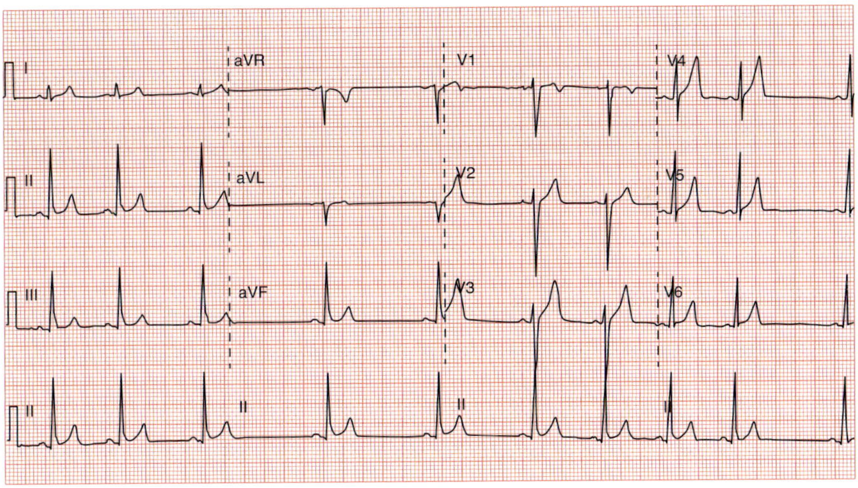

- Answer to EKG 21: The most important finding here is diffuse ST-segment elevation without the upward bowing you typically see with an STEMI. This patient had acute pericarditis.

EKG 22:

A 21-year-old patient who experienced an episode of tachycardia and syncope this morning. He now feels better, but his friends urged him to come to the emergency department.

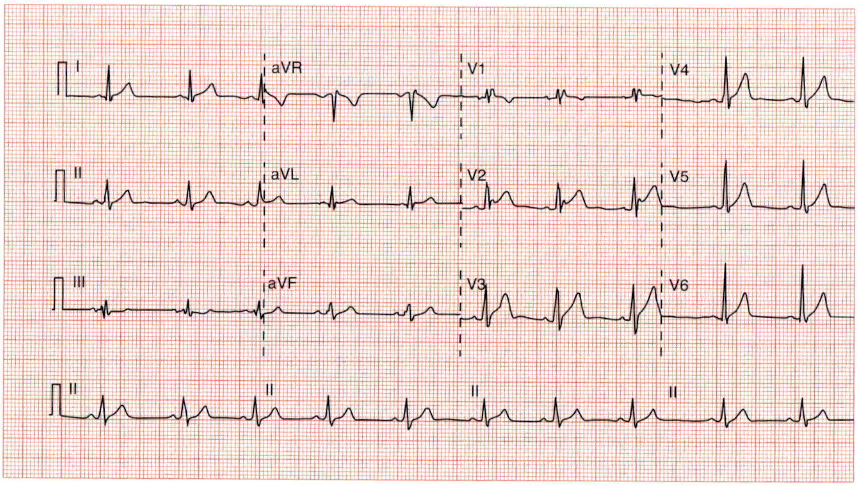

- Answer to EKG 22: Let's finish up with this one. Did you catch the right bundle-branch pattern with an inverted T wave in lead VI and ST-segment elevation most prominent in lead V2? This patient has Brugada syndrome.

Index

Note: Page numbers followed by '*f*' indicate figures.

C

D

M

N

O

P

Q

R

S

T